THE THEORY AND TREATMENT OF DEPRESSION
TOWARDS A DYNAMIC INTERACTIONISM MODEL

FIGURES OF THE UNCONSCIOUS 5

The Theory and Treatment of Depression: Towards a Dynamic Interactionism Model

Edited by

Jozef Corveleyn
Patrick Luyten
Sidney J. Blatt

Published jointly by

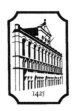

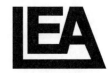

LEUVEN UNIVERSITY PRESS
BELGIUM

LAWRENCE ERLBAUM ASSOCIATES
MAHWAH, NEW JERSEY, LONDON

Published 2005 by

Leuven University Press
Europahuis
Blijde-Inkomststraat 5
B 3000 Leuven

ISBN 90 5867 425 8
D/2005/1869/5
NUR: 777

and

Lawrence Erlbaum Associates, Inc.
10 Industrial Avenue
Mahwah, New Jersey 0 7430

Library of Congress Cataloging-in-Publication Data

The theory and treatment of depression: towards a dynamic interactionism model / edited by
    Jozef Corveleyn, Patrick Luyten, Sidney J. Blatt.
    p. cm.
    Includes bibliographical references and index.
    ISBN 0-8058-5669-2 (alk. paper)
    1. Depression, Mental. 2. Depression, Mental–Treatment. I. Corveleyn, Jozef. II. Luyten,
    Patrick. III. Blatt, Sidney J. (Sidney Jules), 1928-

RC537.T478 2005
616.85'2706–dc22   2005040632

Design Cover: Lejon Tits

Printed in Belgium

About the editors

Jozef Corveleyn, PhD, is Professor of Psychology, Department of Psychology, Faculty of Psychology and Educational Sciences at the Catholic University of Leuven (Belgium) and part-time professor, Faculty of Psychology and Educational Sciences at the Free University of Amsterdam (The Netherlands), psychoanalyst (Belgian School of Psychoanalysis), and clinical psychologist. He teaches courses on psychoanalysis, psychodynamic psychology, qualitative research methodology and clinical psychology of religion. Professor Corveleyn is also Profesor Honorario of the Universidad de Lima (Peru) and of the Universidad Nacional Mayor de San Marcos (Lima, Peru), and Honorary member of the Center for Psychoanalytic Psychotherapy of Lima, Peru. His main research interests concern psychodynamic approaches of psychosis, moral emotions and religious psychopathology.

Patrick Luyten, PhD, is Postdoctoral Fellow of the Fund for Scientific Research-Flanders (FWO) (Belgium) at the Center for Research in Psychoanalysis and Psychodynamic Psychology (Department of Psychology, University of Leuven, Belgium). He is particularly interested in empirical research of psychodynamic concepts and theories and in the interface between psychodynamic, cognitive-behavioral, and neurobiological research. Currently, his main research interest focuses on the relationship between personality, life stress, and depression. Other research interests include psychotherapy research, emotion research, Chronic Fatigue Syndrome, eating disorders, and the (clinical) psychology of religion.

Sidney J. Blatt, PhD, is Professor of Psychiatry and Psychology at Yale University and Chief of the Psychology Section in the Department of Psychiatry at the Yale University School of Medicine. He is also a member of the faculty of the Western New England Institute of Psychoanalysis in New Haven, Connecticut (USA). His primary interests are in the psychological development of mental representations, or cognitive-affective schemas, of self and significant others; the differential impairments of these representations in various forms of psychopathology (especially schizophrenia and depression); and the differential change in the content and cognitive organization of these representations in the therapeutic process. In addition to his interest in mental representation in individual psychological development, Professor Blatt is also interested in the cultural development of mental representation, particularly the development in Western Civilization of the capacity to represent a three-dimensional reality on a two-dimensional surface in the development of art. Dr. Blatt is the recipient of awards for Distinguished Scientific Contributions from The Association of Medical School Professors of Psychology (1995); and from two divisions of the American Psychological Association — Division of Psychoanalysis (2000) and the Division of Clinical Psychology (2004).

List of contributors

Sidney J. Blatt, PhD, Departments of Psychiatry and Psychology, Yale University, New Haven, Connecticut (USA)

Stephan J. Claes, MD, Department of Molecular Genetics, Flanders Interuniversity Institute for Biotechnology (VIB); Department of Psychiatry, University of Antwerp, Antwerpen (Belgium)

Gaston Cluckers, PhD, Department of Psychology, University of Leuven, Leuven (Belgium)

Jozef Corveleyn, PhD, Department of Psychology, University of Leuven, Leuven (Belgium)

Jürgen De Fruyt, MD, Department of Psychiatry, St.-Jan Hospital, Brugge (Belgium)

Koen Demyttenaere, MD, Department of Psychiatry, University Hospital Gasthuisberg, Leuven (Belgium)

Paul Eelen, PhD, Department of Psychology, University of Leuven, Leuven (Belgium)

Dirk Hermans, PhD, Department of Psychology, University of Leuven, Leuven (Belgium)

Patrick Luyten, PhD, Postdoctoral Fellow of the Fund for Scientific Research-Flanders (FWO) (Belgium), Department of Psychology, University of Leuven, Leuven (Belgium)

Patrick Meurs, PhD, Department of Psychology, University of Leuven, Leuven (Belgium)

Charles B. Nemeroff, MD, PhD, Department of Psychiatry, Emory University, Atlanta, Georgia (USA)

Filip Raes, Research Assistant of the Fund for Scientific Research-Flanders (FWO) (Belgium), Department of Psychology, University of Leuven, Leuven (Belgium)

Golan Shahar, PhD, Department of Psychiatry, Yale University School of Medicine, New Haven, Connecticut (USA); and Department of Behavioral Sciences, Ben Gurion University of the Negev, Israel

Lukas Van Oudenhove, MD, Research Assistant of the Fund for Scientific Research-Flanders (FWO) (Belgium), Department of Psychiatry, University Hospital Gasthuisberg, Leuven (Belgium)

Nicole Vliegen, Department of Psychology, University of Leuven, Leuven (Belgium)

Contents

X

Foreword

Robert S. Wallerstein, MD

Depression, in its various manifestations, is the chief symptom, and complaint, that brings its sufferers into the mental health care system. In this it is the counterpart of physical pain, which plays the same central role in propelling individuals into the general medical care system. But what is made very clear in this impressively comprehensive volume about the totality of the depressive phenomena and the depressive experience, from the most subtle subclinical dispositions to the most profoundly crippling and even life-threatening illness pictures, is that we have been living in a world of vastly insufficient and even misleading understandings of this major symptom and character complex, as well as of insufficient awareness of the conceptual, diagnostic, and therapeutic implications of the chronic, recurrent, and often progressive, nature of so much depressive illness.

An implicit message of this volume is that the chief basis for these misunderstandings and skewed conceptualizations has been the dominance over these past several decades of the a-theoretical and a-etiological framework imposed upon diagnosis and therapy recommendations within the realm of mental and emotional disorders by the American Psychiatric Association's Diagnostic and Statistical Manual of Mental Disorders (DSM). Valuable as that compendium has been for categorization for statistical (epidemiological) purposes, and for reliability and comparability in empirical research study, DSM has, by its insistence on precision in compartmentalized categorization of distinct entities, as created by number counts and intensities of symptom clusters, but devoid of meanings or conditions of onset and development in the individual patients, has led, by this insistence, to grossly inadequate understandings of depression, and in many ways has rendered more difficult the kind of study and research needed to truly enhance our knowledge of the conditions of onset and development, and the most effective treatment of depression, in all its variant forms.

What this volume so convincingly demonstrates by its multi-pronged and dynamic interactional consideration of epidemiological, psychodynamic (psychoanalytic), cognitive-behavioral, developmental, psychopathological and neurobio-logical factors, is that depression, in its predispositions and in its various overt expressions, is profoundly dimensional, not categorical, in nature. Its various features and manifestations are intertwined and mutually interactive, not orthogonally separated as distinctive entities. And it is above all the outcome of a long developmental process, in which in-built (genetic) vulnerabilities and quality of life circumstance, most profoundly in the earliest mother-infant caregiver relationship, but also throughout the lifetime developmental trajectory, further accentuated by the traumata, losses and disappointments that can impact any life, all lead together in dialectically and recursively interacting ways to the significant distortions and deviations in the normal developmental process. These distortions can be expressed – even early in life, if severe enough – as a depressive personality disposition, or as mild or transient depressive symptomatic episodes in response to readily identifiable life crisis and distress (such as loss, illness, work failures or disappoint-ments, etc.). Alternatively, these distortions can also be expressed as more severe, and at times, recurrent, chronic, and progressive severe-enough depressive illness outbreaks, often of increasing intensity and diminishing interval states, or all the way to what have been classically designated as major unipolar or bipolar de-pressions. In later years, involutional melancholias may result, with profound disruptions in life functioning, necessary hospitalizations, and marked suicidal propensities that need to be vigorously guarded against.

A major theoretical organizing framework for this volume has been provided by the work of Sidney Blatt of Yale University, one of the co-editors, as well as one of the co-authors of chapters in this volume, and has been further developed and then brought together in all its ramifying and mutually interacting expressions by a gifted and dedicated group of clinicians and researchers headed by Professor Jozef Corveleyn of the University of Leuven in Belgium, chief editor and also co-author of chapters in this volume, with most but not all contributing authors members of his strongly psychoanalytically-informed research group at the Department of Psychology, including his chief collaborator in this overall enterprise, Patrick Luyten, the third co-editor and co-author. The very persuasive conceptual frame-work, elaborated and brought together by this whole cooperating group, is based on that developed originally by Blatt and his many collaborators at Yale, over an entire professional lifetime, and recently brought together in comprehensive and compel-ling exposition in Blatt's own 2004 magisterial volume, *Experiences of Depression: Theoretical, Clinical, and Research Perspectives.*

What is the originating essence of this elaborated organizing framework? It is simply and fundamentally that clinical depression and/or the depressive character formation do not represent a unitary, coherent, illness and character pattern. Rather, both out of his clinical psychoanalytic experience, and his thirty years of empirical research study (along with an array of gifted colleagues), Blatt separated out two significantly different depressive diatheses, designated by him anaclitic and introjective, differing in their character attributes and in their presenting symptomatology, differing in the formative early life experiences that create their predispositions, and differing in the implications for prognosis and for psychothera-peutic course.

The anaclitic (or dependent) depression is marked by interpersonal issues of care and connectedness and relatedness. A central fear is of abandonment and loss, and of a state of helplessness as a consequence. There is a desperate need to maintain supporting and nurturant links, and to ward off feelings of being unwanted and unloved. At its life threatening extremes in infancy and toddlerhood, it can be manifested as hospitalism and marasmus, as has been chronicled by Spitz and the Robertsons. And it occurs more frequently in females, who are declared to be more oriented to issues of relatedness than are males. Blatt locates the infantile proto-types of this disorder in the deformative experiences of the earliest, oral, develop-mental stage.

Contrariwise, the introjective (self-critical) depression is marked by issues of self-definition, separateness, and autonomy, with often a coercive characterological perfectionism. The central concerns are with self-criticism, self-worth, and self-doubt. There is a profound fear of failure to measure up to one's own exalted standards (internally felt, or presumably externally imposed), with consequent guilt and either self blame or blame aggressively projected onto one's most important objects. In the Engel-Schmale formulations, this engenders a feeling of hopeless-ness. This species of depression occurs more frequently in males, who are declared to be more oriented to issues of self-definition, ambition, and achievement. And it is located by Blatt at a higher developmental level, built around the deviant experiences of Mahler's separation-individuation phase, and then the superego issues of guilt and blame.

Given this originating theoretical frame, the overall thrust of this volume by Corveleyn and his many colleagues is not to explore further the many similarities and differences between these two variant forms of depression, nor the linkages to intermediate states which partake of both and border on both, but rather to explore them as alternative deviations from the normal developmental path with, in each instance, an abnormal preoccupation with the issues and conflicts of one or the other side of this dichotomy (and possibly a concomitant excessive avoidance of, or defense against, the issues and conflicts of the other side), and then to set all of these etiological and developmental considerations that can give rise to the variant expressions of the depressive experience and illness, conceptualized thus psychoanalytically, into conjunction with, and in dialectical interaction with, all the other realms of accruing knowledge of the depressive condition already mentioned, the epidemiological, the cognitive-behavioral, the developmental, the psychopatho-logical, and the neurobiological – each of these developed very comprehensively and convincingly, in each instance by a chapter co-authored by experts in that arena, mostly Belgian co-authors, but also with two cooperating American workers beyond Blatt, Golan Shahar at Yale (now at Ben Gurion University in Israel), and Charles Nemeroff at Emory University in Atlanta.

The treat awaiting the reader of this volume is to witness the unfolding interplay of these multiple considerations of the many-sided complexity of the totality of the depressive experience, as illuminated from these many disparate vantage points, variously clinical or empirical, psychosocial or neurobiological, nomothetic or idiosyncratic, etc., as they are all mutually interacting, and at each moment exist at various points of convergence or divergence. Examples abound and recur, throughout the text, for example, the various convergences seen among psychological theoretical perspectives grounded in seemingly antithetical assumptions about the nature of mental activity, like the quite classically psychoanalytic perspectives of Blatt, the behavioral theory perspectives of Beck, the attachment formulations of Bowlby, and the interpersonal propositions of Arieti and Bemporad; or like the inner-outer interplay of a depressive character disposition (itself an outcome of the interplay of genetic vulnerabilities and adverse developmental life experience) and its "depressogenic" impact in shaping continuing environmental contingency in ways that reinforce the depressive outlook and confirm the depressive character expectation.

Perhaps the best conclusion to this foretelling to the readers is to quote from the very last paragraph of this volume. Overall, "an etiologically-based, dynamic interactionism view of depression, emphasizing interactions among genetics, early adversity, current life stress, and relatively stable cognitive-affective schemas or personality dimensions, emerges as a model that may facilitate the integration of various theoretical, methodological, and clinical approaches to depression. At the same time, much work remains to be done." The entire volume propounds very convincingly all the evidence that buttresses this conclusion, all the work done by so many that has brought us to this point, and that points enticingly to all the many opened avenues of continuing clinical and research endeavor awaiting our collective attention. As such, it is a tribute to this group of primarily Belgian clinicians and researchers who have collaboratively written it. Reading it should be a journey of pleasure and of widening perspective. Bon voyage!

Introduction

Patrick Luyten, Sidney J. Blatt, & Jozef Corveleyn

Depression: Changing Views

Depression, with a lifetime prevalence of approximately 15% (Blazer, Kessler, McGonagle, & Swartz, 1994), is one of the most prevalent disorders worldwide (NIMH, 2001). By the year 2020, depression is expected to be the second most serious disorder with respect to global disease burden (Murray & Lopez, 1996). The personal and social costs associated with this disorder are immense. Depression seriously affects both intrapersonal and interpersonal functioning (Beach, 2001), not only for those suffering from depression, but also for those in their immediate environment. Moreover, these negative effects are not limited to an episode of depression, but may extend over years, as is for instance shown by the fact that children of depressed parents are at elevated risk for psychopathology in later life (Blatt & Homann, 1992; Goodman & Gotlib, 2002). In addition, depression has also a serious economic cost. For instance, the National Institute of Mental Health estimated the total cost of depression in the U.S.A. to be $30-44 billion annually (NIMH, 1999).

Until recently, it was believed that depression, though prevalent, was a relatively "benign" disorder, because it was thought to be associated with a good prognosis, even when untreated. Depression therefore was often called the "common cold" of psychopathology. However, over the past two decades, our view on the natural course and the treatment of depression has dramatically changed (Costello et al., 2002; Hollon et al., 2002). Research concerning the natural course of depression has made increasingly clear that depression is a recurrent and for a considerable number of patients even a chronic disorder (Frank et al., 2002; Segal, Pearson, & Thase, 2003). Recent estimates suggest relapse rates after a first episode of 20-30% within 3 years, and 70-80% within the same period in subjects who have had three depressive episodes or more (Judd, 1997; Segal et al., 2003; Solomon et al., 2000). The risk for at least one other episode after a first episode is estimated at almost 90% (Kupfer & Frank, 2001), and the average depressed patient, during their life time, will experience four episodes, each of about 20 weeks duration (Judd, 1997). Also, research has shown that with each new episode, the time between two next episodes shortens (Solomon et al., 2000). Moreover, in about 10% to 30% of the cases, depression becomes chronic (Verheul, 2003). Finally, adding to the growing realization that depression is not a relatively benign and isolated disorder, research indicates that comorbidity of depression with other Axis I and especially Axis II disorders is the rule rather than the exception. Estimates of comorbitity between depression and personality disorders, for instance, vary in psychiatric populations between 50-60% (Klein & Hayden, 2000; Mulder, 2002). And it is now well established that comorbid Axis I and Axis II disorders have a negative impact on the prognosis and treatment of depression (Mulder, 2002; Westen, Novotny, & Thompson-Brenner, 2004).

This leads us to a second domain in which our view of depression has dramatically changed. The treatment of depression by both psychotherapeutic and pharmacological means has proved much more difficult and less successful then once was hoped for. In the 1980's, many researchers and clinicians believed that depression could be effectively treated with short-term (standardized) psychotherapeutic treatments, such as Cognitive-Behavioral Therapy (CBT) or Interpersonal Therapy (IPT), and/or pharmacological treatment (e.g., see Dobson, 1989; APA, 2000).

This optimism has been seriously tempered. A growing body of research has shown important limitations of these brief treatments for many depressed patients (Hollon et al., 2002; Luyten, Lowyck, & Corveleyn, 2003; Parker, Roy, & Eyers, 2003; Rush & Thase, 2002; Westen & Morrison, 2001; Westen et al., 2004). For instance, in what is probably the most prestigious and extensive Randomised Clinical Trial (RCT) to date, the National Institute of Mental Health (NIMH)-sponsored Treatment of Depression Collaborative Research Program (TDCRP; Elkin, Parloff, Hadley, & Autry, 1985), only about half of the patients that received 16 weeks of treatment with either Cognitive-Behavioral Therapy (CBT), Interpersonal Therapy (IPT), or antidepressant medication (Imipramine plus Clinical Management; IMI-CM), met criteria for remission at termination (Elkin et al., 1989) and only about 20% of the patients were considered as fully recovered (remission without relapse) at a follow-up assessment conducted 18-months after the termination of treatment (Shea et al., 1992).

Westen and Morrison (2001) estimated from well-designed randomized clinical trials (RCTs) of so-called Empirically Supported Treatments (ESTs) of depression, such as Cognitive-Behavioral Therapy (CBT) and Interpersonal Therapy (IPT), that only about 50% of depressed patients who completed such treatments showed improvement. For the Intent-To-Treat (ITT) sample, this figure was only 37%. Moreover, because of high exclusion rates in outcome studies, patients in routine practice might show even less response to these treatments. Congruent with this hypothesis, Westen and Morrison (2001) found that there was a high correlation between outcome and exclusion criteria ($r=.41$), indicating that the more stringent the exclusion criteria (the greater the exclusion rate), the more likely it was for the study to have a greater number of patients who showed improvement. In addition, it is important to note that the average patient who shows improvement after these brief treatments, remains symptomatic and thus does not show full recovery (Westen & Morrison, 2001; see also Elkin et al., 1989; Shea et al., 1992).

Besides these modest effects of short-term treatments at termination, there is also a lack of controlled studies on the long-term effects of ESTs of depression. Westen and Morrison (2001), for instance, could locate only 4 studies published in the 1990's in which the long-term effects (from 12 to 18 months) of ESTs of depression were investigated. The average percentage of patients showing no relapse after 12-18 months was 36.6%. For instance, in the NIMH TDCRP-study, at follow-up after 18 months, only 20% of the patients were fully recovered (Blatt, Zuroff, Bondi, & Sanislow, 2000; Shea et al., 1992). Westen and Morrison (2001) could only locate one study with follow-up data of 2 years or more. The results of this study demonstrated that as little as 27% of the patients who were in treatment and 8% of all patients initially screened, showed no relapse. Westen and Morrison (2001, p. 886) rightfully conclude from these and similar findings: "By any standards, it is difficult to construe these data as evidence for the hypothesis that these treatments show genuine efficacy for the treatment of depressive disorders".

Similar response rates of about 50% (compared to 30-35% placebo response) have been reported for the pharmacotherapeutic treatment of depression (e.g., Williams et al., 2002). More critical reviews, which also include non-published negative studies, have even claimed that drug-placebo differences are minimal and "of questionable clinical significance" (Kirsch & Sapirstein, 1998; Kirsch, Moore, Scoboria, & Nicholls, 2002; see also Khan & Khan, 2003). In addition, a recent meta-analysis has shown that approximately 40 years of research on drug treatment of depression has only led to progression concerning the side effects of medication, but not concerning its efficacy (Barbui & Hotopf, 2001). Thus, so-called "older" antidepressants are at least as effective as "newer" ones, but they show more side effects. And although research has shown that the long-term treatment of depression with antidepressants leads to a significant reduction in relapse rates (e.g., see Kupfer & Frank, 2001), there is no relationship between the duration of drug treatment and the probability of relapse after discontinuation of the drug (Viguera, Baldessarini, & Friedberg, 1998; see also Fava, 2002).

The Search for More Effective Treatments and the Need for Integration in Research on Depression

The findings just reviewed clearly suggest that further research on depression, its origins, the factors influencing its course, and particularly its treatment, are important future tasks from a scientific, clinical, as well as from a national mental health perspective. We clearly have an important responsibility to find better treatments for this disabling disorder, and also to develop primary and secondary prevention strategies. Moreover, these prevention and treatment strategies need to be made more available to the public because research has shown that very few depressed persons – estimates vary between 19-37% – ever seek treatment (Grote & Frank, 2003). In addition, the modal patient who does seek treatment, either is not treated or inadequately treated or drops out early from treatment (Grote & Frank, 2003).

Not surprisingly, these findings concerning the recurrent and often chronic course of depression, the high rates of comorbidity of depression with personality disorders, and the growing awareness of the limits of brief treatments of depression, have led to a renewal of interest in theories and techniques that are based on long-term treatments of depression, such as psychodynamic theories (Jones & Pulos, 1993; Kwon, 1999; Shapiro et al., 1994), and especially in theoretical models that focus on the relationship between personality and depression (Gunderson, Triebwasser, Philips, & Sullivan, 1999; Klein, Kupfer, & Shea, 1993; Kupfer & Frank, 2001; Verheul, 2003).

The convergence among psychodynamic and more recent cognitive-behavioral theories of depression plays an important role in this evolution (Blatt, 2004; Blatt & Maroudas, 1992; Robins, 1993). Most research in this domain has concentrated on the psychodynamic conceptions of Sidney J. Blatt (Yale University) and the cognitive-behavioral formulations of Aaron T. Beck (University of Pennsylvania). Both Blatt (e.g., Blatt, 1974, 1998, 2004; Blatt, D'Afflitti, & Quinlan, 1976; Blatt, Quinlan, Chevron, McDonald, & Zuroff, 1982) and Beck (e.g., Beck, 1983, 1999) have proposed that two personality dimensions, i.e., interpersonal dependency or sociotropy and self-critical perfectionism or autonomy, are vulnerability factors for clinical and nonclinical forms of depression. According to Blatt and Beck, these personality dimensions are associated with different personality structures, a different relational and attachment style, a vulnerability for specific life events (loss vs. failure), a different clinical presentation, and a different response to psycho-therapy and pharmacotherapy. Moreover, Blatt has proposed that these personality dimensions are also associated with different developmental factors and biological vulnerabilities (Blatt & Homann, 1992; Blatt, Cornell, & Eshkol, 1993). Support for these formulations has come from three decades of empirical research (Blatt, 2004; Blatt & Zuroff, 1992; Clark & Beck, 1999). Yet, this research is often little known, even among experts in research on depression.

This is only one example that shows that the field of research on depression is still relatively fragmented. Different theoretical and research traditions concerning depression have often developed separately from each other. The time seems overdue to bring these different views together with the aim of developing a more comprehensive theoretical framework for depression. It is our firm conviction that only then more effective treatments of this serious and disabling disorder can be developed and implemented. This has also been recognized recently by the National Institute of Mental Health Strategic Plan for Mood Disorders Research (NIMH, 2003). This Strategic Plan, which will guide the NIMH's research initiatives in the coming years, identified several routes and barriers towards integration among approaches towards depression with the aim of enhancing both theoretical insights in depression and treatment strategies. Although this initiative from the NIMH deserves utmost praise, in our view it misses out on some important developments in mood disorders research (Luyten et al., 2003). This is in part due to the fragmented state of research in this field, but also to different theoretical and research traditions within the U.S.A., and between the U.S.A. and other parts of the world, especially in Europe.

This led us to the idea of organizing a conference on depression, inviting several scholars from a wide variety of different fields in depression research. Professor Sidney J. Blatt (Yale University, New Haven, USA), who was, at that time, Visiting Professor at the University of Leuven (Belgium), was invited as the main speaker. The aim of this conference was not only to present a "state of the art" of depression research, but also, and perhaps more importantly, to formulate possible avenues for integration between different approaches of depression. In addition, it seemed crucial to identify important barriers towards integration among various psychological and biological approaches of depression. Subsequently, on March 14, 2003, a conference on the integration of psychological and biological approaches towards depression was held at the St. Jozef University Psychiatric Clinic in Kortenberg (Leuven), Belgium.

The chapters in this book are based on the presentations at this conference. However, most chapters have been rewritten based on the interactions and discussion among the participants. In preparing their chapter for this volume, we asked the authors (1) to review the current state of research in their area and (2) to also identify possible routes and barriers towards the integration among different approaches in depression research. In the epilogue, we have made an attempt at an "integration of the integration", summarizing possibilities and barriers towards integration, spelling out future lines of investigation, and discussing clinical implications of the recent research on depression from the various perspectives presented in this volume.

Overview of the Book

The first chapter by Demyttenaere, Van Oudenhove and De Fruyt sets the stage for this volume by summarizing and discussing recent epidemiological studies, including the recent European Study on Mental Disorders (ESEMeD), which have dramatically changed our view of depression. Among the many interesting findings they discuss, two seem particularly important. First, recent epidemiological studies do not support the categorical view of depression promulgated by the Diagnostic and Statistic Manual for Mental Disorders (DSM; APA, 1994). Instead, a dimensional view appears to more adequately fit to the data. Second, these epidemiological studies also clearly show that depression is not an isolated, state-like disorder, but a recurrent disorder that becomes chronic in a considerable amount of patients, and one that can lead to considerable and lasting changes in functioning, even on the neurobiological level.

In the second chapter, Hermans, Raes and Eelen review recent developments in cognitive behavioral theory and research on depression. Their contribution is noteworthy in many respects, including their emphasis on the need for more experimental research to inform research on depression. In this context, they emphasize the relevance of cognitive psychological research on memory in general and on autobiographical memory in particular for understanding depression. In addition, this chapter is also an excellent example of how fundamental experimental research can inform clinical practice. Hermans and colleagues, for example, demonstrate how research on mood congruent encoding and recall might help understand the vicious cycles of negative thoughts typical of depressed patients. Equally important is their emphasis on relapse prevention. They note that the fact that depression tends to be a recurrent disorder should lead to a focus in both research and treatment on the prevention of future relapses. In this context, Hermans and colleagues discuss the integration between cognitive research on (autobiographical) memory and more recent cognitive-behavioral treatments for depression such as Mindfulness-Based Cognitive Therapy (MBCT; Segal, Williams, & Teasdale, 2002).

The next three chapters are devoted to the convergence among psychodynamic and cognitive-behavioral theories of depression. In Chapter 3, Luyten, Blatt and Corveleyn provide an overview of the convergence in psychodynamic and cognitive-behavioral theorizing concerning depression. In particular, they focus on the conceptualizations of Sidney J. Blatt and Aaron T. Beck concerning Dependency/Sociotropy and Self-Critical Perfectionism/Autonomy as primary vulnerability factors for depression. As this overview shows, there are many similarities and thus much common ground between psychodynamic and cognitive-behavioral theories of depression. However, at the same time, Luyten and colleagues note that there are also some important barriers towards further integration because of major differences in the underlying view of human nature in these two models.

In Chapter 4, Luyten, Corveleyn and Blatt review empirical research concerning the three most central assumptions of the theories of Blatt and Beck as well as research concerning the clinical implications of these theories. The review in this chapter demonstrates that the central assumptions of Blatt and of Beck have received considerable empirical support. However, Luyten and colleagues also identify several areas for further research. Their review also shows that Blatt's and Beck's views have not only led to considerable integration between psychodynamic and cognitive-behavioral formulations, but also between psychodynamic and cognitive-behavioral theories and research in the fields of personality, social psychology, developmental psychology, and neurobiology, clearly illustrating the vitality of these theoretical models in generating integrative research.

Subsequently, in Chapter 5, Blatt and Shahar address recent developments in research on Dependency/Sociotropy and Self-Critical Perfectionism/Autonomy. In particular, Blatt and Shahar argue that depression should be situated within a general theory of personality development. Depression should not be viewed categorically as a disease, but as a distortion of normal personality development. In addition, a dynamic interactionism model is proposed that involves reciprocal interactions between adaptive and maladaptive dimensions of self-definition (identity) and interpersonal relatedness, life stress, social support, and depression. According to this dynamic interactionism model, individuals are not just the passive recipients of their stressful environment, but actively, though often unwittingly, interpret and generate, in part, their own (social) environment. Finally, Blatt and Shahar also discuss recent research exploring the dynamics of patients showing mixed dependent and self-critical characteristics.

Whereas until recently many even doubted whether children could experience depression, today the question is rather how many adults have their first onset of depression in childhood (Costello et al., 2002). Developmental research on depression is therefore a most important task for the future. In Chapter 6, Vliegen, Meurs and Cluckers review research in developmental psychopathology on depression in childhood and adolescence. This research has not only shown that depression in childhood and adolescence is not uncommon, but that developmental factors appear to play an important role in the etiology and pathogenesis of depression. Moreover, Vliegen, Meurs and Cluckers also stress the need for broad, comprehensive, developmentally-based theories of depression in childhood and adolescence. Such comprehensive theories are needed to develop prevention programs and treatments strategies that are developmentally sensitive. The next chapter, Chapter 7, provides the outlines for such an overarching, psychodynamically inspired developmental psychopathological framework to understand the origins of depression. In particular, in this chapter, Meurs, Vliegen and Cluckers delineate several developmental tasks and stages that might be involved in the development of depression. Their views are illustrated by a detailed discussion of excerpts of the treatment of a depressed boy.

Chapter 8 by Claes and Nemeroff addresses what can be considered to be the greatest future challenge for research on depression and perhaps psychopathology in general, namely the integration between biological and psychological approaches. This integration is of high relevance for both researchers and clinicians alike. From a research perspective, with each new study, it becomes increasingly clear that genes, neurobiological processes, psychological, and environmental factors constantly interact, and that any theory that assumes a neat distinction between "nature" and "nurture" is incapable of capturing these intrinsic and recursive interactions between biological, psychological, and social factors. Clinicians, in turn, are faced with difficult questions such as the decision on whether and how they should combine pharmaceutical and psychotherapeutic treatments of depression. At present, no theoretical rationale that is firmly grounded in empirical research exists for such decisions. Hence, the need for integrative research and theories is clear and urgent. According to Claes and Nemeroff, such integrative research has already begun in the domain of neurobiological research on stress. In particular, they argue that this area of research could provide an important framework for bridging the gap between psychological and biological theories of depression. However, they also point to the tremendous problems associated with this research. Not only is such research very costly and time-consuming, it also assumes the existence of interdisciplinary research teams, consisting of geneticists, neurobiologists, psychiatrists, and psychologists.

This volume concludes with an epilogue in which we have tried to answer three basic sets of questions. Our first set of questions concerns identifying the current possibilities and barriers to the integration between psychological and biological approaches of depression. Is there sufficient "common ground" between these approaches? If so, can we determine more precisely what these approaches have in common? And what are important barriers towards such integration? Our second set of questions is even more challenging. Taking into account existing possibilities as well as barriers to integration among various approaches of depression, can we delineate important research tasks for the future that could foster further dialogue and enhance integration between psychological and biological approaches of depression? With the third and final set of questions, we returned to our starting point. How can "old" and "new" knowledge that has accumulated over the years concerning depression be used to improve our treatment of patients suffering from this disorder? In other words: what are the clinical implications? Our answers to these three sets of questions led us to propose an etiologically-based, transdiagnostic dynamic interactionism model as an alternative for the DSM view of depression.

When we embarked on the adventure of writing this book, we were already convinced that we had much to learn about depression. Yet, while working on this book, we came to realize that our knowledge of depression and its treatment is even more limited than we initially assumed. It has therefore not only been a pleasure, but also a privilege to work with all of the authors that have contributed to this book, and with all those who participated in the discussions on the conference in Kortenberg (Leuven, Belgium) that gave the impetus for this volume. Their expertise and openness towards perspectives often very different from their own are exemplary. In addition, although they sometimes must have tired of our continuous questions, they never failed to provide us with what we asked from them, often within very short time spans.

It is also a pleasure to thank those people who have contributed to our preparation of this book. First of all, we want to thank all our colleagues – too many to list individually – that have either directly or indirectly contributed to this volume. We are indebted to Benedicte Lowyck, Catherine Estas, Bart Soenens (all from the Department of Psychology, University of Leuven), and Raymond Paloutzian (Westmont College, California), who read portions of the manuscript for this book and provided us with many insightful suggestions. We are also indebted to Marleen Devijver for her dedication in preparing this manuscript, to Hilde Lens, our publisher at Leuven University Press, and to Susan Milmoe and Kristen Depken at Lawrence Erlbaum Associates, for their expertise and patience. In addition, we wish to thank Larry Erlbaum, for his interest, support, and generosity, and Barbara Lavrysen for compiling the author and subject index.

This volume was made possible, in part, by a grant to Patrick Luyten and Jozef Corveleyn from the Research Advisory Board (RAB) of the International Psychoanalytic Association (IPA). We gratefully acknowledge their support. We also want to express our gratitude to Peter Fonagy, Drew Westen, John Clarkin, Linda Mayes, Manfred Beutel, Marianne Leuzinger-Bohleber, George Gergely, and Rudi Vermote for their support and encouragement. Special thanks to Bernard Sabbe, Sieglinde Meganck, Bart Jansen, Carmen De Grave, Marck Swinnen, and the whole team from the Psychiatric Center St. Norbertushuis in Duffel (Belgium), for their collaboration and friendship over the years. We also thank the Director of the St. Jozef University Psychiatric Clinic in Kortenberg (Leuven), Jozef Peuskens, for hosting the conference on depression that led to this volume. And, finally, we want to thank our patients, because they constantly remind us that we have still much to learn about the nature of depression.

References

American Psychiatric Association (1994). *Diagnostic and statistical manual of mental disorders* (4th ed.). Washington, DC: Author.

American Psychiatric Association (2000). *Practice guidelines for the treatment of patients with major depression.* Retrieved September 3, 2004, from http://www.psych.org/psych_pract/treatg/pg/Depres sion2e.book.cfm

Barbui, C., & Hotopf, M. (2001). Amitriptyline *v.* the rest: Still the leading antidepressant after 40 years of randomised controlled trials. *British Journal of Psychiatry, 178,* 129-144.

Beach, S. R. H. (Ed.). (2001). *Marital and family processes in depression: A scientific foundation for clinical practice.* Washington, DC: American Psychological Association.

Beck, A. T. (1983). Cognitive therapy of depression: New perspectives. In P. J. Clayton & J. E. Barrett (Eds.), *Treatment of depression: Old controversies and new approaches* (pp. 265-290). New York: Raven Press.

Beck, A. T. (1999). Cognitive aspects of personality disorders and their relation to syndromal disorders: A psychoevolutionary approach. In C. R. Cloninger (Ed.), *Personality and psychopathology* (pp. 411-429). Washington, DC/London: American Psychiatric Press.

Blatt, S. J. (1974). Levels of object representation in anaclitic and introjective depression. *The Psycho-analytic Study of the Child, 29,* 107-157.

Blatt, S. J. (1998). Contributions of psychoanalysis to the understanding and treatment of depression. *Journal of the American Psychoanalytic Association, 46,* 722-752.

Blatt, S. J. (2004). *Experiences of depression: Theoretical, clinical and research perspectives.* Washington, DC: American Psychological Association.

Blatt, S. J., Cornell, C. E., & Eshkol, E. (1993). Personality style, differential vulnerability and clinical course in immunological and cardiovascular disease. *Clinical Psychology Review, 13,* 421-450.

Blatt, S. J., D'Afflitti, J. P., & Quinlan, D. M. (1976). Experiences of depression in normal young adults. *Journal of Abnormal Psychology, 85,* 383-389.

Blatt, S. J., & Homann, E. (1992). Parent-child interaction in the etiology of dependent and self-critical depression. *Clinical Psychology Review, 12,* 47-91.

Blatt, S. J., & Maroudas, C. (1992). Convergence among psychoanalytic and cognitive-behavioral theories of depression. *Psychoanalytic Psychology, 9,* 157-190.

Blatt, S. J., Quinlan, D. M., Chevron, E. S., McDonald, C., & Zuroff, D. C. (1982). Dependency and self-criticism: Psychological dimensions of depression. *Journal of Consulting and Clinical Psychology*, *63*, 125-132.

Blatt, S. J., & Zuroff, D. C. (1992). Interpersonal relatedness and self-definition: Two prototypes for depression. *Clinical Psychology Review*, *12*, 527-562.

Blatt, S. J., Zuroff, D. C., Bondi, C. M., & Sanislow III, C. A. (2000). Short- and long-term effects of medication and psychotherapy in the brief treatment of depression: Further analyses of data from the NIMH TDCRP. *Psychotherapy Research*, *10*, 215-234.

Blazer, D. G., Kessler, R. C., McGonagle, K. A., & Swartz, M. S. (1994). The prevalence and distribution of major depression in a national community sample: The National Comorbidity Survey. *American Journal of Psychiatry*, *151*, 979-986.

Clark, D. A., & Beck, A. T. (1999). *Scientific foundations of cognitive theory and therapy of depression*. New York: John Wiley & Sons.

Costello, E. J., Pine, D. S., Hammen, C., March, J. S., Plotsky, P. M., Weissman, M. M., Biederman, J., Goldsmith, H. H., Kaufman, J., Lewinsohn, P. M., Hellander, M., Hoagwood, K., Koretz, D. S., Nelson, C. A., & Leckman, J. F. (2002). Development and natural history of mood disorders. *Biological Psychiatry*, *52*, 529-542.

Dobson, K. S. (1989). A meta-analysis of the efficacy of cognitive therapy for depression. *Journal of Consulting and Clinical Psychology*, *57*, 414-419.

Elkin, I., Parloff, M. B., Hadley, S. W., & Autry, J. H. (1985). NIMH Treatment of Depression Collaborative Research Program. *Archives of General Psychiatry*, *42*, 305-316.

Elkin, I., Shea, M. T., Watkins, J. T., Imber, S. D., Sotsky, S. M., Collins, J. F., Glass, D. R., Pilkonis, P. A., Leber, W. R., Docherty, J. P., Fiester, S. J., & Parloff, M. B. (1989). NIMH treatment of depression collaborative research program: General effectiveness of treatments. *Archives of General Psychiatry*, *46*, 971-983.

Fava, G. A. (2002). Long-term treatment with antidepressant drugs: The spectacular achievements of propaganda. *Psychotherapy and Psychosomatics*, *71*, 127-132.

Frank, E., Rush, A. J., Blehar, M., Essock, S., Hargreaves, W., Hogan, M., Jarrett, R., Johnson, R. L., Katon, W. J., Lavori, P., McNulty, J. P., Niederehe, G., Ryan, N., Stuart, G., Thomas, S. B., Tollefson, G. D., & Vitiello, B. (2002). Skating to where the puck is going to be: A plan for clinical trials and translation research in mood disorders. *Biological Psychiatry*, *52*, 631-654.

Goodman, S., & Gotlib, I. (2002). *Children of depressed parents. Mechanisms of risk and implications for treatment*. Washington, DC: American Psychological Association.

Grote, N. K., & Frank, E. (2003). Difficult-to-treat depression: The role of contexts and comorbidities. *Biological Psychiatry*, *53*, 660-670.

Gunderson, J. G., Triebwasser, J., Philips, K. A., & Sullivan, C. N. (1999). Personality and vulnerability to affective disorders. In C. R. Cloninger (Ed.), *Personality and psychopathology* (pp. 3-32). Washington, DC/London: American Psychiatric Press.

Hollon, S. D., Munoz, R. F., Barlow, D. H., Beardslee, W. R., Bell, C. C., Bernal, G., Clarke, G. N., Franciosi, L. P., Kazdin, A. E., Kohn, L., Linehan, M. M., Markowitz, J. C., Miklowitz, D. J., Persons, J. B., Niederehe, G., & Sommers, D. (2002). Psychosocial intervention development for the prevention and treatment of depression: Promoting innovation and increasing access. *Biological Psychiatry*, *52*, 610-630.

Jones, E. E., & Pulos, S. M. (1993). Comparing the process of psychodynamic and cognitive-behavioral therapies. *Journal of Consulting and Clinical Psychology*, *61*, 306-316.

Judd, L. J. (1997). The clinical course of unipolar major depressive disorders. *Archives of General Psychiatry*, *54*, 989-991.

Khan, A., & Khan, S. (2003). Placebo in mood disorders: The tail that wags the dog. *Current Opinion in Psychiatry*, *16*, 35-39.

Kirsch, I., Moore, T. J., Scoboria, A., & Nicholls, S. S. (2002). The emperor's new drugs: An analysis of antidepressant medication data submitted to the U.S. Food and Drug Administration. *Prevention & Treatment*, *5*, Article 23. Retrieved September 3, 2004, from http://journals.apa.org/prevention/volume5/pre0050023a.html

Kirsch, I., & Sapirstein, G. (1998). Listening to Prozac but hearing placebo: A meta-analysis of antidepressant medication. *Prevention & Treatment*, *1*, Article 0002a. Retrieved September 3, 2004, from http://journals.apa.org/prevention/volume1/pre0010002a.html

Klein, D. N., & Hayden, E. P. (2000). Dysthymic disorder: Current status and future directions. *Current Opinion in Psychiatry*, *13*, 171-177.

Klein, M. H., Kupfer, D. J., & Shea, M. T. (1993). *Personality and depression. A current view*. New York/London: The Guilford Press.

Kupfer, D. J., & Frank, E. (2001). The interaction of drug- and psychotherapy in the long-term treatment of depression. *Journal of Affective Disorders, 62*, 131-137.

Kwon, P. (1999). Attributional style and psychodynamic defense mechanisms: Toward an integrative model of depression. *Journal of Personality, 67*, 645-658.

Luyten, P., Lowyck, B., & Corveleyn, J. (2003). Teoria y tratamiento de la depression: Hacia su integracion? [Theory and treatment of depression: Towards integration?]. *Persona, 6*, 81-97.

Mulder, R. T. (2002). Personality pathology and treatment outcome in major depression: A review. *American Journal of Psychiatry, 159*, 359-371.

Murray, C. J. L., & Lopez, A. D. (Eds.) (1996). *The global burden of disease: A comprehensive assessment of mortality and disability from diseases, injuries and risk factors in 1990 and projected to 2020*. Cambridge, MA: Harvard University Press.

National Institute of Mental Health (1999). *The effects of depression in the workplace*. Retrieved September 3, 2004, from http://www.nimh.nih.gov/publicat/workplace.cfm

National Institute of Mental Health (2001). *The numbers count. Mental disorders in America*. Retrieved September 3, 2004, from http://www.nimh.nih.gov/publicat/numbers.pdf

National Institute of Mental Health (2003). *Breaking ground, breaking through: The Strategic Plan for Mood Disorders Research*. Retrieved September 3, 2004, from http://www.nimh.nih.gov/strategic/mooddisorders.pdf

Parker, G., Roy, K., & Eyers, K. (2003). Cognitive behavior therapy for depression? Choose horses for courses. *American Journal of Psychiatry, 160*, 825-834.

Robins, C. J. (1993). Implications of research in the psychopathology of depression for psychotherapy integration. *Journal of Psychotherapy Integration, 3*, 313-330.

Rush, A. J., & Thase, M. E. (2002). Psychotherapies for depressive disorders: A review. In M. Maj & N. Sartorius (Eds.), *Depressive disorders* (2nd ed.) (pp. 161-206). Chichester: Wiley.

Segal, Z. V., Pearson, J. L., & Thase, M. E. (2003). Challenges in preventing relapse in major depression. Report of a National Institute of Mental Health Workshop on state of the science of relapse prevention in major depression. *Journal of Affective Disorders, 77*, 97-108.

Segal, Z. V., Williams, J. M .G., & Teasdale, J. D. (2002). *Mindfulness-based Cognitive Therapy for depression. A new approach to preventing relapse*. New York: Guilford Press.

Shapiro, D. A., Barkham, M., Rees, A., Hardy, G. E., Reynolds, S., & Startup, M. (1994). Effects of treatment duration and severity of depression on the effectiveness of cognitive-behavioral and psychodynamic interpersonal psychotherapy. *Journal of Consulting and Clinical Psychology, 62*, 522-534.

Shea, T., Elkin, I., Imber, S. D., Sotsky, S. M., Watkins, J. T., Collins, J. F., et al. (1992). Course of depressive symptoms over follow-up: Findings from the National Institute of Mental Health Treatment of Depression Collaborative Research Program. *Archives of General Psychiatry, 49*, 782-787.

Solomon, D. A., Keller, M. B., Leon, A. C., Mueller, T. I., Lavori, P. W., Shea, M. T., Coryell, W., Warshaw, M., Turvey, C., Maser, J. D., & Endicott, J. (2000). Multiple recurrences of major depressive disorder. *American Journal of Psychiatry, 157*, 229-233.

Verheul, R. (2003). Chronische depressie en persoonlijkheidsstoornis. Overeenkomsten, onderscheid en consequenties [Chronic depression and personality disorder. Similarities, distinctions and consequences]. In M. B. J. Blom, J. Spijker & R. van Dyck (Eds.), *Behandelingsstrategieën bij chronische depressie en dysthymie* [Treatment strategies for chronic depression and dysthymic disorder] (pp. 27-44). Houten/Mechelen: Bohn Stafleu Van Loghum.

Viguera, A. C., Baldessarini, R. J., & Friedberg, J. (1998). Discontinuing antidepressant treatment in major depression. *Harvard Review of Psychiatry, 5*, 293-306.

Westen, D., & Morrison, K. (2001). A multidimensional meta-analysis of treatments for depression, panic, and generalized anxiety disorder: An empirical examination of the status of empirically supported therapies. *Journal of Consulting and Clinical Psychology, 69*, 875-899.

Westen, D., Novotny, C. M., & Thompson-Brenner, H. (2004). The empirical status of empirically supported psychotherapies: Assumptions, findings, and reporting in controlled clinical trials. *Psychological Bulletin, 130*, 631-663.

Williams, J. W., Jr., Mulrow, C. D., Chiquette, E., Hitchcock Noël, P., Aguilar, C., & Cornell, J. (2000). A systematic review of newer pharmacotherapies for depression in adults: Evidence report summary. *Annals of Internal Medicine, 132*, 749-756.

Chapter 1

The Lifecycle of Depression

Koen Demyttenaere, Lukas Van Oudenhove, & Jürgen De Fruyt

Mood disorders in general and major depressive disorder (MDD) in particular are common, disabling psychiatric disorders with an estimated lifetime prevalence for MDD of around 17% in the community (Angst, 1997). The Belgian ESEMeD (European Study of Epidemiology of Mental Disorders) results confirm this estimate (lifetime prevalence of MDD 10.4% and 18.9% in males and females, respectively) (Alonso, Angermeyer, Bernert, Bruffaerts, et al., 2004).

Furthermore, the prevalence rates of MDD seem to have increased considerably over the past decades. A substantial increase in the rates in cohorts born after World War II and a decrease in the age of onset have been found in several large epidemiologic and family studies (Klerman & Weissman, 1989). There is some evidence that these changes are at least partly artifactual, though. Identification phenomena, memory effects and differential mortality, among others, can explain why these findings may be to some extent due to artifacts (Klerman & Weissman, 1989).

Over the past fifteen years, there has been increasing interest in the longitudinal course of MDD in the scientific literature. The discovery of psychotropic drugs in general and antidepressants in particular certainly made it possible to treat the acute phase of MDD more appropriately, but did this influence the long-term naturalistic outcome of the disorder? Nowadays, it is becoming more and more clear that MDD should be seen as a disorder that is chronic, progressive and recurrent in nature (Angst, 1997; Mueller et al., 1999; Solomon et al.,

2000; Kessing, Andersen, Mortensen, & Bolwig, 1998). In this review, we'll try to clarify some important aspects concerning the longitudinal course of depressive illness, in particular the recent evidence on the differences between first and recurrent episodes.

Finally, there has been a growing amount of research on the validity of the concept of MDD as defined by DSM-IV diagnostic criteria. Until a few years ago, little was known about the significance of subthreshold depressive symptoms or "subsyndromal depression". Some recent research provides support for the hypothesis that the "cut-off" of five symptoms or two weeks duration as required by DSM-IV is rather arbitrary: conventional limits put on a continuum of depressive symptoms of varying severity and duration. In other words, the key question is: should the diagnosis of MDD be seen in a categorical or a dimensional perspective (Judd et al., 1998a, 1998b; Kendler & Gardner, 1998)?

Increasing Rates of Depression: Fact or Fiction?

In 1989, Klerman and Weissman (1989) commented on the results of several large epidemiologic and family studies, suggesting important temporal changes in the rate of major depression. In the cohorts born after World War II, an increasing rate is found, as well as a decrease in the age of onset (with an increase in the late teenage and early adult years), an increase between 1960 and 1975 in the rates of depression for all ages, a persistent gender effect (with the risk of depression consistently two to three times higher among women than men across all adult ages) and finally a persistent family effect, with the risk about two to three times higher in first-degree relatives as compared with controls.

Undoubtedly, the use of standardized diagnostical instruments in large community-based studies and the application of modern statistical techniques to the large data sets from these studies have made more reliable research on the temporal changes in rates of mental disorders possible. The results from this kind of studies, especially those with a longitudinal design, can provide some important information regarding syndromal validity, natural course and, more indirectly, etiology, pathogenesis and finally treatment of mental disorders. For instance, the combination of familial aggregation and temporal changes suggests that gene-environment interaction plays an important role in the pathogenesis of MDD (Klerman & Weissman, 1989). It is important, though, to mention that the reported studies have a cross-sectional instead of a longitudinal design, which plays a considerable role in some of the issues discussed below.

Some of the findings mentioned above, like the higher rate among women and first-degree relatives of depressed patients, are consistently reported in the literature (Klerman & Weissman, 1989). Others, especially the increasing rate in recent birth cohorts are more controversial and merit some further clarification. First, the cohort effect in MDD is not universally reported. For example, community-based

18

epidemiological studies in Puerto Rican, Mexican-American and Korean populations do not report these temporal changes, whereas comparable American, German and Canadian studies consistently find a cohort effect (Klerman & Weissman, 1989). Furthermore, there are some possible explanations why these findings of temporal changes may be artifactual rather than reflecting real changes in the rate of MDD. We will discuss three of the most interesting ones in detail.

Identification Phenomenon

An identification phenomenon can be an important confounding factor, as the studies mentioned above relied mainly on subjects' retrospective reports. Hasin and Link (1988) set up a study to test the hypothesis that there is an interaction between age and recognition. In other words, they expected that older individuals are less likely to recognize depression as a mental disorder, compared to younger adults, who might have a more "psychological" view to their experiences. The subjects in the study, 152 randomly selected citizens living in a suburban area of New York, were asked to imagine themselves in the situation described by the following vignette, describing a DSM-III major depressive episode with a duration of a month. A statement reflecting impairment in functioning was inserted after the vignette. Furthermore, subjects were requested to fill in a questionnaire. The questions asked whether the subjects regarded the situation described by the vignette as emotional/psychological in nature, and whether they considered the situation to be a problem or not:

"During the last month, even though nothing has gone wrong that you can think of, you have been feeling depressed. You have not been able to get enough sleep at night, you haven't had much appetite, and you have lost over five pounds. You have felt tired much of the time, and haven't been able to concentrate as well as usual. You have also noticed that you aren't enjoying things the way you would normally..." (Hasin & Link, 1988).

The results after analysis of the answers were quite clear. Age had a highly significant effect that did not change after controlling for vignette types, education and gender. The chance of recognizing the vignette as major depression was 3.78 times higher for a 25-year old than for a 60-year old. Thus, older people are less likely to remember depressive episodes or report them when asked for in a questionnaire regarding mental health. The authors conclude that there is a cohort effect in the perception rather than in the real rate of depression (Hasin & Link, 1988).

Memory effects can provide a second possible explanation for a cohort effect in rates of major depression as found in cross-sectional studies: older adults are more likely to forget previous depressive episodes compared to younger ones. Giuffra and Risch (1994) set up a simulation study to examine the effect of forgetting on differences between cohorts. The results suggest that small, constant annual rates of forgetting applied to successive birth cohorts generate cohort-like effects. These findings confirm the hypothesis that diminished recall in older cohorts is one of the possible confounding factors involved in the reported cohort effect in major depression rates. More generally, we have to take into account the somewhat limited value of cross-sectional studies when doing research on temporal changes in prevalence.

Moreover, work by Rice et al. indicates that a lifetime diagnosis of major depression is not stable over time, although the error decreases as severity increases. They assessed a population of 2,226 first-degree relatives of 612 probands who participated in another study at two time points, with an interval of 6 years. A substantial proportion of the assessed subjects were considered as having a lifetime diagnosis of major depression at one of the two time points, but not at the other. This could be due to suboptimal repeatability of the diagnostic instrument (reliability), diminished recall or limited validity of the underlying diagnostic construct, however (Rice, Rochberg, Endicott, Lavori, & Miller, 1992). Anyway, these findings provide some further evidence for the role of memory effects as a confounding factor in cohort effects found in cross-sectional studies.

Differential Mortality

Finally, the findings of temporal changes could be at least partly explained by a difference in mortality between healthy subjects and depressive subjects. If depression is associated with a higher mortality, the older birth cohorts would have lost more depressed subjects by death compared to younger birth cohorts. This could decrease the rate of depression in interviewed older populations (Klerman & Weissmann, 1989).

The relationship between MDD and mortality is complex and there have been some conflicting studies concerning this issue. In a recent systematic review regarding this topic, Wulsin, Vaillant and Wells (1999) found 57 studies. Twenty-nine of these (51%) found a positive association, 13 (23%) were negative and the results of the remaining 15 studies (26%) were mixed. In general, most of the studies on the link between depression and early death varied widely in methodology (sample selection, comparison groups, control for confounding variables, etc.), making comparisons between the different studies rather difficult. Furthermore, publication bias certainly is a problem. Some of the mentioned studies were well designed however. For these reasons, "the evidence that depression increases mortality may not be strong enough to answer the question definitively" (Wulsin et al., 1999).

However, some conclusions can be drawn from this review. 16% to 19% of the mortality in psychiatric samples of depression is due to suicide, which is consistent with the often reported suicide rate of 15% in MDD. By contrast, in most studies based on depressive samples recruited from the community or medical settings, no more than 1% of deaths are caused by suicide. Apart from suicide and other non-natural causes of death, a quite strong link between depression and cardiovascular mortality was found (Wulsin et al., 1999).

Although the important and interesting discussion on possible mechanisms linking depression and mortality lies beyond the scope of this review, we will mention two hypotheses briefly. First, depression may cause early death in an indirect way, for example due to poor self-care (including unhealthy food habits but also compliance with medical treatment). Second, there may be a more direct, pathophysiological link between depression and mortality. For example, there has been considerable evidence that depression is associated with important changes in endocrinological and immune systems. These changes make depressive individuals more vulnerable to cardiovascular and other diseases (Whooley & Browner, 1998). There is some evidence from well-designed studies that even subsyndromal depressive symptoms are associated with both higher mortality and immunological activation, which suggests a possible link (Glaser, Robles, Sheridan, Malarkey, & Kiecolt-Glaser, 2003; Whooley & Browner, 1998). We will discuss the importance of subsyndromal depressive symptoms more thoroughly further on. Dysfunction of the autonomous nervous system or abnormal platelet aggregation could also cause higher cardiovascular mortality among depressed individuals (Whooley & Browner, 1998; Ösby, Brandt, Correia, Ekbom, & Sparen, 2001).

As already mentioned above, there have been some studies on the association between depression and mortality in all kinds of populations and samples and it is important to take this into account when looking at the result of those studies.

Bruce, Leaf, Rozal, Florio and Hoff (1994) examined the relationship between psychiatric illness and mortality over 9 years in the community sample from the New Haven Epidemiologic Catchment Area Study, consisting of 3,560 subjects. Subjects who reported a recent episode of MDD at the first interview had a 9-year relative mortality risk of 2.01. There was a significant interaction with gender: recently depressed men were 4.22 times more likely to die during the follow-up period compared to men without recent depressive episode; for women, the relative mortality risk was 1.65 (Bruce et al., 1994).

In a recent study by Ösby et al. (2001), the cause of death of all Swedish inpatients with a diagnosis of bipolar (N=15,386) or unipolar mood disorder (N=39,182) between 1973 and 1995 was determined. All patients were followed from their first hospital admission, using the Swedish psychiatric inpatient register.

The date and the cause of death were found in the national cause-of-death register. The standardized mortality ratios (SMRs) for suicide in unipolar disorder were 20.9 and 27.0 for males and females, respectively. These rates are particularly high, which can be explained by the population studied, consisting of severely ill inpatients. The risk of suicide was particularly high for younger patients during the first years after the first diagnosis, findings that are important when looking for prevention strategies. The SMRs for all natural causes of death in unipolar disorder were 1.5 and 1.6 for males and females, respectively (Östby et al., 2001). In a longitudinal study of psychiatric inpatients, Angst et al. found higher suicide rates compared to a control population, as well as a higher cardiovascular mortality rate. Moreover, pharmacological treatment lowered the suicide rate (Angst, Stassen, Clayton, & Angst, 2002).

Bingefors, Isacson, Knorring, Smedby and Wicknertz (1996) conducted a community-based study in a primary and psychiatric ambulatory care setting. They identified all first-incidence antidepressant users in ambulatory care and analyzed their mortality during a nine year follow-up period. They found that in patients aged 65 and older, antidepressant treatment at index was a significant predictor of higher 9-year mortality. A hazard ratio of 1.52 was found, controlling for potential confounding variables like chronic medical disease at baseline. Regarding cardiovascular death, antidepressant treatment was not an independent risk factor, but patients with both ischemic heart disease and antidepressant treatment at baseline had a significantly higher risk of death compared to individuals with ischemic heart disease or antidepressant treatment alone. The implications of this study are somewhat limited, though. First, not all individuals taking antidepressants suffer from MDD. Second, the higher mortality rate among patients suffering from ischemic heart disease and taking antidepressants at baseline could be due to the widespread use of tricyclic antidepressants at the time this study was conducted, as those agents are known to have adverse cardiac effects (Bingefors et al., 1996).

As a part of the recent Dutch Amsterdam Study of the Elderly (AMSTEL), Schoevers et al. (2000) examined the influence of major depression, but also minor depressive symptoms, on risk of death. The study is longitudinal in design and the large sample consists of non-institutionalized, older persons who are living in the community and consult their GP. The follow-up period was 6 years, with an average of 55.5 months. The overall prevalence of depression was 12.9%, with 6.9% in men and 16.5% in women. These findings are in line with other studies on the prevalence of depression in community-living elderly people. Severe depression with psychotic features was significantly associated with higher mortality in both men and women, with unadjusted relative risks of 3.77 and 2.43, respectively. After adjustment for potential other explanatory variables, the relative risks were 1.64 and 1.66 respectively, which was still statistically significant. However, at the end of the follow up period 75% of the men suffering from psychotic depression had died, as compared to 41.4% of the women. For less serious "neurotic depression", the relative mortality risk reached statistical significance only in men, before and after controlling for potential confounding factors (2.67 and 1.90, respectively). In "neurotically depressed" women, an unadjusted relative risk of 1.14

was found. After adjustment, the RR was 1.02. It is noteworthy that not only MDD but also "milder" depression (not meeting the full DSM-IV diagnostic criteria) has an impact on mortality in old men. As a consequence, more attention should be paid to the diagnosis and treatment of this kind of depression in elderly men. Some possible explanations for the differential mortality between men and women are provided by Schoevers et al. (2000) but will not be discussed further here.

Finally, the association between depression and mortality in a nursing home population was investigated by Rovner et al. (1991). Newly admitted patients were followed prospectively for one year. First, the rates of depression in nursing homes were higher than those reported in the general population. A lot of factors, both psychosocial and medical, contribute to these higher rates. However, this will not be addressed further here. Second, the majority of cases of MDD were not recognized nor treated by nursing home physicians. Finally, MDD but not subsyndromal depressive symptoms, was a significant predictor of mortality, independent of other risk factors like medical disease, with a relative risk of 1.59 (Rovner et al., 1991).

Conclusion

In summary, the cohort effect of MDD reported in several, but not all, large cross-sectional epidemiologic studies is at least partly due to artifacts. We discussed some potential explanations, including identification phenomena, memory effects and differential mortality.

Long Term Course of MDD: First Versus Recurrent Episode

*"The attacks begin not infrequently after the illness
or death of near relatives...
We must regard all alleged (psychic) injuries as possible sparks
for the discharge of individual attacks, but the real cause of the malady
must be sought in permanent internal changes...
In spite of the removal of the discharging cause,
the attack follows its independent development...
But finally, the appearance of wholly similar attacks on
wholly dissimilar occasions or quite without external
occasion shows that even there where there has been
external influence, it must not be regarded as a necessary
presupposition for the appearance of the attack"*

E. Kraepelin (1921)

*"Single episodes are extremely rare if the period of observation
is significantly extended"*

J. Angst (1973)

These two quotes illustrate that there has been interest in the long-term course of affective disorders for many years, from the beginning of the 20th century onward. However, the amount of research on this topic has considerably increased over the past two decades. As it is now generally accepted that mood disorders are often chronic, recurrent and progressive in nature, attention has partly shifted from treatment of the acute phase to prevention of relapse/recurrence. In other words, the high rates of relapse, recurrence and chronicity reported in the literature made clear that the search for effective and efficacious strategies of continuation or maintenance treatment for affective disorders is one of the most important challenges of contemporary psychiatry.

When comparing different studies on the longitudinal course of MDD, the terms "response", "recovery", "relapse" and "remission" are not always defined in the same way, which may make comparisons between studies difficult. However, these terms are conceptualized by Frank et al. (1991). The term "response" indicates a decrease in depressive symptoms without returning to baseline, as opposed to "remission". The difference between "remission" and "recovery" is based on a rather arbitrarily chosen time criterion (6 months) and not on a pathophysiological basis. This is also true for the distinction between "relapse" and "recurrence". Moreover, not all studies use the same time criterion.

We will discuss some of the most relevant topics regarding the long-term course of MDD in the following paragraphs.

High Risk of Recurrence in MDD

There is a growing consensus that the risk of relapse and/or recurrence in MDD is generally high. Lavori, Dawson and Mueller (1994) followed depressive patients longitudinally after recovery from their first lifetime episode. The recurrence rate was 13% after six months, 28% after one year, 62% after five years, 75% after ten years and finally 87% after fifteen years. These findings clearly provide further evidence for the 30-year-old quote by Angst (1973), cited above.

In the NIMH Collaborative Program on the Psychobiology of Depression – Clinical Studies, a cohort of 380 depressed patients from five university psychiatric clinics has been prospectively followed after recovery from the index episode over a period of fifteen years. Müller et al. (1999) report on the results of this unique longitudinal, naturalistic study. The cumulative proportion of recurrence (by

Kaplan-Meier estimate) at the end of the follow-up period was 85%, with a median time to recurrence (well interval) of 132 weeks. The group who experienced a recurrence and the group who remained well received similar low levels of antidepressant treatment during both the index episode and the subsequent well interval. During this period of remission/recovery the amount and extent of antidepressant treatment decreased further. In addition, the authors focused on the subgroup of patients who remained well for five years after the index episode (n=105). In this subgroup, 58% suffered from a recurrent episode of MDD during the subsequent 10 years of follow-up. This indicates that the risk of recurrence decreases with the length of the well interval after an index episode, but there remains a considerable risk of relapse even after lengthy well intervals. It is important to take this finding into account when making clinical decisions on maintenance treatment (Mueller et al., 1999).

Predictors of Early Relapse/Recurrence

First of all, having experienced more prior episodes is strongly associated with a higher risk of relapse/recurrence. It is consistently reported in the literature that risk of recurrence increases by some 15% with each successive recurrence (Mueller et al., 1999; Solomon et al., 2000; Kessing & Andersen, 1999), although this is not found in all studies (Kessing, Andersen, & Mortensen, 1998).

Sociodemographic variables like gender, age at onset and marital status predict recurrence only in the earlier episodes (Kessing et al., 1998; Post, 1992). This seems to be the case for comorbid alcoholism too (Kessing, 1999). We will return to this issue later on.

Moreover, the risk of recurrence decreases progressively as the "well interval" (duration of recovery) increases (Mueller et al., 1999; Solomon et al., 2000). However, even after a well interval of five years, recurrence rates as high as 58% over the subsequent 10 years are reported in the above-mentioned well-designed naturalistic NIMH study (Mueller et al., 1999). Therefore, long enough courses of maintenance treatment with antidepressants (and/or psychotherapy) are strongly recommended, especially in patients with a history of highly recurrent depression. The optimum duration of maintenance treatment is less clear, though, and remains often a clinical rather than a really evidence-based decision. Durations varying from two to five years or even lifelong are suggested in the literature (Angst, 1997). Despite these recommendations, in a naturalistic setting, many patients do not receive adequate antidepressant maintenance therapy. As already mentioned above, in the NIMH study doses were low and duration was short (Mueller et al., 1999).

Finally, incomplete remission/recovery (the presence of residual subsyndromal depressive symptoms) is strongly associated with early relapse or recurrence. This is an important finding as it questions the validity of the boundaries of MDD as defined by DSM-IV diagnostic criteria. Patients suffering from residual subsyndromal depression (SSD) relapsed three times faster to a major depressive episode compared to patients who fully recovered after the index episode. This association is stronger than the association between the number of prior episodes and time to relapse or recurrence (Judd et al., 1998a, 1998b). Of course, these findings have important implications regarding treatment too. Residual SSD will be discussed more extensively later on in this review.

Duration of Episodes

In a longitudinal, prospective, naturalistic study conducted in tertiary care centers, Solomon et al. followed a cohort of 258 subjects suffering from unipolar major depressive disorder over 10 years from the index episode on. The median duration of illness was around 20 weeks and this was highly consistent across multiple recurrent mood episodes (Solomon et al., 1997). Although consistent with several other studies in the literature (Angst, 1986; Kessing & Mortensen, 1999), this finding does not support the often quoted clinical impression that duration increases with each recurrent episode. That impression may be at least partly due to decreasing well intervals between each subsequent episode (however see below). Moreover, the results described are applicable to the whole cohort, whereas in individual patients consistency in the duration of illness across multiple episodes was low to moderate (Solomon et al., 1997). No sociodemographic or clinical factors were associated with the duration of episodes. This uniform duration of recurrent depressive episodes suggests that the rate of recovery from a depressive episode does not change in the course of illness. In other words, recurrent episodes are equally "treatable" compared to earlier episodes. However, the level of treatment increased with each recurrent episode, which could have influenced the duration (Solomon et al., 1997). Also, compliance is higher in recurrent episodes (Demyttenaere & Bruffaerts, 2003a). Some of our own unpublished data challenge the above-mentioned findings and indicate that recurrent episodes are more difficult to treat compared to first episodes, despite the higher treatment adherence (Demyttenaere & Bruffaerts, 2003b).

Furthermore, the population studied is an important issue when looking at data regarding duration of depressive episodes. The above mentioned studies all consisted of patients seeking help at tertiary care centers, which had an influence on the results. As part of the Dutch NEMESIS study, Spijker et al. (2002) examined the duration of major depressive episodes in the general Dutch population. In this study, the median duration of depressive episodes in the whole study was 3 months and recurrent episodes were shorter in duration compared to first episodes. Severity of the index episode predicted longer episode duration. However, the level of care influenced the duration of episodes (median duration was 3 months for those without professional care, 4.5 months in primary care and 6 months in mental health care), although the differences did not reach statistical significance (Spijker et al., 2002). Other longitudinal community-based studies like the Epidemiologic

Catchment Area study report similar durations around 12 weeks (Eaton et al., 1997; Spijker et al., 2002).

Time to Recurrence

A substantial number of patients experience a progressive course of illness, characterized by "cycle acceleration". In other words, in this group of patients, the "well interval" (or time to recurrence) decreases with each recurrent episode (Kessing et al., 1998; Post, 1992). This finding is in line with most previous studies on this topic, although some studies did not find such a pattern of cycle acceleration. These discrepancies may be explained by methodological differences or problems (Kessing et al., 1998).

Moreover, patients with an initial course of illness characterized by decreasing time intervals between the first three lifetime episodes had a 33% increased risk of experiencing further recurrence, compared with patients who did not follow such a pattern of initial illness (Kessing, Mortensen, & Bolwig, 1998).

The Role of Psychosocial Stress and Life Events. "From Precipitated to Spontaneous Episodes": The Kindling Hypothesis

Several studies suggest that the etiologic role of stressful life events in major depression is more important in first-onset episodes compared to recurrent episodes, at least in an important subgroup of patients. In other words, early episodes are more likely to be triggered by psychosocial stressors, whereas recurrent episodes are more likely to occur spontaneously, i.e., not related to any important life event (Post, 1992). As noted, this pattern was already described by Kraepelin in the early 1920s (Kraepelin, 1921). Nowadays the term "kindling hypothesis" is used to describe this evolution from precipitated to spontaneous episodes. The term "kindling" is derived from epileptology (see below). There is quite a lot of evidence supporting this hypothesis. For example, the effect of never being married decreases during the course of depression (Kessing, Andersen, & Andersen, 2000). Moreover, in the National Institute of Mental Health collaborative study on the psychobiology of depression, the mean number of prior episodes in patients with an "environment-sensitive" episode was 3.7, whereas the mean number of episodes in patients with an "autonomous" episode was 13.4 (Post, 1992; Swann et al., 1990). In a meta-analysis of studies on this topic, 57% of first episode patients experienced a major life event prior to the onset of their depressive episode, compared to 32% of later episode patients (Post, 1992). Although the studies were methodologically quite different, their findings were rather consistent. A recent study by Mitchell et al. (2003) suggested that this differential effect of life events in first compared to recurrent episodes may be specific to non-melancholic depression (Mitchell et al., 2003).

Kendler, Thornton and Gardner (2000) argue that several previous studies on this "kindling" hypothesis suffer from several methodological limitations (clinical

27

populations, cross-sectional studies, etc.). Moreover, the fact that depressive subjects may generate more life events compared to non-depressive controls has to be taken into account (Kendler et al., 2000; Harkness, Monroe, Simons, & Thase, 1999). In a longitudinal population-based twin study (N=2,395), Kendler and colleagues (2000) interviewed participants four times over a period of nine years. Only life events that were clearly independent of the respondent's own behavior were included in the analyses in order to determine "whether the change in sensitivity to the effects of stressful life events over episodes varied within as well across individuals" (Kendler et al., 2000). The results of this study were largely consistent with the kindling hypothesis: the number of previous episodes had a strong effect on the association between stressful life events and depressive onsets, but this relation was biphasic. A strong negative interaction between previous depressive episodes and stressful life events in the prediction of risk for a successive depressive episode was found, especially in the first nine episodes. After the ninth episode, the interaction became weaker. In other words, the odds ratio (OR) for depressive onset given at least one stressful life event decreased significantly with an increasing number of previous depressive episodes for the first nine episodes. From the tenth episode on, the OR remained more or less constant. The authors conclude: "these findings suggest that, whatever the biological or psychological process that underlies this phenomenon, it is 'saturable'" (Kendler et al., 2000).

In another well designed study the same authors examined the impact of genetic risk factors on this "kindling" phenomenon (Kendler, Thornton, & Gardner, 2001). The results were consistent with a model of "prekindling" in those at high genetic risk (defined by presence of a history of depression in the co-twin). Kendler et al. (2001) found that subjects at high genetic risk reached the "kindled" stage (i.e., the stage of spontaneous rather than triggered episodes) after significantly less depressive episodes compared to subjects who were not at high genetic risk. For example, a first depressive onset was associated with a significant life event in 59.7% of the low genetic risk group but only in 38.2% of the high genetic risk group. In summary, "the decline in the association between stressful life events and risk for major depression as the number of previous depressive episodes increases was strongest in those at low genetic risk and weaker in those at high genetic risk. Therefore, there may be potentially distinct environmental and genetic pathways to a "kindled" or "sensitized" state in which the mind/brain is predisposed to spontaneous depressive episodes".

Robert M. Post was the first to apply the models of kindling (originally described in epileptology) and behavioral sensitization (derived from psychopharmacology) to the longitudinal course of affective disorders (Post, Rubinow, & Ballenger, 1986). Kindling can be defined as "the development of major motor seizures in response to repeated intermittent electrical stimulation of the brain with insufficient current to produce overt behavioral effects" (Racine, 1978). This phenomenon seems to be caused by long-lasting, possibly permanent changes in neural excitability induced by the repeated application of a "subthreshold" current to the neuron. Moreover, after many repetitions of kindled seizures, spontaneous seizures may develop (Post et al., 1986). Behavioral sensitization refers to the progressive changes in behavioral response to psychomotor stimulants (like cocaine) after repeated administration of a constant dose. In a sensitized state, the behavioral response is developing with a faster onset, increased intensity and longer duration. Conditioning seems to be important in behavioral sensitization, as for example response to cocaine is highly dependent on the environment in which cocaine is administered. Thus, "the underlying changes in brain biochemistry may be conditioned" (Post et al., 1986).

Post argues that these kindling and sensitization paradigms provide nonhomologous models that can help us understand the longitudinal course of affective disorders in general and the differential impact of psychosocial stressors in first versus subsequent episodes in particular. These are nonhomologous paradigms because kindled seizures and behavioral responses to cocaine do not clinically resemble affective episodes, although the sensitized response to cocaine does share some features with dysphoric mania. However, both repeated psychosocial stress and depressive episodes themselves may induce long lasting cognitive and neurobiological changes, making the subject more vulnerable to subsequent episodes. Just as kindled seizures appear spontaneously after repeated stimulation during a long enough period of time, affective episodes eventually occur without environmental triggers (Post, 1992). Type, magnitude and frequency of the stressor are critical to its long-term effects. For example, stressors involving psychosocial losses may induce a set of cognitive, behavioral and neurobiological consequences making an individual more vulnerable to depressive episodes, whereas acute life-threatening stressors may induce another set of long-lasting changes more likely to cause post-traumatic stress syndrome (Post, 1992; Post et al., 1986).

There is widespread evidence for cortisol hypersecretion both in situations of psychosocial stress and in depressive episodes (for recent reviews, see Sapolsky, 2000; Raison & Miller, 2003). These elevated levels of cortisol could initiate a neurobiological cascade of second, third, etc. messenger systems ending in changes in gene transcription that cause the already mentioned long-lasting neurobiological changes. From a cognitive point of view, both stressors and depressive episodes could cause long-lasting changes in cognitive structures. Associations between previous triggers and their symbolic components may be learned or conditioned so that the symbolic representation of the stressor is eventually able to cause a recurrent depressive episode in the absence of a real stressor or loss. However, the neurobiological and cognitive points of view are not mutually exclusive. The neurobiological changes induced by stressors and depressive episodes may be the cause of alterations in memory and cognitive patterns (Post, 1992; Post et al., 1986).

In summary, like Nobel Prize winner Eric Kandel (Kandel, 1998), the work of Post and collaborators tries to build a bridge between neurobiological and psychosocial theories of depression, providing support for a widely accepted biopsychosocial stress-vulnerability model of MDD. Nonetheless, further research is needed as many of the aspects in this kindling theory, especially regarding the underlying neurobiological mechanisms involved in learning and memory, remain rather speculative.

There have so far been quite a lot of contradictory findings in the literature on cognitive functioning in depression. The importance of cognitive (dys)functioning in professional and social functioning can hardly be overestimated, though. In an excellent review on this topic, Austin et al. try to summarize the results and hypotheses regarding this issue (Austin, Mitchell, & Goodwin, 2001).

Before discussing the pattern of cognitive dysfunction in MDD, it is important to mention that there are quite a lot of confounding factors that make comparisons between different studies quite difficult (Austin et al., 2001). First, studies on the effect of depression severity on cognitive function are conflicting. The observation that depressive individuals scored lower on verbal recall tasks and normal on verbal recognition tasks led to the hypothesis that the cognitive dysfunction in depression is secondary to a motivational deficit, causing lower scores on "effortful" and not on "automatic" tasks (Austin et al., 2001). However, this hypothesis has been undermined by several studies that found abnormal performance on "automatic" as well as on "effortful" tasks. Some tasks may be more sensitive to motivation effects than others. Similarly, some neuropsychological functions are highly dependent on current mood, others are not (Austin et al., 2001). Porter, Gallagher, Thompson and Young (2003) suggest that executive functions are relatively stable, whereas memory functions vary more with severity of depression. In conclusion, there may be an important interaction between motivation, depressed affect and cognitive function; further study is needed to clarify this interaction more precisely (Austin et al., 2001). Second, subtype of depression (e.g., melancholic versus atypical) could be associated with a specific pattern of cognitive dysfunction (Austin et al., 2001). Third, the role of medication in cognitive deficits has not been sufficiently studied. Agents with anticholinergic properties, like most tricyclic antidepressants (TCA), are particularly known for their negative effects on cognition (Porter, Gallagher, Thompson, & Young, 2003). Even the mild anticholinergic effect of the selective serotonin reuptake inhibitor (SSRI) paroxetine causes subtle cognitive deficits (impaired delayed recall on a word-learning task) in young healthy volunteers (Schmitt, Kruizinga, & Riedel, 2001). Finally, age can be an important confounding factor (Austin et al., 2001). Moreover, the role of the microvascular cerebral changes that are often found in (geriatric) depression remains to be determined (Austin et al., 2001).

There is quite good evidence that depression is associated with deficits in episodic memory and learning (Austin et al., 2001). Both explicit verbal and visual memory are impaired, whereas performance on implicit memory tasks is spared. Temporal lobe lesions, especially loss of hippocampal volume potentially caused by glucocorticoid toxicity, may be responsible for these particular cognitive dysfunctions (Austin et al., 2001). We will discuss this extensively further on. The presence and the pattern of executive dysfunction, mediated by the prefrontal cortex, is less clear, however. Attentional set-shifting (as measured by the Trail Making B and Digit Symbol Substitution tests) is most consistently reported to be impaired, with more important dysfunction as severity of depression increases (Austin et al., 2001).

In a study under drug-free conditions, Schatzberg et al. (2000) found that patients suffering from depression with psychotic features show more substantial cognitive impairment compared to non-psychotic depressive controls, including deficits in attention, response inhibition (measured by the Stroop test) and explicit verbal memory. These results are in line with the results of an earlier study by Basso and Bornstein (1999a).

In another study by Basso and Bornstein (1999b), 20 single episode (SE) and 46 recurrent episode (RE) young depressed inpatients were administered a comprehensive neuropsychological test battery. After controlling for age, severity of depression, sedation rate and anticholinergic blocking rate, the SE group showed no significant cognitive impairment. The RE group, on the contrary, showed a significantly impaired recall on the California Verbal Learning Test compared to the SE group and published norms. For example, they recalled fewer words during the five learning trials and also long-delay free and cued recall was impaired. There was no difference in benefit of recognition cueing relative to long-delay free recall. Furthermore, the groups showed equivalent performance on the index comparing long-delay free recall to short-delay free recall. These findings suggest a pattern of deficient acquisition rather than retrieval or retention. There were no significant differences in measures of intelligence (subscales of the WAIS), attention (digit span forwards), visuospatial attention and motor speed (Trail Making Test A) and various frontal-executive functions (FAS verbal fluency, digit span backwards and Trail Making Test B) (Basso & Bornstein, 1999b).

Furthermore, there are some studies which examined cognitive functions in euthymic patients with a history of one or more depressive episodes. First, Tham et al. (1997) found that the group with a history of depression performed significantly worse on several tests of cognitive functions (general intelligence, memory, attention, frontal functions). Moreover, there was a significant association between number of previous hospitalizations for mood disorder and some of these tests (reasoning, general intelligence, Trail Making A, set-shifting as measured by Trail Making B). Second, Kessing (1998) performed a retrospective controlled cohort study based on the Danish psychiatric case register. Cognitive impairment was significantly higher in patients with a history of recurrent depressive episodes, whereas the performance of patients with a history of only one episode did not differ from normal controls. Moreover, intra-individual analyses showed that the number of prior episodes correlated with the degree of cognitive impairment. Third, Paradiso, Lamberty, Garvey and Robinson (1997) found significant cognitive impairment in euthymic patients with a chronic history of depression. Mainly attentional and executive functions were impaired, as well as immediate memory. Finally, Austin et al. (2001) reviewed the literature regarding cognitive deficits during the euthymic phase of MDD. They concluded that, although the few longitudinal studies that tested cognitive functions before and after recovery from depressive episodes suffer from methodological limitations, at least a subgroup of patients suffers from residual deficits in memory and/or executive functions during "well intervals". The exact relationship between these deficits and crucial clinical and sociodemographic variables like number of previous episodes, age, treatment and chronicity needs further research though (Austin et al., 2001).

In summary, the above-mentioned studies provide evidence for the hypothesis that recurrent depressive episodes cause some kind of "cognitive scar", lasting during episodes of recovery. However, the exact relationship between MDD and cognitive functions remains to be studied, preferably in longitudinal studies.

As already mentioned above, loss of hippocampal volume in recurrent depression is an important neurobiological correlate of those residual cognitive (memory) deficits. This will be discussed more thoroughly in the next paragraph.

Neurobiological Correlates of (Cognitive Deficit in) Depression: Hippocampus and Amygdala

In a Magnetic Resonance Imaging (MRI) study conducted in 1996, Sheline, Wang, Gado, Csernansky and Vannier (1996) found a significant negative association between left and right hippocampal volume and total duration of illness in euthymic patients with a history of depression compared to matched control subjects. These results were confirmed by another study by Sheline, Sanghavi, Mintun and Gado (1999): hippocampal volume decreased as total duration of depression increased. Moreover, subjects with a history of depression performed significantly worse on explicit verbal learning tasks. Interestingly, these tasks are known to be highly hippocampus-dependent. Furthermore, no correlation between hippocampal volume and age, which could be a confounding factor, was found (Sheline et al. (1999). Sheline, Gado and Price (1998), in turn, found a 17% decrease in amygdala core nuclei volume in previously depressed subjects who were in remission at the time of the study. As the amygdala plays an important role in emotional processing and memory, these findings are in line with earlier studies that found impaired performance on emotional tasks in depressed subjects (Sheline et al., 1998). Finally, Sheline, Gado and Kraemer (2003) found a significant relationship between degree of hippocampal volume loss and duration of untreated depressive episodes. These findings provide some more evidence for the hypothesis that antidepressants provide a neuroprotective effect, which is in line with studies by Bremner and colleagues in both depression and post-traumatic stress disorder (PTSD) (Bremner et al., 2000; Vermetten, Vythilingam, Southwick, Charney, & Bremner, 2003).

MacQueen et al. (2003) compared hippocampal volume and hippocampal function (as measured by a recollection memory task) of never-treated first-episode patients, patients with a history of recurrent episodes and matched healthy controls. First, the authors found impaired performance on several recollection memory tasks in first and recurrent-episode patients compared to controls. Measures of habit memory did not differ between the three groups, which is important as habit memory is not hippocampus-dependent. These findings indicate that hippocampal dysfunction is present from the first episode on. Second, loss of hippocampal volume on MRI was found in recurrent-episode patients and not in first-episode patients or controls. Moreover, the relation between illness duration and hippocampal volume was best described by a logarithmic curve, indicating that hippocampal volume loss occurs rather early in the course of the disease, although it is not yet detectable in first-episode patients (MacQueen et al., 2003).

There are several possible pathophysiological mechanisms that could lead to hippocampal volume loss in depression. First, hippocampal neuronal cell death due to glucocorticoid toxicity is important (Sheline, 2000; Sheline et al., 1999; Sapolsky, 2000; Sapolsky, Krey, & McEwen, 1986). It is widely accepted that dysfunctional feedback mechanisms of the HPA axis cause elevated levels of cortisol in at least an important subgroup of depressive subjects (Sapolsky, 2000; Sheline, 2000). Similarly, exposure to repeated stressors causes elevated levels of cortisol. Both animal and human research has provided substantial evidence for a toxic effect of glucocorticoids on hippocampal neurons (Sapolsky, 2000; Sapolsky et al., 1986; Sheline, 2000; Sheline et al., 1998, 1999). For example, patients with primary Cushing's syndrome (who are exposed to highly elevated glucocorticoid levels for a long period of time) are found to have both lower hippocampal volume and impaired hippocampal (memory) functions. Moreover, these changes are reversible after treatment, resulting in normalization of cortisol levels (Starkman, Giordani, Berent, Schork, & Schteingart, 2001; Starkman, Giordani, Gebarski, & Schteingart, 2003). Glucocorticoid toxicity in hippocampal neurons may be mediated by enhanced vulnerability to the excitotoxic effect of excitatory amino acids like glutamate (Sheline, 2000). Furthermore, Corticotrophin Releasing Factor (CRF) also has a direct or indirect neurotoxic effect. Several studies found elevated levels of CRF in depression and CRF antagonists are neuroprotective (Sheline et al., 1999). Second, loss of glial cells could be a potential mechanism, again resulting in increased vulnerability to glutamate (Sheline, 2000; Sheline et al., 1999). Third, stress-induced reduction in neurotrophic factors like Brain-Derived Neurotrophic Factor (BDNF) could play a role in volume loss. Stress decreases the expression of BDNF and antidepressants reverse this decrease in expression. This may be one potential mechanism for the above-mentioned neuroprotective potential of these agents (Sheline, 2000, 2003; Sheline et al., 1999).

However, many questions remain to be answered. For example, it is not known whether depression is the cause or the result of the above mentioned structural changes, or even both (Sheline, 2003). Modern high-resolution brain imaging techniques like Positron Emission Tomography (PET) and functional Magnetic Resonance Imaging (fMRI) will undoubtedly contribute to a better knowledge of the neurobiological correlates of depression and their evolution during the long-term course of depressive illness.

A DSM-IV diagnosis of major depressive episode (MDE) requires five depressive symptoms or more, clinically significant impairment and at least 2 weeks duration. This definition reflects a categorical view of major depression: either you suffer from MDE, or you do not, depending on criteria defining a "cut-off". Similarly, DSM-IV defines criteria for some other depressive syndromes like minor depressive episode (MinDE). However, there has been increasing debate about these rather arbitrarily chosen criteria over the past few years. The key question is whether these "boundaries" set by DSM-IV criteria reflect "real" limits of distinct depressive syndromes. Alternatively, depressive illness can be seen as a continuum of depressive symptoms with variable severity and duration over the course of illness (dimensional diagnosis). In other words: does major depression differ qualitatively or just quantitatively from minor depression or "subsyndromal" depressive symptoms? A qualitative difference means that the different unipolar mood disorders as defined by DSM-IV (MDD, minor depression, dysthymic disorder) do represent different clinical entities, each with different clinical characteristics and pathophysiology. In contrast, if the difference between these depressive syndromes is only quantitative, depression should be seen as a single disease characterized by a continuum of different and variable levels of symptoms, but with a single, although multifactorial, etiology and pathogenesis. Recently, there have been quite a number of studies which tried to answer this important question.

Judd and colleagues have done a lot of work on this topic. They define subsyndromal symptomatic depression (SSD) as "depressive symptoms beneath the diagnostic threshold for minor, dysthymic or major depressive disorder" (Judd et al., 1998a). In community samples, high prevalences of SSD are found, causing significant psychosocial impairment. Moreover, some studies indicate that residual SSD after recovery of an index major depressive episode is a significant predictor of relapse or recurrence, as we already briefly mentioned (Judd et al., 1998a). To test this hypothesis, Judd et al. (1998a) followed a large cohort of patients prospectively for 10 years after recovery from an index episode of MDD, with special interest in the influence of SSD on duration of recovery. First, asymptomatic recovery (AR) patients had significantly shorter intake MDEs and significantly more AR patients did not suffer from a recurrent episode during the 10 years of follow-up. Second, MDE relapse was more than three times faster for residual SSD recovery patients. Moreover, SSD recovery patients relapsed 5.5 times faster to any depressive episode (MinDE or MDE). AR patients remained well for a median of 231 weeks, whereas residual SSD recovery patients had a median time to recurrence of only 68 weeks. Furthermore, recovery status (AR versus SSD) was a stronger predictor of relapse/recurrence than history of previous recurrent depressive episodes. SSD patients received more antidepressants during their first well interval, but not during the index episode, indicating that the higher relapse rates in SSD recovery patients are not due to differences in antidepressant treatment

(Judd et al., 1998a). These findings are in line with several earlier studies and confirm the hypothesis that SSD is an active state of depressive illness rather than some kind of recovery (Judd et al., 1998a). In other words, the results of this study provide some evidence for a dimensional rather than a categorical approach to depressive illness. Furthermore, this study illustrates the need for treatment until full recovery is reached rather than partial remission. It is possible that SSD recovery patients need higher doses or combinations of antidepressants, more frequent psychotherapy or some other forms of intensive treatment to reach asymptomatical status (Judd et al., 1998a). Fava, Rafanelli, Grandi, Conti and Belluardo (1998) found cognitive behavioral therapy (CBT) to be significantly more effective than clinical management in reducing residual symptoms and preventing relapse after remission from an index MDE. In this study, antidepressants were tapered and finally discontinued during the 2-year follow-up period. After two years, the CBT group had a relapse rate of 25% compared to 80% in the clinical management group.

In another article, Judd et al. (1998b) report on the weekly symptomatic course of MDD in a cohort of patients from the same naturalistic study. Patients were followed prospectively over a period of 12 years and weekly depressive symptoms were recorded and divided into 4 levels of severity. The first level was defined as depressive symptoms at or above the DSM-IV threshold for MDE, the second level as depressive symptoms at the threshold for MinDE, the third as SSD below the thresholds for MDE or MinDE and the fourth level was defined as no depressive symptoms (asymptomatic). Patients were divided into 3 subgroups: first lifetime MDE, recurrent episode and "double depression" (MDE superimposed on dysthymia). The authors found that patients presented with multiple levels of symptoms over time: 59% of patients spent time at each of the 4 levels and only 1% of patients spent their entire follow-up period at one symptom level. Moreover, symptom levels changed relatively quickly and often, with an average total of 17.1 changes during follow-up. Furthermore, patients suffering from their first lifetime MDE at intake were significantly more often symptom-free than the two other groups in the sample and they had significantly fewer changes, suggesting a more benign course in first-episode patients. Finally, MinD and SSD symptoms were 3 times more common than MD symptoms (Judd et al., 1998b). This is an important finding as we have to consider SSD as an active state of illness that highly predicts MDE relapse, as mentioned above (Judd et al., 1998a). These results provide further support for the "single clinical illness" (i.e., dimensional) hypothesis of unipolar depression. Judd et al. (1998b) conclude: "We believe a growing confluence of scientific evidence supports the hypothesis that unipolar MDD is a clinically homogeneous illness in which major, minor and subsyndromal depressive symptoms commonly alternate as different manifestations and levels of illness activity". This was confirmed by a more recent study from the same group (Judd et al., 2000).

Kendler and Gardner (1998) examined the relationship between three key features of the major depressive syndrome and the risk of future episodes of major depression in both the subject and his/her co-twin, two widely used validating criteria for psychiatric disorders. The twin pairs were ascertained from a population-based registry; they were followed longitudinally at two time points after the first interview. The three evaluated features were: numbers of symptoms listed under DSM-IV criterion A for MDE (at least five required by DSM-IV), level of severity or impairment (DSM-IV requires either significant distress or significant impairment in functioning) and duration (minimum of 2 weeks required by DSM-IV). The risk of major depression in both the subject and his/her co-twin increased with an increasing number of criterion A symptoms, without any discontinuity between four and five symptoms, as hypothesized by DSM-IV. Similarly, subjects who reported five or more depressive symptoms leading to only mild or moderate impairment still had a significantly greater risk of major depression compared to subjects who did not report five or more depressive symptoms. The same was true in the co-twins. However, the increased risk was substantially greater for those who reported five or more symptoms leading to severe impairment. Finally, major depressive episodes lasting less than two weeks proved to increase the risk of future major depression in both subjects and their co-twins, compared to those who did not report a depressive episode of any duration. In summary, the authors failed to find empirical evidence for a discontinuity at the boundaries proposed by DSM-IV (Kendler & Gardner, 1998).

Moreover, our own unpublished data provide some more evidence for a "differential weight" of the different DSM-IV depressive symptoms, without any discontinuity between four or five symptoms. Depressed mood, diminished interest and loss of energy are the most consistently reported symptoms, even at "subsyndromal" level (Demyttenaere & Bruffaerts, 2002).

In a longitudinal, prospective cohort study of 7,518 older women with a follow-up of 7 years, Whooley and Browner (1998) found an increased risk of death by both cardiovascular and non-cancer, non-cardiovascular diseases in patients who reported "only" subsyndromal or mild depressive symptoms on the 15-item Geriatric Depression Scale. Moreover, mortality increased with number of depressive symptoms.

As already mentioned, the relationship between depressive symptoms and mortality is likely to be multifactorial. One hypothesis is that immunological changes make depressive patients more vulnerable to "somatic" diseases. In a recent study, Glaser et al. found that even subsyndromal depressive symptoms in older adults are associated with higher blood levels of the proinflammatory cytokine interleukin-6 (IL-6) at baseline. Moreover, subjects reporting depressive symptoms had an increase in IL-6 levels 2 weeks after influenza vaccination, whereas the IL-6 levels of non-depressives did not change (Glaser, Robles, Sheridan, Malarkey, & Kiecolt-Glaser, 2003).

In conclusion, there is a growing body of scientific evidence supporting a dimensional rather than a categorical concept of MDD. However, we have to take into account that "disease concepts are always pragmatic in character" (Sadler, Hulgus, & Agich, 1994). This is especially true in psychiatry because quantifiable objective measures of disease activity are lacking. Therefore, current psychiatric classification systems are based on clinical rather than pathophysiological criteria. Given the above-mentioned body of evidence, scientific rigor may demand a dimensional view of depression but a categorical disease concept may be more practically useful. We should not forget that comparisons between large studies were simply not possible before DSM diagnostic criteria, because not everybody spoke the same "diagnostic language". Moreover, a categorical diagnosis makes the use of outcome measures in large studies easier, which is important for both clinicians doing clinical trials and of course for pharmaceutical companies that want to prove the efficacy of their psychotropic drugs in randomized controlled trials (RCTs). RCTs are nowadays the "gold standard" in outcome research and they need some kind of quantification or cut-off that sets the "boundaries" of a certain disease. This does not mean, however, that the current diagnostic criteria for MDD do set the "real" boundaries of depression as a discrete disease entity. Therefore, debate and discussion about diagnostic criteria and validity of disease concepts are useful and needed to ascertain that these criteria and concepts change over time rather than remain static. Epidemiological research (especially prospective studies with a long follow-up period) can teach us a lot about natural course, risk factors, etiology, pathogenesis and finally validity of the current psychiatric syndromes. Thus, the results of this kind of research should be taken into account when diagnostic criteria are evaluated, discussed and/or changed.

Conclusions

This review of the "lifecycle of depression" is far from comprehensive, mainly because of the complex and multifactorial nature of the topic and the growing number of publications on different aspects of the long-term course of MDD. Nowadays, it seems quite well established that the reciprocal interaction between biological, psychological and social factors plays an important role in both the onset and long-term course of MDD. The exact mechanisms by which these different pathophysiological factors interact to cause depression remain to be determined, however.

Some important conclusions can be drawn, though. First, the increasing prevalence of MDD is at least partly due to psychological biases and differential mortality. Second, in at least an important subgroup of patients, the course of MDD deteriorates over time. We discussed some key features of this deteriorating course such as cycle acceleration, evolution from precipitated to spontaneous episodes and the induction of psychological/biological scars that possibly deteriorate after each successive episode. Finally, there is some ongoing scientific debate concerning the categorical or dimensional approach to MDD, which may have important implications for the validity of the disease concept of depression as currently defined by DSM-IV criteria.

References

Alonso, J., Angermeyer, M. C., Bernert, S., Bruffaerts, R., Brugha, T. S., Bryson, H., Girolamo, G., Graaf, R., Demyttenaere, K., Gasquet, I., Haro, J. M., Katz, S. J., Kessler, R. C., Kovess, V., Lepine, J. P., Ormel, J., Polidori, G., Russo, L. J., Vilagut, G., Almansa, J., Arbabzadeh-Bouchez, S., Autonell, J., Bernal, M., Buist-Bouwman, M. A., Codony, M., Domingo-Salvany, A., Ferrer, M., Joo, S. S., Martinez-Alonso, M., Matschinger, H., Mazzi, F., Morgan, Z., Morosini, P., Palacin, C., Romera, B., Taub, N., Vollebergh, W. A. The ESEMeD/MHEDEA 2000 Investigators (2004). Prevalence of mental disorders in Europe: Results from the European Study of the Epidemiology of Mental Disorders (ESEMeD) project. *Acta Psychiatrica Scandinavica, 420 (Suppl)*, 21-27.

Angst, F., Stassen, H. H., Clayton, P. J., & Angst, J. (2002). Mortality of patients with mood disorders: Follow-up over 34-38 years. *Journal of Affective Disorders, 68*, 167-181.

Angst, J. (1986). The course of affective disorders. *Psychopathology, 19 (Suppl)*, 47-52.

Angst, J. (1997) Fortnightly review. A regular review of the long-term follow up of depression. *British Medical Journal, 315*, 1143-1146.

Angst, J., Baastrup, P., Grof, P., Hippius, H., Poldinger, W., & Weis, P. (1973). The course of monopolar depression and bipolar psychoses. *Psychiatry, Neurology & Neurochirurgy, 76*, 489-500.

Austin, M. P., Mitchell, P., & Goodwin, G. M. (2001). Cognitive deficits in depression: Possible implications for functional neuropathology. *British Journal of Psychiatry, 178*, 200-206.

Basso, M. R., & Bornstein, R. A. (1999a). Neuropsychological deficits in psychotic versus nonpsychotic unipolar depression. *Neuropsychology, 13*, 69-75.

Basso, M. R., & Bornstein, R. A. (1999b). Relative memory deficits in recurrent versus first-episode major depression on a word-list learning task. *Neuropsychology, 13*, 557-563.

Bingefors, K., Isacson, D., Knorring, L. V., Smedby, B., & Wicknertz, K. (1996). Antidepressant-treated patients in ambulatory care. Mortality during a nine-year period after first treatment. *British Journal of Psychiatry, 169*, 647-654.

Bremner, J. D., Narayan, M., Anderson, E. R., Staib, L. H., Miller, H. L., & Charney, D. S. (2000). Hippocampal volume reduction in major depression. *American Journal of Psychiatry, 157*, 115-118.

Bruce, M. L., Leaf, P. J., Rozal, G. P., Florio, L., & Hoff, R. A. (1994). Psychiatric status and 9-year mortality data in the New Haven Epidemiologic Catchment Area Study. *American Journal of Psychiatry, 151*, 716-721.

Demyttenaere, K., & Bruffaerts, R. (2002). *Differential weight of DSM-IV symptoms in major and minor depression.* Technical Report, Department of Psychiatry, KU Leuven.

Demyttenaere, K., & Bruffaerts, R. (2003a). *Evolution of adherence in first and recurrent episode depressive patients.* Technical Report, Department of Psychiatry, KU Leuven.

Demyttenaere, K., & Bruffaerts, R. (2003b). *Evolution of symptom scores in first and recurrent episode depressive patients.* Technical Report, Department of Psychiatry, KU Leuven.

Eaton, W. W., Anthony, J. C., Gallo, J., Cai, G., Tien, A., Romanoski, A., Lyketsos, C., & Chen, L. S. (1997). Natural history of Diagnostic Interview Schedule/DSM-IV major depression. The Baltimore Epidemiologic Catchment Area follow-up. *Archives of General Psychiatry, 54*, 993-999.

Fava, G. A., Rafanelli, C., Grandi, S., Conti, S., & Belluardo, P. (1998). Prevention of recurrent depression with cognitive behavioral therapy: Preliminary findings. *Archives of General Psychiatry, 55*, 816-820.

Frank, E., Prien, R. F., Jarrett, R. B., Keller, M. B., Kupfer, D. J., Lavori, P. W., Rush, A. J., & Weissman, M. M. (1991). Conceptualization and rationale for consensus definitions of terms in major depressive disorder. Remission, recovery, relapse, and recurrence. *Archives of General Psychiatry, 48*, 851-855.

Giuffra, L. A., & Risch, N. (1994). Diminished recall and the cohort effect of major depression: A simulation study. *Psychological Medicine, 24*, 375-383.

Glaser, R., Robles, T. F., Sheridan, J., Malarkey, W. B., & Kiecolt-Glaser, J. K. (2003). Mild depressive symptoms are associated with amplified and prolonged inflammatory responses after influenza virus vaccination in older adults. *Archives of General Psychiatry, 60*, 1009-1014.

Harkness, K. L., Monroe, S. M., Simons, A. D., & Thase, M. (1999). The generation of life events in recurrent and non-recurrent depression. *Psychological Medicine, 29*, 135-144.

Hasin, D, & Link, B. (1988). Age and recognition of depression: Implications for a cohort effect in major depression. *Psychological Medicine, 18*, 683-688.

Judd, L. L., Akiskal, H. S., Maser, J. D., Zeller, P. J., Endicott, J., Coryell, W., Paulus, M. P., Kunovac, J.

L., Leon, A. C., Mueller, T. L., Rice, J. A., & Keller, M. B. (1998a). Major depressive disorder: A prospective study of residual subthreshold depressive symptoms as predictor of relapse. *Journal of Affective Disorders, 50*, 97-108.

Judd, L. L., Akiskal, H. S., Maser, J. D., Zeller, P. J., Endicott, J., Coryell, W., Paulus, M. P., Kunovac, J. L., Leon, A. C., Mueller, T. L., Rice, J. A., & Keller, M. B. (1998b). A prospective 12-year study of subsyndromal and syndromal depressive symptoms in unipolar major depressive disorders. *Archives of General Psychiatry, 55*, 694-700.

Judd, L. L., Paulus, M. J., Schettler, P. J., Akiskal, H. S., Endicott, J., Leon, A. C., Maser, J. D., Mueller, T., Solomon, D. A., & Keller, M. B. (2000). Does incomplete recovery from first lifetime major depressive episode herald a chronic course of illness? *American Journal of Psychiatry, 157*, 1501-1504.

Kandel, E. R. (1998). A new intellectual framework for psychiatry. *American Journal of Psychiatry, 155*, 457-469.

Kendler, K. S., & Gardner, C. O., Jr. (1998). Boundaries of major depression: An evaluation of DSM-IV criteria. *American Journal of Psychiatry, 155*, 172-177.

Kendler, K. S., Thornton, L. M., & Gardner, C. O. (2000). Stressful life events and previous episodes in the etiology of major depression in women: An evaluation of the "kindling" hypothesis. *American Journal of Psychiatry, 157*, 1243-1251.

Kendler, K. S., Thornton, L. M., & Gardner, C. O. (2001). Genetic risk, number of previous depressive episodes, and stressful life events in predicting onset of major depression. *American Journal of Psychiatry, 158*, 582-586.

Kessing, L. V. (1998). Cognitive impairment in the euthymic phase of affective disorder. *Psychological Medicine, 28*, 1027-1038.

Kessing, L. V. (1999). The effect of comorbid alcoholism on recurrence in affective disorder: A case register study. *Journal of Affective Disorders, 53*, 49-55.

Kessing, L. V., & Andersen, P. K. (1999). The effect of episodes on recurrence in affective disorder: A case register study. *Journal of Affective Disorders, 53*, 225-231.

Kessing, L. V., Andersen, E. W., & Andersen, P. K. (2000). Predictors of recurrence in affective disorder. Analyses accounting for individual heterogeneity. *Journal of Affective Disorders, 57*, 139-145.

Kessing, L. V., Andersen, P. K., & Mortensen, P. B. (1998). Predictors of recurrence in affective disorder. A case register study. *Journal of Affective Disorders, 49*, 101-108.

Kessing, L. V., Andersen, P. K., Mortensen, P. B., & Bolwig, T. G. (1998). Recurrence in affective disorder. I. Case register study. *British Journal of Psychiatry, 172*, 23-28.

Kessing, L. V., & Mortensen, P. B. (1999). Recovery from episodes during the course of affective disorder: A case-register study. *Acta Psychiatrica Scandinavica, 100*, 279-287.

Kessing, L. V., Mortensen, P. B., & Bolwig, T. G. (1998). Clinical definitions of sensitisation in affective disorder: A case register study of prevalence and prediction. *Journal of Affective Disorders, 47*, 31-39.

Klerman, G. L., & Weissman, M. M. (1989). Increasing rates of depression. *Journal of the American Medical Association, 261*, 2229-2235.

Kraepelin, E. (1921). *Manic-Depressive Insanity and Paranoia*. Edinburgh: E & S Livingstone.

Lavori, P. W., Dawson, R., & Mueller, T. B. (1994). Causal estimation of time-varying treatment effects in observational studies: Application to depressive disorder. *Statistics in Medicine, 13*, 1089-1100.

MacQueen, G. M., Campbell, S., McEwen, B. S., Macdonald, K., Amano, S., Joffe, R. T., Nahmias, C., & Young, L. T. (2003). Course of illness, hippocampal function, and hippocampal volume in major depression. *Proceedings of the National Academy of Sciences of the United States of America, 100*, 1387-1392.

Mitchell, P. B., Parker, G. B., Gladstone, G. L., Wilhelm, K., & Austin, M. P. (2003). Severity of stressful life events in first and subsequent episodes of depression: The relevance of depressive subtype. *Journal of Affective Disorders, 73*, 245-252.

Mueller, T. I., Leon, A. C., Keller, M. B., Solomon, D. A., Endicott, J., Coryell, W., Warshaw, M., & Maser, J. D. (1999). Recurrence after recovery from major depressive disorder during 15 years of observational follow-up. *American Journal of Psychiatry, 156*, 1000-1006.

Osby, U., Brandt, L., Correia, N., Ekbom, A., & Sparen, P. (2001). Excess mortality in bipolar and unipolar disorder in Sweden. *Archives of General Psychiatry, 58*, 844-850.

Paradiso, S., Lamberty, G. J., Garvey, M. J., & Robinson, R. G. (1997). Cognitive impairment in the euthymic phase of chronic unipolar depression. *Journal of Nervous and Mental Disease, 185*, 748-754.

Porter, R. J., Gallagher, P., Thompson, J. M., & Young, A. H. (2003). Neurocognitive impairment in drug-free patients with major depressive disorder. *British Journal of Psychiatry, 182*, 214-220.

Post, R. M., Rubinow, D. R., & Ballenger, J. C. (1986). Conditioning and sensitisation in the longitudinal course of affective illness. *British Journal of Psychiatry, 149*, 191-201.

Post, R.M. (1992). Transduction of psychosocial stress into the neurobiology of recurrent affective disorder. *American Journal of Psychiatry, 149*, 999-1010.

Racine, R. (1978). Kindling: The first decade. *Neurosurgery, 3*, 234-252.

Raison, C. L., & Miller, A. H. (2003). When not enough is too much: The role of insufficient glucocorticoid signaling in the pathophysiology of stress-related disorders. *American Journal of Psychiatry, 160*, 1554-1565.

Rice, J. P., Rochberg, N., Endicott, J., Lavori, P. W., & Miller, C. (1992). Stability of psychiatric diagnoses. An application to the affective disorders. *Archives of General Psychiatry, 49*, 824-830.

Rovner, B. W., German, P. S., Brant, L. J., Clark, R., Burton, L., & Folstein, M. F. (1991). Depression and mortality in nursing homes. *Journal of the American Medical Association, 265*, 993-996. Erratum in *Journal of the American Medical Association, 265*, 2672.

Sadler, J. Z., Hulgus, Y. F., & Agich, G. J. (1994). On values in recent American psychiatric classification. *Journal of Medicine and Philosophy, 19*, 261-277.

Sapolsky, R. M. (2000). Glucocorticoids and hippocampal atrophy in neuropsychiatric disorders. *Archives of General Psychiatry, 57*, 925-935.

Sapolsky, R. M., Krey, L. C., & McEwen, B. S. (1986). The neuroendocrinology of stress and aging: The glucocorticoid cascade hypothesis. *Endocrine Reviews, 7*, 284-301.

Schatzberg, A. F., Posener, J. A., DeBattista, C., Kalehzan, B. M., Rothschild, A. J., & Shear, P. K. (2000). Neuropsychological deficits in psychotic versus nonpsychotic major depression and no mental illness. *American Journal of Psychiatry, 157*, 1095-1100.

Schmitt, J. A., Kruizinga, M. J., & Riedel, W. J. (2001). Non-serotonergic pharmacological profiles and associated cognitive effects of serotonin reuptake inhibitors. *Journal of Psychopharmacology, 15*, 173-179.

Schoevers, R. A., Geerlings, M. I., Beekman, A. T., Penninx, B. W., Deeg, D. J., Jonker, C., & Van Tilburg, W. (2000). Association of depression and gender with mortality in old age. Results from the Amsterdam Study of the Elderly (AMSTEL). *British Journal of Psychiatry, 177*, 336-342.

Sheline, Y. I. (2000). 3D MRI studies of neuroanatomic changes in unipolar major depression: The role of stress and medical comorbidity. *Biological Psychiatry, 48*, 791-800.

Sheline, Y. I. (2003). Neuroimaging studies of mood disorder effects on the brain. *Biological Psychiatry, 54*, 338-352.

Sheline, Y. I., Gado, M. H., & Kraemer, H. C. (2003). Untreated depression and hippocampal volume loss. *American Journal of Psychiatry, 160*, 1516-1518.

Sheline, Y. I., Gado, M. H., & Price, J. L. (1998). Amygdala core nuclei volumes are decreased in recurrent major depression. *Neuroreport, 9*, 2023-2028. Erratum in *Neuroreport, 9*, 2436.

Sheline, Y. I., Sanghavi, M., Mintun, M. A., & Gado, M. H. (1999). Depression duration but not age predicts hippocampal volume loss in medically healthy women with recurrent major depression. *Journal of Neuroscience, 19*, 5034-5043.

Sheline, Y. I., Wang, P. W., Gado, M. H., Csernansky, J. G., & Vannier, M.W. (1996). Hippocampal atrophy in recurrent major depression. *Proceedings of the National Academy of Sciences of the United States of America, 93*, 3908-3913.

Solomon, D. A., Keller, M. B., Leon, A. C., Mueller, T. I., Lavori, P. W., Shea, M. T., Coryell, W., Warshaw, M., Turvey, C., Maser, J. D., & Endicott, J. (2000). Multiple recurrences of major depressive disorder. *American Journal of Psychiatry, 157*, 229-233.

Solomon, D. A., Keller, M. B., Leon, A. C., Mueller, T. I., Shea, M. T., Warshaw, M., Maser, J. D., Coryell, W., & Endicott, J. (1997). Recovery from major depression. A 10-year prospective follow-up across multiple episodes. *Archives of General Psychiatry, 54*, 1001-1006.

Spijker, J., de Graaf, R., Bijl, R. V., Beekman, A. T., Ormel, J., & Nolen, W. A. (2002). Duration of major depressive episodes in the general population: Results from The Netherlands Mental Health Survey and Incidence Study (NEMESIS). *British Journal of Psychiatry, 181*, 208-213.

Starkman, M. N., Giordani, B., Berent, S., Schork, M. A., & Schteingart, D. E. (2001). Elevated cortisol levels in Cushing's disease are associated with cognitive decrements. *Psychosomatic Medicine, 63*, 985-993.

Starkman, M. N., Giordani, B., Gebarski, S. S., & Schteingart, D. E. (2003). Improvement in learning associated with increase in hippocampal formation volume. *Biological Psychiatry, 53*, 233-238.

Swann, A. C., Secunda, S. K., Stokes, P. E., Croughan, J., Davis, J. M., Koslow, S. H., & Maas, J. W.

(1990). Stress, depression, and mania: Relationship between perceived role of stressful events and clinical and biochemical characteristics. *Acta Psychiatrica Scandinavica, 81*, 389-397.

Tham, A., Engelbrektson, K., Mathe, A. A., Johnson, L., Olsson, E., & Aberg-Wistedt, A. (1997). Impaired neuropsychological performance in euthymic patients with recurring mood disorders. *Journal of Clinical Psychiatry, 58*, 26-29.

Vermetten, E., Vythilingam, M., Southwick, S. M., Charney, D. S., & Bremner, J. D. (2003). Long-term treatment with paroxetine increases verbal declarative memory and hippocampal volume in posttraumatic stress disorder. *Biological Psychiatry, 54*, 693-702.

Whooley, M. A., & Browner, W. S. (1998). Association between depressive symptoms and mortality in older women. Study of Osteoporotic Fractures Research Group. *Archives of Internal Medicine, 158*, 2129-2135.

Wulsin, L. R., Vaillant, G. E., & Wells, V. E. (1999). A systematic review of the mortality of depression. *Psychological Medicine, 61*, 6-17.

Chapter 2

Mood and Memory: A Cognitive Psychology Perspective

on Maintenance of Depressed Mood

and Vulnerability for Relapse

Dirk Hermans, Filip Raes, & Paul Eelen

Depression is a seriously disabling disorder with high incidence and prevalence rates. The National Comorbidity Study revealed a lifetime prevalence of 17.1% in the general American population (Blazer, Kessler, McGonagly, & Swartz, 1994). Similar results have been found in the Belgian and Dutch community (Bayingana, Drieskens, & Tafforeau, 2002; Bijl, van Zessen, & Ravelli, 1997; see also Chapter 1, this volume). An important difference with anxiety disorders is that even without treatment most depressive episodes disappear after a number of months. But at the same time, depression is associated with a relatively high risk of relapse/recurrence. Patients who recovered from a first depressive episode have about a 50% chance of developing a new episode, whereas this risk of recurrence is already 70-80% for those who have a history of two or more depressive episodes (Belsher & Costello, 1988). Also, for about 6% to 13% of the patients depression becomes chronic, and every new episode entails a new risk of chronicity.

These figures indicate that interventions should not only target the treatment of current depressive episodes, but also, or even more so, the primary and secondary prevention of depression. Such prevention programs require solid knowledge of the vulnerability factors associated with the development of depression, as well as of the mechanisms that maintain (chronic) depression or that put individuals at risk of relapse/recurrence. Thus, in accordance with the changing view of depression as a recurrent, highly disabling and often chronic or life-long disorder (e.g., Judd, Akiskal, & Paulus, 1997), throughout this chapter our focus will be on the prevention of relapse/recurrence and on the study of vulnerability factors of depression. If researchers from different disciplines or different theoretical paradigms strive towards integration in the conceptualization and treatment of depression, we believe that the area of relapse prevention and vulnerability research is an important domain in which this integration could be pursued.

One of the models that has attracted a lot of attention during the last three decades, and that has proven fruitful in developing and testing hypotheses concerning the risk factors and mechanisms of depression, is the cognitive-behavioral model developed by Beck (Beck, Rush, Shaw, & Emery, 1979). Although this model has always in the first place been a clinical theory, it has been heavily inspired by experimental cognitive psychology from the start. This is most evident from the concepts used to describe the model's crucial constructs and mechanisms (e.g., memory schemata, automatic negative thoughts, dysfunctional beliefs). In spite of this obvious inspiration by cognitive science, research concerning the cognitive-behavioral model of depression has largely relied on self-report and correlational research designs. Quite simultaneously, there has been a research tradition that was less clinically inspired, but more experimental in nature, and more rooted in the general study of human behavior and cognition. These studies primarily aimed at revealing the information-processing characteristics of depression and depressed mood (for an overview, see Williams, Watts, MacLeod, & Mathews, 1997). Examples of such research topics are: the study of mood and memory, depression and selective attention, processes of interpretation and reasoning, learning mechanisms in depression, and processes of social cognition. As a matter of fact, this field of research turned out to be quite fruitful, and not without clinical implications. It is thus not surprising that during the last decade this more experimental approach got increasingly integrated within the cognitive-behavioral theory (and to a lesser extent also therapy) of depression (e.g., Clark & Beck, 1999). An experimental cognitive psychology approach surely represents in our opinion a valuable adjunct to other approaches in the study of depression and its vulnerability factors (e.g., psychodynamic or personality psychology approaches, neurobiology, etc.). Biological, genetic, social and psychological factors interact, and do not just act as independent factors that simply add up to the complex picture of depression (e.g., Weiss, Longhurst, & Mazure, 1999). Thus, the respective approaches studying these different factors have to be seen as more than just adjuncts to one another, given the complexity of depression in general and of all mechanisms and processes underlying its etiology and course. Future research should then aim at truly integrating these different approaches, and not just place them along side one another.

In the present chapter we will focus on one particular topic in the domain of information processing in depression and depressed mood, namely the study of memory processes in depression. In particular, we will cover research on explicit memory. The study of implicit memory in depression, which has attracted a lot of attention during the last ten years, falls outside the scope of our discussion (for a review, see Watkins, 2002). Two separate but related lines of research will be highlighted. First, we will discuss the experimental research tradition on the interaction between mood and memory. In the second part we will discuss more recent work on autobiographical memory specificity. In doing so, we will pay particular attention to the clinical implications of this research with respect to the maintenance of depression and vulnerability for relapse.

Mood and Memory

In 1981, Gordon Bower published an influential article in *American Psychologist* that can be regarded as the seminal paper for all mood and memory research. Bower opened his overview of research with a quite pleasant anecdote (Bower, 1981, p. 129). It referred to the movie *City Lights* in which Charlie Chaplin played the role of a little tramp and saved a drunk from leaping to his death. The drunk, who turned out to be a millionaire, befriends Charlie, and the two spend the evening together drinking. The next day, when he was sober, the millionaire does not recognize Charlie and ignores him. Later, when the millionaire got drunk again, he spotted Charlie and treats him as his long-lost companion. The two get drunk again and Charlie stays over to sleep in the millionaire's mansion. But, the next morning, the sober millionaire again does not recognize Charlie, treats him as an intruder and has the butler kick him out. The scene ends with the little tramp telling the audience his opinion of high society and the evils of drunkenness.

For Gordon Bower, the story exemplified an interesting case of "context-dependent memory". This more general phenomenon of context dependency was already known from the work of Godden and Baddeley (1975) who asked subjects to learn lists of words either on the beach or under approximately 4.5 meters of water. They were then asked to recall the list learned in one context (e.g., on the beach) while in the same context on some occasions (i.e., on the beach) and while in a different context on other occasions (in this case, under water). Godden and Baddeley observed that there was a decrement in recall of words of over 30% if the context was changed between learning and recall. The important difference between the study of Godden and Baddeley and the tale of Charlie Chaplin and his millionaire friend is that, in the former case, context was defined as an external situation (on the beach vs. under water), whereas in the latter, context could be regarded as an internal state (drunk vs. sober). Bower's work aimed at the question of *state-dependent memory*, and more specifically of whether moods and emotions can also act as internal contexts that facilitate or inhibit memory retrieval.

As we will argue later, this question has important clinical relevance with respect to the understanding of the mechanisms involved in the maintenance of depression and the vulnerability of depressive relapse (see also Gotlib & Krasnoperova, 1998). Hence, our discussion of the "mood and memory" literature will be specifically focused on the studies that address this very issue of depression.

In this context, Williams (1992) gives an interesting case example. He quotes the case of a patient who, at one therapy session, recalled a swimming event as particularly pleasant. At that moment, she was in a good mood. At a later session, however, when she was in a more depressed mood, she remembered different elements of the same swimming event which made it seem rather unpleasant. She described that she was afraid of making herself look ridiculous, and that it had been embarrassing to see herself in a swimsuit because of her weight problem. This case probably illustrates a more general experience that is shared by many patients suffering from depression and undoubtedly also by many nondepressed persons: when you feel down, you seem to remember more negative experiences from your past than when you feel elated. It is as if a depressed mood is a filter that sifts your personal memories.

If one takes a closer look at the swimming example, one will notice that it is conceptually somewhat different from the state-dependent memory phenomenon. Mood state dependency refers to the fact that stimuli are recalled better if the mood during recall is the same as the mood during encoding. This is independent of the affective nature of the stimuli that are encoded and retrieved. The swimming event example essentially differs from state dependency in that the emotional tone of the retrieved events is now relevant. Events that are congruent with the current mood are retrieved more easily. We will refer to this latter pheno-menon as *mood congruency*. In fact, two types of mood congruency can be distinguished: *mood congruent encoding* and *mood congruent recall*. After we have briefly discussed Bower's theory on mood and memory, we will illustrate both types of mood congruency, as well as mood state dependency, and we will highlight how these might play a role in the maintenance and exacerbation of depression.

Mood and the Associative Memory Network

Theories of human memory have been diverse. In addition to more recent connectionist models, the associative network view of emotion has been one of the most important and fruitful ways of conceptualizing the way in which knowledge is stored in memory (Schwartz & Reisberg, 1991). According to the associative network view, memory is a vast web or network of ideas. The network is built up of units of knowledge (remembered episodes, remembered facts, sights, etc.), referred to as "nodes", and associations or associative links between these nodes. The way this network is structured is different for each individual and will be dependent upon the learning experiences throughout the individual's life. Some associative links will be relatively weak, whereas repeated experience (e.g., co-occurrence) will have made other associations quite strong. When a unit of knowledge is activated – for instance the node "cat" upon seeing a cat – one can become aware of the content of that node if it has received sufficient input. Also, through spreading of activation to associatively related nodes, one can become aware of other things. For instance, seeing a cat might "remind" you to buy food for your own cat. In that case, spreading of activation has made other mental contents more accessible to awareness. The activated concept "cat" might have spread activation to the related concept "cat food" which activated the stored autobio-graphical event that you ran out of cat food.

Contexts can exert an influence on memory if they are encoded together with specific knowledge. The accessibility of this knowledge for retrieval might be enhanced if the context is again present during retrieval. This is because, through spreading of activation, the context-nodes will already pre-activate the relevant knowledge. This pre-activation is absent when the context is absent and, hence, retrieval shall be somewhat less successful. This is basically how the associative network deals with observations like those of Godden and Baddeley (1975).

The crux of Bower's theory (1981) is that emotions (mood) can be considered as individual nodes in the associative memory network. They are embedded in memory representations of semantic knowledge, autonomic activity and muscular activity. Information that is encoded during emotional states will likely be encoded in association with the related "emotion node". Through the spreading of activation, emotions can then serve as "contexts" and thus influence memory performance.

For a more detailed description of Bower's "Network Theory of Affect" we refer to Bower (1981, 1991) and Gilligan and Bower (1984). For the present purposes it suffices to recapitulate the three most important hypotheses that were derived from this theory. In subsequent paragraphs we will discuss experimental evidence for each.

1. *State-dependent learning*: Emotions serve as contextual cues in learning and recall. Memory is facilitated when mood state at learning matches mood at recall.
2. *Mood congruent recall*: Material with affective tone that is congruent with current mood is most easily retrieved from memory.
3. *Mood congruent encoding*: Material with affective tone that is congruent with current mood is most easily learned (i.e., encoded in memory).

State-dependent Learning

One of the first studies that demonstrated state-dependent learning – sometimes referred to as "state-dependent memory", given the relevance of both encoding and retrieval in this phenomenon – stems from Bower, Monteiro and Gilligan (1978; Experiment 3). In this study a group of 24 participants was asked to study two lists of 16 words. When studying the first list (List A) a positive mood was induced for half of the participants, whereas a sad mood was induced for the other participants. The mood induction procedure employed in this study consisted of hypnosis combined with self-generated imagery. Subsequently, they were asked to study a second list (List B) while under the same or the opposite mood. After these two learning phases, participants were asked to recall as many words as possible from List A. During this free recall phase, participants were again induced with either a sad or happy mood. Results showed that retention was statistically superior when memory during the test phase matched the mood they were in when studying List A. As compared to mood controls, retention was impaired when mood during studying and testing List A mismatched. These results provided clear support for the hypothesis that mood can act as a context for the retrieval of memories. A crucial aspect of this experiment was that participants were asked to study two different lists, which is why it is also referred to as the "interference paradigm". Other studies that only employed one word list failed to demonstrate a state-dependency effect. This points to the fact that the emotional mood was a helpful feature in distinguishing the target material (List A) from interfering material (List B). This multiple-list situation seems a closer analogue to real life, where one stores a multitude of experiences while in different moods.

Later studies have replicated the mood state-dependent effect as well as the importance of the interference paradigm in obtaining this effect (e.g., Share, Lisman, & Spear, 1984). Singer and Salovey (1988) provide an overview of these studies and conclude that the existing data support the mood state-dependency hypothesis. When translated to the understanding of depression, these data suggest that information that was encoded during a depressive episode will be more accessible when one is in a negative mood again later on. Given that experiences during an episode of depression are more often than not negatively toned, the higher accessibility of their memory traces during a subsequent negative mood will most likely fuel this negative emotional state.

Given that the majority of studies on state-dependency have employed procedures like hypnosis or imagery to induce moods, and have used stimulus materials like neutral words, phrases, nonsense syllables or pictures of neutral objects, one can question the ecological validity of this phenomenon. A study by Weingartner, Miller and Murphy (1977) is worth mentioning in this respect. They asked a group of patients with bipolar disorder to freely associate to two nouns in states of depression or mania. Later, they had to recall these associations in states that were the same or different from which they were originally generated. These patients showed superior recall when in the same state as their learning state.

Mood Congruent Recall

Several investigations have examined the relation between depression and the time taken to retrieve personal memories. Lloyd and Lishman (1975) presented neutral cue words to a group of 40 depressed inpatients and instructed them to think of either a pleasant or unpleasant memory, and to signal to the experimenter when a suitable memory came to mind. The time taken to retrieve memories was recorded by stopwatch. They observed that the more severe the depression, as measured by the Beck Depression Inventory (BDI), the faster the patient retrieved an unpleasant memory (relative to the pleasant memories). Furthermore, more depressed patients retrieved more intense negative memories.

Although these data fit nicely with Bower's theory, there are at least two interpretative problems associated with this study. First, it can not be excluded that the more severely depressed patients may have had more genuinely depressing experiences during their life, and, hence, find it easier to retrieve any one of them. Second, the more severely depressed patients may simply be interpreting more of their neutral or ambiguous experiences as more depressive, thus inflating the number of memories to choose from. In this latter case the data would be supporting an interpretational bias rather than a memory bias.

These alternative explanations were taken into account in an elegant study by David Clark and John Teasdale (1982). They selected depressed patients for the presence of diurnal variation of mood. At several moments they asked these patients to respond with the first personal memory that came to mind. These memories were later rated for pleasantness. It was observed that happy memories were less probable (and depressing memories more probable) when patients were more depressed. However, when the same patients were at the less depressed point in their cycle, the picture was reversed. These results cannot be explained in terms of differential frequencies of depressive experiences, because the data stem from the same person at different moments. With respect to the possibility of an interpretational bias, the pleasantness ratings were indeed also mood-dependent. The more depressed the current mood, the more negative these ratings, but this effect was by itself not sufficient to explain the memory bias.

Other studies have approached the mood congruent recall hypothesis using experimentally induced moods within the laboratory. These studies have the advantage that they can more easily control for mood during encoding. One such example is a study by Teasdale and Russell (1983). In this study, nondepressed college students were asked to study a list of positive and negative trait words. During the second phase of the study an elated or depressed mood was induced, during which participants were asked to recall as many words as possible from the list. The memory data showed a clear effect of mood congruent retrieval: "depressed" participants recalled more negative than positive words, whereas the elated participants recalled more positive than negative words. This mood congruency effect has been replicated numerous times and has proven to be a quite robust phenomenon (for overviews, see Blaney, 1986; Matt, Vázquez, & Campbell, 1992; Singer & Salovey, 1988). One particular finding is that these effects are stronger when the stimuli are self-referent. It is possible that self-reference induces more elaborate processing, which would be necessary for the effect to come to light. Recent research also indicates that mood congruency cannot be reduced to a heuristic response bias, but truly reflects an increased sensitivity to mood congruent information (Fiedler, Nickel, Muehlfriedel, & Unkelbach, 2001).

Still, how do the findings on mood congruent retrieval relate to the suggestion that people suffering from depression are often more accurate in perceptions and judgments than nondepressed people? Actually, it is sometimes suggested that the bias resides in nondepressed people, who would tend to look at life through rose-colored glasses. According to this theory of "depressive realism", depressed people would be more even-handed, more realistic. Results from a meta-analysis of mood congruency studies by Matt et al. (1992) shed some light on this proposal. They concluded that nondepressed persons recall between 6% and 8% more positive than negative stimuli. Subclinically depressed persons turn out to be even-handed; they show a balanced recall of affectively valenced stimuli. For clinically depressed patients, however, a negatively toned bias can be observed, that is estimated at up to 10% more negative than positive memories.

Given these figures, it is not unrealistic to assume that the process of mood congruent recall has an important role in maintaining and intensifying depressed mood. The depressed patient might get stuck in a vicious circle in which depressed mood heightens the accessibility of negative memories, which in turn amplify the depressed mood.

Mood Congruent Encoding

Besides mood congruency during retrieval, mood might also influence the type of information that is encoded. According to the "mood congruent encoding" hypothesis, material with affective tone that is congruent with current mood is most easily learned. This too might be part of a vicious circle, in which the depressed patient spirals between a disproportionate encoding of negative memories and an escalating negative mood.

Because of the difficulty of control over naturally occurring moods at encoding, most of the studies on mood congruent encoding have been conducted in the laboratory. In these experiments, moods are induced followed by a task involving the reading of a story or the learning of a word list. Then, after the induced mood has worn off, participants are tested for recognition or recall of this previously learned material. A good example of mood congruent encoding can be found in the work of Bower, Gilligan and Monteiro (1981). The mental health professionals and college students who participated in this study read some simulated psychiatric interviews. The patient in the narrative briefly describes a series of unrelated happy and sad incidents from his life. During reading, participants were either in a happy or sad mood, which was experimentally induced. Later, in a neutral mood, they were asked to recall the narrative. The results were clear-cut: "happy" readers recalled about one and a half times as many happy incidents as sad events, whereas "sad" readers recalled about one and one third times as many sad as happy incidents. Thus, it can be concluded that being in a sad or happy mood significantly influences the type of information that is encoded. Later studies have repeatedly replicated this effect.

One particular problem associated with some of these studies is that their effects might (in part) be dependent on experimenter demand (Bower, 1987). When participants are induced to feel happy or sad by an autosuggestion technique (using either hypnosis, guided fantasy or the Velten technique), they may believe that to maintain that mood throughout the subsequent learning phase they should attend more to mood-sustaining material; and as a consequence they learn it better. However, the data of several studies can not readily be explained by this alternative explanation. In these studies, mood was induced in a subtle manner, so that demand effects cannot be invoked to explain the results (e.g., Forgas & Bower, 1987).

Mood and Memory: Some Concluding Remarks

The seminal work of Gordon Bower has been an impetus for several productive lines of research concerning the interaction between explicit memory and mood. These studies have particular relevance for the study of depression. The phenomena of state dependency and mood congruency, when active, will contribute to the perpetuation or exaggeration of existing mood states. It seems likely that mnemonic selectivity occurs in depressed persons and that it contributes to the vicious cycle of deepening depression (Blaney, 1986). When depressed, state dependency will make information that was encoded during previous depressive episodes more accessible. Specific memories and feelings that were associated with these preceding episodes come to mind more easily. It might seem that feelings and thoughts that were previously encoded in this depressed state seem to "return". This is sometimes obvious in the experiences of patients who experience relapse and from the first moment on have the feeling that "everything seems to come back".

In addition to state dependency, mood congruency will further darken a depressed individual's mood. When depressed, mood congruent retrieval will color the type of memories that are remembered. This may make one's past life seem much more negative than it actually was. Negative experiences with others will be selectively remembered over positive encounters, affecting social behavior. One's own qualities will be interpreted against a predominant accessibility of memories of failures over successes, impacting self-esteem and amplifying feelings of hopelessness. And finally, mood congruent encoding will further increase this imbalance. Selective learning of negative materials will make a person more vulnerable because this process actually leads to an objectively higher amount of negative memories in long-term memory. Each of these processes may lead to a vicious circle, and each circle can further feed into each of the other cycles (Wachtel, 1994, 1997).

It will be clear that these processes will only account for part of the processes that are responsible for the maintenance and amplification of depressed moods. Moreover, the existence of other regulatory processes is necessary. If not, one would have to predict that once one starts to drift away from a neutral mood, there will be an unstoppable spiral towards a more and more negative mood, ending up in severe depression. This is surely not the case, and even the most severe of clinical depressions will ameliorate at some point. The study of "mood repair" provides insight in the processes that regulate mood. Under normal circumstances different types of processes will keep mood changes within an acceptable range. The discussion of these processes, however, falls outside the scope of this chapter. For a recent discussion of mood-regulation strategies and mood-congruent memory, we refer to Rusting and DeHart (2000). In the remainder of this chapter, we will focus on the study of the specificity of autobiographical memory, which is a research tradition that was originally rooted in mood and memory research.

Autobiographical Memory Specificity

In the context of mood and memory research, Williams and Broadbent (1986) studied patients within the first few days after they were hospitalized because of a severe suicide attempt by overdose. For most of these patients the suicide attempt had taken place against the background of a depressive disorder. During this study, they were asked to retrieve specific autobiographical memories to positive or negative cue words (e.g., happy, angry). Response latencies to retrieve these memories were compared with those of a group of nondepressed patients from the same hospital, most of whom were hospitalized for physical investigations, as well as with a group of nondepressed volunteers who were not hospitalized. Results from this cuing task showed that the parasuicide patients took longer than controls to retrieve a memory when given a positive word. This was in line with the mood congruency hypothesis in that memories that were incongruent with the current mood were less accessible.

Upon closer inspection of their data, Williams and Broadbent discovered a striking *qualitative* difference in the memories produced by the depressed and nondepressed groups, in addition to the more quantitative differences in response speed. Despite the fact that they were asked to retrieve specific memories, the overdose patients tended, as a first response to the cues, to retrieve inappropriately general memories. Whereas controls produced specific memories, like "When I passed my driving license (successful)" or "With my supervisor on Monday (angry)", the depressed patients typically reported overgeneral memories, e.g., "In my job (successful)" or "When I have had a row (angry)". The difference in memory specificity between depressed and nondepressed persons was observed for both positive and negative cue words. Also, this effect could not be attributed to pharmacological effects of the overdose, because no differences were observed between both groups on two other measures of semantic memory that are known to be sensitive to the effects of drugs.

A few years later, in 1988, the Williams research group published three separate papers that replicated and extended these findings. In the first paper, Williams and

Dritschel (1988) tested a group of 24 overdose patients within the first four days following the self-poisoning. The procedure was similar to the procedure employed by Williams and Broadbent (1986), except that participants were now given only 30 instead of 60 seconds to retrieve a specific memory. If the first response was not a specific memory, the participants were prompted to produce one ("Can you think of a specific time – one particular event?"). After each subsequent inappropriately overgeneral memory the participant was prompted again. As compared to the control group, the overdose patients again produced less specific autobiographical memories. A similar effect was observed in a second "overdose" group that took part in this study. These participants were tested 3 to 14 months after deliberate self-poisoning and were included to test whether lack of memory specificity was related to the presence of an ongoing emotional crisis. This group, however, displayed a lack of autobiographical memory specificity comparable to the "recent overdose" group. Although both overdose groups displayed similar elevated levels of depressed mood, these patients were not selected on the basis of a current depressive disorder. In a subsequent study, autobiographical memory was investigated in a group of patients who met criteria of Major Depressive Disorder according to DSM-III-R (Williams & Scott, 1988). This study provided clear evidence for a lack of memory specificity in clinically diagnosed depressed patients. Similar results were observed by Moore, Watts and Williams (1988).

The cue word paradigm first used by Williams and Broadbent (1986) has become known as the Autobiographical Memory Test (AMT). Subsequent studies by other research groups employed variants of this procedure, typically involving the presentation of 10 or more cue words, alternating in valence (positive or negative). For each cue word, the participant is asked to retrieve a specific memory that refers to an event that happened once and lasted not longer than one day (de Decker, Hermans, Raes, & Eelen, 2003). Different ways of categorizing the responses have been employed. In our own research, the first response is coded as either a *specific memory* or a *non-specific memory*. The analyses are based on the number of specific first responses. For exploratory reasons, non-specific memories are further qualified as either a *categoric memory* (referring to events that occurred more often, and are difficult to date exactly, e.g., "Watching my favourite talk show on Friday evenings"), an *extended memory* (referring to events that last longer than one day, e.g., "My holiday in Senegal two years ago"), *no memory* (e.g., a verbal association to the cue, thoughts about the future), *no response* (no response is given to the cue, "?", "I don't know", etc.), or *same event* (a response referring to the same event already mentioned in response to a previous cue). Using this scoring procedure, Raes, Hermans, de Decker, Eelen and Williams (2003) obtained a very good inter-rater agreement of 98.8% (kappa coefficient of .957) for the categorization of specific vs. non-specific responses. Other researchers have focused on the number of categoric memories and refer to a relatively higher proportion of these non-specific memories as "overgeneral autobiographical memory".[1] Therefore, we will

---

[1] It is important to note that increased overgenerality in clinical groups is typically attributable to an excess of categoric memories, and less of extended memories. This is also important with respect to the theoretical models concerning the processes involved in overgeneral memory retrieval (e.g., Williams, 1996).

use the terms "overgeneral memory" and "lack of memory specificity" interchangeably to refer to these related results.

Since the seminal work by Williams and colleagues, several studies employing the AMT replicated the lack of memory specificity in groups of (clinically) depressed adults (e.g., Brewin, Watson, McCarthy, Hyman, & Dayson, 1998; Goddard, Dritschel, & Burton, 1996; Kuyken & Dalgleish, 1995; Puffet, Jehin-Marchot, Timsit-Berthier, & Timsit, 1991; Wessel, Meeren, Peeters, Arntz, & Merckelbach, 2001). Recent research has replicated this finding in adolescents with major depressive disorder (Park, Goodyer, & Teasdale, 2002).

Besides the studies that focused on depression, other studies have investigated autobiographical memory specificity in anxiety disorders. However, to date, overgenerality does not seem to be a characteristic of anxiety disorders such as obsessive-compulsive disorder (Wilhelm, McNally, Baer, & Florin, 1997) and generalized anxiety disorder (Burke & Matthews, 1992). The fact that overgenerality is linked to major depressive disorder rather than anxiety disorder was recently confirmed by Wessel et al. (2001). On the basis of this latter study it could also be concluded that overgeneral memory is related to the presence of a diagnosis of depressive disorder but not to the level of depression. Besides the strong link between autobiographical memory specificity and depression, there also seems to be a strong association with trauma. Several studies have shown that lack of specificity (or overgenerality) is inversely related to different forms of past trauma experience (e.g., sexual, physical, and parental abuse) (Dalgleish et al., 2003; de Decker et al., 2003; Henderson, Hargreaves, Gregory, & Williams, 2002; Hermans et al., 2004). This particular relation with trauma will be further discussed later on.

In the following sections we will focus on the possible clinical relevance of reduced autobiographical memory specificity in depression. Is it merely a by-product of depression, or does it represent a more stable characteristic of persons vulnerable to depression? Does it have any clinical diagnostic relevance? How is overgeneral memory engaged in the maintenance and relapse of depression?

Lack of Memory Specificity as a Trait Marker for Depression?

If one could identify the factors that make people vulnerable to depression or depressive relapse, screening and primary and secondary prevention interventions could be more efficiently implemented. In the past, a number of psychological characteristics have been assessed for whether they represent stable characteristics of depressed patients and place individuals at risk of depressive onset or relapse. Many of these studies have compared individuals in remission from depression with groups of currently depressed and never depressed persons. Most of these cognitive factors (e.g., dysfunctional attitudes), however, turned out to be state-dependent. Together with remission of the depressive symptoms, these candidate risk factors disappeared and no longer differentiated between previously depressed and never depressed individuals. With respect to the study of cognitive schemas as vulnerability factor for depression, these findings of normalization have led some researchers to hypothesize that these dysfunctional schemas are "latent" and need to be activated before they can be measured. Activation by priming techniques (most often mood induction) generally demonstrates that formerly depressed individuals differ from nondepressed in the negativity of their responses on information-processing tasks or questionnaires (Hammen, 2001). But only a few studies (e.g., Segal, Gemar, & Williams, 1999) have actually demonstrated the association between such negativity and a risk of subsequent depression.

Within the study of autobiographical memory specificity, several studies have indicated that the presence of overgeneral memory specificity is not state-dependent, but represents a relatively stable characteristic. In the previously discussed study by Williams and Dritschel (1988), for instance, memory specificity of the overdose patients that were tested several months after the suicide attempt could not be distinguished at all from the results of the "recent overdose" group. However, this study was cross-sectional and no strong inferences can be drawn because a number of the "ex-patients" were still depressed. In a later longitudinal study by Brittlebank, Scott, Williams and Ferrier (1993) depressed patients were tested on admission, 3 months and 7 months later. Although the depressive symptomatology, as measured by the Hamilton Rating Scale for Depression (HRSD), did significantly improve over time, the responses to the AMT's cue words did not become significantly more specific. More recently, Mackinger, Pachinger, Leibetseder and Fartacek (2000) compared two groups of women who were not depressed at the time of study, one of which had a history of depression. This group of women in remission from major depression was significantly more overgeneral than the group without a lifetime prevalence of depression. The never-depressed group retrieved about twice as many specific autobiographical memories and half the number of categoric descriptions than the group in remission.

Together with the finding that overgeneral memory is related to the diagnosis of depression but not with depression severity (Wessel et al., 2001) these studies indicate that, in contrast to many other cognitive characteristics of depression, lack of autobiographical memory specificity is quite stable and does not disappear during remission. In this respect it seems to be a good candidate for being considered as a vulnerability factor for depression. But, before one can firmly conclude that it does represent a vulnerability factor for the onset of depression, more longitudinal research is needed that investigates whether less specific persons do indeed have an increased probability of developing a first onset of depressive disorder. A study by Mackinger, Loschin and Leibetseder (2000) represents a first step in this direction. They followed a group of 50 pregnant women and assessed postpartum affective changes, using the Edinburgh Postnatal Depression Scale with one test during pregnancy and a second test 3 months after delivery. The AMT was also assessed during pregnancy. Regression analysis showed that the number of categoric responses to negative cues allowed a significant prediction of affective changes. The more overgeneral, the greater the extent of affect change in the negative direction. A weakness of this study was, however, that it did not control for the presence of possible depressive episodes before pregnancy. Hence, there remains a need for methodologically strong prospective studies to investigate whether overgeneral memory is more than just a stable "consequence" of depression, and represents a true vulnerability factor for the development of depressive disorder.

Lack of Memory Specificity and Poor Long-Term Outcome

Irrespective of whether overgeneral memory represents a vulnerability factor for the onset of depression, one can also investigate to what extent overgeneral memory contributes to the maintenance of a current depressive episode or to relapse after remission. A study by Brittlebank et al. (1993) has revealed quite impressive results relevant to these questions. In this study, a group of patients was tested at admission and 3 and 7 months later. During the first test session, besides the AMT, patients had to complete two traditional measures of depression severity (the HRSD and the BDI), as well as a measure of dysfunctional attitudes. This testing was repeated at the two follow-up moments. Overgeneral memory at baseline (test session 1) significantly predicted outcome at 3 and 7 months. Multiple regression analysis revealed that overgeneral responses to positively toned words significantly predicted outcome and accounted for 33% of the variance of the final HRSD score. Hence, more overgeneral responses were strongly associated with a poorer long-term outcome. It was also found that only 11% of those who could be considered as "overgeneral to positive cues" were recovered at seven months, whereas 80% in the "specific to positive cues" group had recovered. These results are even more remarkable when compared with those of the traditional depression measures (HRSD and BDI) for which no significant predictive power was observed.

Although some researchers failed to find a similar predictive power of the AMT (e.g., Brewin, Reynolds, & Tata, 1999; see also Scott, Williams, Brittlebank, & Ferrier, 1995), a number of more recent studies did replicate the findings of Brittlebank et al. (1993). For instance, Dalgleish, Spinks, Yiend and Kuyken (2001) examined autobiographical memory in patients with seasonal affective disorder (SAD). These patients completed the AMT during winter, when depressed. Symptom levels were reassessed during the summer, when participants were in remission. The number of overly general memories to positive cues generated when depressed predicted symptom levels when in remission, over and above initial symptom levels during winter. A second study demonstrated that, although the number of overgeneral responses predicted outcome, the SAD patients were not more overgeneral than a control group without a history of depression. This indicates that even when levels of general memories are no greater in a given target group than in controls, the absolute level of general memories (to positive cue words) is still independently related to symptom outcome. Another study that demonstrated the predictive power of the AMT with respect to long term outcome in depression stems from Peeters, Wessel, Merckelbach and Boon-Vermeeren (2002). Finally, Harvey, Bryant and Dang (1998) made similar observations in the context of acute stress disorder. On the basis of these studies one can conclude that overgeneral memory might play an important role in the course of depression, with lack of specificity being related to less positive outcomes. At the moment there are several hypotheses about how this relationship could be conceptualized. We will briefly discuss them in the following paragraph.

Memory Specificity, Social Problem Solving, Imageability of the Future and Emotional Processing

A number of studies have demonstrated that overgeneral memory is associated with poor social problem solving. Evans, Williams, O'Loughlin and Howells (1992) examined the relation between AMT performance and interpersonal problem solving, using the Means-Ends Problem Solving test (MEPS; Platt & Spivack, 1975). This test gives a problem scenario together with a positive ending to the story (e.g., moving to a new neighborhood and having few friends; the story ends with the person having successfully made some friends). Participants have to propose solutions to complete the middle of the story. The participants in the study of Evans and colleagues were 12 overdose patients within their first 36 hours of admission. Although it was to be expected that these depressed and suicidal persons would be less effective in this type of social problem solving than control persons, these authors additionally observed that the effectiveness of the solutions proposed by the overdose group was significantly related to the specificity of autobiographical memory. The less specific, the less effective were the solutions (see also Pollock & Williams, 2001; Sidley, Whitaker, Calam, & Wells, 1997). Similar results were observed in groups of depressed students and clinically depressed patients (Goddard, Dritschel, & Burton, 1996, 1997) and persons suffering from bipolar disorder (Scott, Stanton, Garland, & Ferrier, 2000). It is hypothesized that adequate problem solving is in part based on the capacity to retrieve specific memories. Specific memories about past situations might function both at the "problem definition" and the "generation of alternatives" stages of problem solving by offering cues from which to build elaborate social problem-solving strategies. The categoric retrieval style imposes a changeless perspective on one's own past problem-solving experiences. This inaccessibility of specific autobiographical memories of previous situations in which one was confronted with similar problems hinders effective problem solving. In turn, this impaired social problem solving might negatively affect depression, as it will give rise to negatively toned social situations and relationships and to a diminished amount of social reinforcement.

A second perspective pertains to the relationship between the specificity of autobiographical memory and imageability of the future. Several studies of our own (de Decker, 2001) as well as other labs (e.g., Williams et al., 1996) have demonstrated that there is a positive relationship between the specificity with which people retrieve episodes from their past and the specificity with which they imagine the future. For persons who are characterized by a more overgeneral memory, images of the future too are less specific. Evidence is not only correlational in nature: experimental work by Williams and colleagues (1996) showed that inducing a generic or specific retrieval style affected the specificity of images of the future accordingly. This might entail important clinical implications, given that reduced specificity in imagining (especially positive aspects of) the future might fuel feelings of hopelessness.

A third way in which overgeneral autobiographic memory might contribute to the maintenance of depression or vulnerability for relapse, relates to a relative absence of exposure to negatively toned memories or feelings. Repeated confrontation with past negative or traumatic events can substantially reduce the negative emotions associated with these events (Littrell, 1998). Because of low specificity of the related autobiographical memories, this naturally occurring exposure effect might be impeded in persons that are characterized by an over-general memory style. In the short run, this lack of exposure might have a positive effect (due to the absence of confrontation with negative memory traces), but in the long run this will have a strongly unfavourable effect on psychological well-being (Hermans & de Decker, 2001).

We can thus conclude that overgeneral autobiographical memory can exert a maintaining influence on depressed mood through impaired social problem solving, reduced imageability of the future and limited exposure to negative memories and feelings.

Memory Specificity and Affect Regulation

Besides depression, a series of studies demonstrates that overgeneral memory can also be observed in persons who have experienced traumatic sexual or physical abuse (e.g., Henderson et al., 2002; for a recent overview, see Hermans et al., 2004). Kuyken and Brewin (1995), for example, investigated the relationship between early adversities and autobiographical memory retrieval style. They found that in a clinical sample of depressed women, those who reported childhood sexual abuse (CSA) retrieved significantly more overgeneral memories on the AMT than those who did not report CSA. These results have recently been extended by Hermans et al. (2004) to the presence of physical abuse. Also, in the group of depressed inpatients investigated by Hermans and colleagues, 10 out of the 18 patients reported being sexually approached before the age of 18. Within this group, the number of specific responses was significantly correlated with the age at which this sexual approach started. The younger the person was when the sexual approaches took place and the more distressing these events, the less specific were the answers on the AMT.

There are several ways in which this relation between trauma and lack of memory specificity can be explained. Besides explanations in terms of the psycho-biological or neuroanatomical impact of trauma on brain functioning, two psychological accounts are viable. First, in cases of traumatic experiences that took place early in childhood (before the age of 5), children might have missed a normal developmental stage during which they learn to inhibit relatively automatic cate-goric descriptions, allowing the child greater strategic control over the recollection process (including accessing specific memory traces). Together with the biological explanation, this account can be considered as a "deficit model". A second, and more functional, account states that being overgeneral might diminish the emotional impact of traumatic or negative events from the past. Persons who experienced traumatic adversities might adopt a generic style in retrieving auto-biographical memories as an affect regulating strategy. Being less specific then reduces the risk of confrontation with painful memories concerning the traumatic experiences. This strategy only works if it is not only applied with respect to the traumatic memories, but to memory in general. This hypothesis, referred to here as the *affect-regulation hypothesis*, has received experimental support from recent research by Raes et al. (2003). They demonstrated that being less specific in the retrieval of autobiographical memories has a positive effect on the affective impact of a negative event. This could be seen as an extension of Williams' original affect-regulation hypothesis (1996): being less specific not only regulates affect associated with past negative events, but also makes one less vulnerable to future adversities. It appears that being less specific in some cases is advantageous – at least in the short run (!) – and might be termed as *functional*, *protective* or *adaptive*. In the long run, however, this reduced specificity may very well prove to be *maladaptive* and to have *detrimental* effects for reasons described above. This more functional approach to the study of autobiographical memory seems to be an appealing route to the understanding of the mechanisms of overgeneral memory in depression.

Autobiographical Memory Specificity: Some Concluding Remarks

The study of autobiographical memory specificity is still in its infancy, but has already proven to be quite fruitful. The fact that depression and the presence of traumatic experiences have a unique linkage with reduced memory specificity has been the impetus for some developmental hypotheses. One possibility is that trauma leads to overgeneral memory as a way of coping with adverse memories. When this strategy loses its flexibility and gets more and more engrained it puts the person at risk for depression for reasons mentioned earlier. Although attractive, this hypothesis is in need of good prospective studies to be put to the test. Irrespective of this developmental issue, reduced memory specificity seems to be a quite stable characteristic of many depressed persons. It is predictive of poor long-term outcome, and it is associated with poor social problem solving and limited imageability of the future. In as much as it represents an affect-regulation strategy it might have positive short-term consequences, but will be detrimental in the long run because it deprives the person of a lot of naturally occurring self-exposure to negative memories and feelings. Although it is most probable that overgeneral memory is a characteristic that prolongs depressed mood and renders the depressed person more vulnerable for relapse, future research will have to unveil its precise role in the onset of depression.

Discussion and Clinical Implications

The present chapter reviewed cognitive psychology research on mood and (explicit) memory. In particular we addressed aspects relevant to the maintenance of depression and vulnerability for depressive relapse. First, the research tradition on the interaction between mood an memory was covered. Next, findings of the related but more recent line of research on autobiographical memory specificity were discussed.

It is interesting to see how paradigms from experimental cognitive psychology, discussed in the present chapter, are being used to further support psychological theories on depression that originated outside experimental cognitive psychology and of which some are reviewed elsewhere in this volume. For example, in Chapter 3 and 4 in this volume, recent theorizing from Beck (Beck, 1987; Beck, Epstein, & Harrison, 1983) on the role of sociotropy and autonomy in precipitating depression is discussed, which relates to Blatt's (1974) ideas on the distinction between anaclitic and introjective depression. Moore and Blackburn (1993) looked for evidence for this sociotropy/autonomy distinction in depressed patients, using a paradigm from experimental cognitive psychology research: the autobiographical memory paradigm. They found that sociotropy, as measured by the Sociotropy Autonomy Scale (SAS; Beck, Epstein, Harrison, & Emery, 1983), was associated with faster retrieval of negative sociotropic autobiographical memories. A similar relationship between autonomy and increased (biased) accessibility of negative autonomous autobiographical events, however, was not found (the authors note that this might be due to validity problems of the Autonomy subscale of the SAS, see also Chapter 4, this volume). These results then partly support the sociotropy/ autonomy distinction and related selective information processing.

Not only in the memory domain, but also in the field of attentional processing, experimental paradigms are being applied to investigate evidence in support of the sociotropy/autonomy idea. Nunn, Mathews and Trower (1997) applied an experimental Stroop task to investigate whether sociotropy and autonomy would be related to selective attentional processing of "sociotropic" and "autonomous" words respectively. Results indicated that there was a bias for all types of negative words and no specific relation between the two domains of concern (sociotropy/

auto-nomy) and biased processing of corresponding word types. These authors too, suggest that psychometric problems of the Sociotropy-Autonomy Scale may partly explain why no such relation was found. It should be clear that these results are not to be regarded as real counter-evidence for the sociotropy/autonomy distinction and related biased cognitive processing. Moreover, the fact that there seems to be some evidence for a biased processing, related to the sociotropy/autonomy distinction, in the memory study (Moore & Blackburn, 1993), and not in the attention study (Nunn et al., 1997), actually should come as no surprise: cognitive biases in memory processes are more commonly found in depression as compared to biased attentional processing, which seems to be more related to anxiety disorders (Williams et al., 1997).

Aside from integrating – or at least relating – different psychological perspectives or approaches to depression, another issue is the coupling of psychological theories with biological, neuroanatomical and neurophysiological approaches. In that respect, brain imaging techniques opened the way to the study of the neuroanatomical and neurophysiological bases of memory in general, and of autobiographical memory retrieval processes in particular (see Conway, 2001; Rugg & Wilding, 2000). A viable route, then, for future studies in the above–mentioned research on autobiographical memory specificity will be the application of brain imaging expertise to study the neurophysiological correlates of the overgenerality phenomenon in the retrieval of autobiographical memories in depressed patients.

Let us now turn to the possible *clinical implications* of the research findings discussed in the present chapter. Irrespective of the input these results provide to the development of new therapeutic techniques and procedures or the improvement of old ones, we believe that the therapeutic relevance of research on depression and memory also lies in its psycho-educational potential. Informing patients about this research, and in particular about the mechanisms at work in depression (e.g., mood-congruent recall, overgeneral memory, etc.) might in itself already be a valuable part (or first step) of treatment. This "first step" also nicely matches patients' first, and at the outset of treatment often most predominant question: "How did it come this far?", rather than "How can I solve my problem?". That way, patients gradually gain insight into depression, in particular into the processes and mechanisms relevant to maintenance of depression and vulnerability for depressive relapse. And in so doing, a preventive way of thinking is introduced and encouraged which will considerably facilitate the task of motivating patients to start working on (relapse) prevention. For example, when depressed patients, at the beginning of a session, are asked to report on the past week, they will often talk about all that went wrong and will articulate a stream of negative thoughts, feelings, experiences, etc. At such a point, a therapist might introduce and explain or – if already discussed in a previous session – again point to the mood congruency mechanisms, and check how they are "at work" here in patients' reports of the preceding week. It is our feeling and experience that when patients are able to look at their symptoms with some background of knowledge concerning the psychological mechanisms involved in depression, this will enable them to take on a meta-perspective (see below) on their depression. Whereas otherwise negative thoughts and feelings are often viewed as objective representations of reality, this meta-perspective will allow them to take distance. For example, negative thoughts about the world and the others are no longer seen as evidence for the fact that the world indeed "is" a bad place, but can now be viewed as products of biased information processing. Or in the words of a patient: "It is my depression that is talking now". Hence, when a patient is in a negative mood and catches himself dwelling on negative thoughts about past failures and losses, he is able to correct himself by realizing that it is his depression that is "misleading" him, or "playing tricks" on him. The more this meta-perspective can be generalized to situations outside the therapeutic sessions, the more a downward spiral might be stopped in an early stage, and a further amplification of depressed mood is averted. Future research will need to establish the therapeutic significance of such psycho-education.

Aside from this psycho-educational aspect, research findings on mood and memory have also led researchers to develop or refine therapeutic methods to counteract the various memory processes involved in the maintenance of depression and depressive relapse. For example, given the evidence reviewed above for the negative impact of autobiographical memory overgenerality on functioning (e.g., poor social problem solving) and on the course of depression, researchers and therapists have pointed to the importance for patients "to go beyond general statements such as 'I've always been a failure' or 'I used to be so happy' to describe the details of particular instances when they had failed or felt fulfilled" (Williams & Dritschel, 1988, p. 232). In this respect, researchers often refer to techniques such as diary keeping and self-monitoring (e.g., Williams & Scott, 1988). A consequence of a tendency to overgeneralize or to not attend to specific details of experiences is that positive events or positive elements of events go unnoticed. For example, Fava (1999), in his "well-being therapy", asks patients to monitor and to write down in a structured diary the detailed circumstances of all events leading to feelings of well-being. Also, positive instances that could counter-argue a more overgeneral negative memory (e.g., "I've always disappointed other people") might go unnoticed, due to this mechanism of overgeneral memory. For example, in response to the cue word "cowardly", a depressed patient in our autobiographical memory research retrieved the following overgeneral "categoric" memory: "Since my depression, I've had no longer the courage to attend any of the weekly meetings at work on Fridays". When he was further prompted to recall a specific instance of that overgeneral memory, he responded: "Oh now wait a minute, two months ago, I did attend the Friday meeting". Further "detailed" elaboration of that memory revealed that he had rather enjoyed that particular meeting (he received a compliment from his boss, and from one of his closest colleagues). This specific memory provided a nice counterexample for the overall "negative" overgeneral memory of not attending the weekly meetings.

Williams, Teasdale, Segal and Soulsby (2000) further showed how a more elaborate treatment package, called "mindfulness-based cognitive therapy" (MBCT; Segal, Williams, & Teasdale, 2002; Teasdale, Segal, & Williams, 1995), significantly reduces overgenerality in formerly depressed patients. MBCT is about making patients aware of specific aspects of their experiences and about promoting the adoption of a different perspective on one's own thoughts and worries, namely a meta-perspective in which one "observes" one's own ruminative thoughts without judging or trying to suppress them. This reflects an attitude of "decentering" or distraction where one no longer actively engages in further dwelling on negative thoughts. It may come as no surprise then, that research has shown ruminative thinking to be involved in the maintenance of overgenerality (e.g., Watkins & Teasdale, 2001). Rumination is a clear manifestation of depressed patients' difficulty with disengaging from all negative material (thoughts, memories, events). As such, this "decentering" philosophy might not only be of use in tackling overgeneral memory, but might also be of importance in countering or breaking through vicious circles such as mood-congruent recall and mood-congruent encoding in the prevention of depression and depressive relapse, as already hinted at above.

Thus, it seems clear that as a response to the changing view of depression as a recurrent and often chronic disorder (see above), treatment of depression is broadening its perspective as well. There is now broad agreement that the focus in treatment of depression should extend beyond treatment of a current depressive episode. More important, treatment should focus also, and maybe even more so, on the prevention of future relapse or recurrence. And this is what MBCT is all about: it is an approach to preventing relapse in depression (Segal et al., 2002). In essence, MBCT could be regarded as a short-term, eight-session, treatment program. But in the end, it has a long-term vision, as it is about providing patients with life-long skills for adequately dealing with negative emotion in the future (Segal et al., 2002). Thus, whether we need short-term or long-term treatment in depression seems to be not the most important issue. What is important is that the focus in treatment lies on relapse prevention, and that it extends beyond treating a single depressive episode.

References

Bayingana, K., Drieskens, S., & Tafforeau, J. (2002). *Depressie. Stand van zaken in België. Richtlijnen voor een gezondheidsbeleid* [Depression. State of the art. Guidelines for mental health policy]. Wetenschappelijk Instituut Volksgezondheid IPH/EPI Reports nr. 2002 –011.

Beck, A. T. (1987). Cognitive model of depression. *Journal of Cognitive Psychotherapy, 1,* 2-27.

Beck, A. T., Epstein, N., & Harrison, R. (1983). Cognitions, attitudes and personality dimensions in depression. *British Journal of Cognitive Psychotherapy, 1,* 1-16.

Beck, A. T., Epstein, N., Harrison, R., & Emery, G. (1983). *Development of the Sociotropy-Autonomy Scale: A measure of personality factors in psychopathology.* Unpublished manuscript, University of Pennsylvania, Philadelphia.

Beck, A. T., Rush, A., Shaw, B., & Emery, G. (1979). *Cognitive therapy of depression.* New York: Guilford Press.

Belsher, G., & Costello, C. G. (1988). Relapse after recovery from unipolar depression: A critical review. *Psychological Bulletin, 104,* 84-96.

Bijl, R. V., van Zessen, G., & Ravelli, A. (1997). Psychiatrische morbiditeit onder volwassenen in Nederland: het NEMESIS-onderzoek II. Prevalentie van psychiatrische stoornissen [Psychiatric morbidity in adults in The Netherlands: The NEMESIS study II: Prevalence of psychiatric disorders]. *Nederlands Tijdschrift voor Geneeskunde, 141,* 2453-2460.

Blatt, S. J. (1974). Level of object representation in anaclitic and introjective depression. *Psychoanalytic Study of the Child, 29,* 107-157.

Blaney, P. H. (1986). Affect and memory: A review. *Psychological Bulletin, 99,* 229-246.

Blazer, D. G., Kessler, R. C., McGonagle, K. A., & Swartz, M. S. (1994). The prevalence and distribution of major depression in a national community sample: The National Comorbidity Survey. *American Journal of Psychiatry, 151,* 979-86.

Bower, G. H. (1981). Mood and memory. *American Psychologist, 36,* 129-148.

Bower, G. H. (1987). Commentary on mood and memory. *Behaviour Research and Therapy, 25,* 443-455.

Bower, G. H. (1991). Mood congruity of social judgements. In J. P. Forgas (Ed.), *Emotion and social judgments* (pp. 31-54). Oxford: Pergamon Press.

Bower, G. H., Gilligan, S. G., & Monteiro, K. P. (1981). Selective learning caused by affective states. *Journal of Experimental Psychology: General, 110,* 451-473.

Bower, G. H., Monteiro, K. P., & Gilligan, S. G. (1978). Emotional mood as a context of learning and recall. *Journal of Verbal Learning and Verbal Behavior, 17,* 573-585.

Brewin, C. R., Reynolds, M., & Tata, P. (1999). Autobiographical memory processes and the course of depression. *Journal of Abnormal Psychology, 108,* 511-517.

Brewin, C. R., Watson, M., McCarthy, S., Hyman, P., & Dayson, D. (1998). Intrusive memories and depression in cancer patients. *Behaviour Research and Therapy, 36,* 1131-1142.

Brittlebank, A. D., Scott, J., Williams, J. M. G., & Ferrier, I. N. (1993). Autobiographical memory in depression: State or trait marker? *British Journal of Psychiatry, 162,* 118-121.

Burke, M., & Mathews, A. (1992). Autobiographical memory and clinical anxiety. *Cognition and Emotion, 6,* 23-35.

Clark, D. A., & Beck, A. T. (1999). *Scientific foundations of cognitive theory and therapy of depression.* New York: John Wiley & Sons.

Clark, D. M., & Teasdale, J. D. (1982). Diurnal variation in clinical depression and accessibility of memories of positive and negative experiences. *Journal of Abnormal Psychology, 91,* 87-95.

Conway, M. A. (2001). Sensory-perceptual episodic memory and its context: Autobiographical memory. *Philosophical Transactions of the Royal Society of London, 356,* 1375-1384.

Dalgleish, T., Spinks, H., Yiend, J., & Kuyken, W. (2001) Autobiographical memory style in seasonal affective disorder and its relationship to future symptom remission. *Journal of Abnormal Psychology, 110,* 335-340.

Dalgleish, T., Tchanturia, K., Serpell, L., Hems, S., Yiend, J., de Silva, P., & Treasure, J. (2003). Self-reported parental abuse relates to autobiographical memory style in patients with eating disorders. *Emotion, 3,* 211-222.

de Decker, A. (2001). *The specificity of the autobiographical memory retrieval style in adolescents with a history of trauma.* Unpublished doctoral dissertation, University of Leuven, Belgium.

de Decker, A., Hermans, D., Raes, F., & Eelen P. (2003). Autobiographical memory specificity and trauma in inpatient adolescents. *Journal of Clinical Child and Adolescent Psychology, 32,* 22-31.

Evans, J., Williams, J. M. G., O'Loughlin, S., & Howells, K. (1992). Autobiographical memory and problem solving strategies of individuals who parasuicide. *Psychological Medicine, 22,* 399-405.

Fava, G. A. (1999). Well-being therapy: Conceptual and technical issues. *Psychotherapy and Psychosomatics, 68,* 171-179.

Fiedler, K., Nickel, S., Muehlfriedel, T., & Unkelbach, C. (2001). Is mood congruency an effect of genuine memory or response bias. *Journal of Experimental Social Psychology, 37,* 201-214.

Forgas, J. P., & Bower, G. H. (1987). Mood effects on person-perception judgments. *Journal of Personality and Social Psychology, 53,* 53-60.

Gilligan, S. G., & Bower, G. H. (1984). Cognitive consequences of emotional arousal. In C. E. Izard, J. Kagan & R. Zajonc (Eds.), *Emotions, cognitions, and behaviour* (pp. 547-588). New York: Cambridge Press.

Goddard, L., Dritschel, B., & Burton, A. (1996). Role of autobiographical memory in social problem solving and depression. *Journal of Abnormal Psychology, 105,* 609-616.

Goddard, L., Dritschel, B., & Burton, A. (1997). Social problem-solving and autobiographical memory in non-clinical depression. *British Journal of Clinical Psychology, 36,* 449-451.

Godden, D. R., & Baddeley, A. D. (1975). Context dependency in two natural environments: On land and underwater. *British Journal of Psychology, 91,* 99-104.

Gotlib, I. H., & Krasnoperova, E. (1998). Biased information processing as a vulnerability factor for depression. *Behavior Therapy, 29,* 603-617.

Hammen, C. (2001). Vulnerability to depression in adulthood. In R. E. Ingram & J. M. Price (Eds.), *Vulnerability to psychopathology. Risk across the life-span* (pp. 226-257). New York: The Guilford Press.

Harvey, A. G., Bryant, R. A., & Dang, S. T. (1998). Autobiographical memory in acute stress disorder. *Journal of Consulting and Clinical Psychology, 66,* 500-506.

Henderson, D., Hargreaves, I., Gregory, S., & Williams, J. M. G. (2002). Autobiographical memory and emotion in a non-clinical sample of women with and without a reported history of childhood sexual abuse. *British Journal of Clinical Psychology, 41,* 129-141.

Hermans, D., & de Decker, A. (2001, December). *Adaptive aspects of overgeneral memory: Part 2.* Paper presented at the Second Autobiographical Memory Workshop, Cambridge, England.

Hermans, D., Van den Broeck, K., Belis, G., Raes, F., Pieters, G., & Eelen, P. (2004). Trauma and autobiographical memory specificity in depressed inpatients. *Behaviour Research and Therapy, 42,* 775-789.

Judd, L. L., Akiskal, H. S., & Paulus, M. P. (1997). The role and clinical significance of subsyndromal depressive symptoms (SSD) in unipolar major depressive disorder. *Journal of Affective Disorders, 45,* 5-17.

Kuyken, W., & Brewin, C. R. (1995). Autobiographical memory functioning in depression and reports of early abuse. *Journal of Abnormal Psychology, 104,* 585-591.

Kuyken, W., & Dalgleish, T. (1995). Autobiographical memory and depression. *British Journal of Clinical Psychology, 34,* 89-92.

Littrell, J. (1998). Is the reexperience of painful emotion therapeutic? *Clinical Psychology Review, 18,* 71-102.

Lloyd, G. G., & Lishman, W. A. (1975). Effect of depression on the speed of recall of pleasant and unpleasant memories. *Psychological Medicine, 5,* 173-180.

Mackinger, H. F., Loschin, G. G., & Leibetseder, M. M. (2000). Prediction of postnatal affective changes by autobiographical memories. *European Psychologist, 5,* 52-61.

Mackinger, H. F., Pachinger, M. M., Leibetseder, M. M., & Fartacek, R. R. (2000). Autobiographical memories in women remitted from major depression. *Journal of Abnormal Psychology, 109,* 331-334.

Matt, G. E., Vázquez, C., & Campbell, K. W. (1992). Mood congruent recall of affectively toned stimuli: A meta-analytic review. *Clinical Psychology Review, 12,* 227-255.

Moore, R. G., & Blackburn, I.-M. (1993). Sociotropy, autonomy and personal memories in depression. *British Journal of Clinical Psychology, 32,* 460-462.

Moore, R. G., Watts, F. N., & Williams, J. M. G. (1988). The specificity of personal memories in depression. *British Journal of Clinical Psychology, 27,* 275-276.

Nunn, J. D., Mathews, A., & Trower, P. (1997). Selective processing of concern-related information in depression. *British Journal of Clinical Psychology, 36,* 489-503.

Park, R. J., Goodyer, I. M., & Teasdale, J. D. (2002). Categoric overgeneral autobiographical memory in adolescent Major Depression. *Psychological Medicine, 32,* 267-276.

Peeters, F., Wessel, I., Merckelbach, H., & Boon-Vermeeren, M. (2002). Autobiographical memory specificity and the course of major depressive disorder. *Comprehensive Psychiatry, 43,* 344-350.

Platt, J. J., & Spivack, G. (1975). *Manual for the Means-Ends Problem-Solving (MEPS): A measure of interpersonal problem-solving skill.* Philadelphia: Hahnemann Medical College and Hospital.

Pollock, L. R., & Williams, J. M. G. (2001). Effective problem solving in suicide attempters depends on specific autobiographical recall. *Suicide and Threatening Behavior, 31,* 386-396.

Puffet, A., Jehin-Marchot, D., Timsit-Berthier, M., & Timsit, M. (1991). Autobiographical memory and major depressive states. *European Psychiatry, 6,* 141-145.

Raes, F., Hermans, D., de Decker, A., Eelen, P., & Williams, J. M. G. (2003). Autobiographical memory specificity and affect-regulation: An experimental approach. *Emotion, 3,* 201-206.

Rugg, M. D., & Wilding, E. L. (2000). Retrieval processing and episodic memory. *Trends in Cognitive Sciences, 4,* 108-115.

Rusting, C. L., & DeHart, T. (2000). Retrieving positive memories to regulate negative mood: Consequences for mood-congruent memory. *Journal of Personality and Social Psychology, 78,* 737-752.

Schwartz, B., & Reisberg, D. (1991). *Learning and memory.* New York: Norton.

Scott, J., Williams, J. M. G., Brittlebank, A., & Ferrier, I. N. (1995). The relationship between premorbid neuroticism, cognitive dysfunction and persistence of depression. *Journal of Affective Disorders, 33,* 67–72.

Scott, J., Stanton, B., Garland, A., & Ferrier, I. N. (2000). Cognitive vulnerability in patients with bipolar disorder. *Psychological Medicine, 30,* 467-472.

Segal, Z. V., Gemar, M. G., & Williams, S. (1999). Differential cognitive response to a mood challenge following successful cognitive therapy or pharmacotherapy for unipolar depression. *Journal of Abnormal Psychology, 108,* 3-10.

Segal, Z. V., Williams, J. M. G., & Teasdale, J. D. (2002). *Mindfulness-based Cognitive Therapy for depression. A new approach to preventing relapse.* New York: Guilford Press.

Share, M. L., Lisman, S. A., & Spear, N. E. (1984). The effects of mood variation on state-dependent retention. *Cognitive Therapy and Research, 8,* 387-408.

Sidley, G. L., Whitaker, K., Calam, R. M., & Wells, A. (1997). The relationship between problem solving and autobiographical memory in parasuicide patients. *Behavioural and Cognitive Psychotherapy, 25,* 195-202.

Singer, J. A., & Salovey, P. (1988). Mood and memory: Evaluating the network theory of affect. *Clinical Psychology Review, 8,* 211-251.

Teasdale, J. D., & Russell, M. L. (1983). Differential effects of induced mood on the recall of positive, negative and neutral words. *British Journal of Clinical Psychology, 22,* 163-171.

Teasdale, J. D., Segal, Z. V., & Williams, J. M. G. (1995). How does cognitive therapy prevent depressive relapse and why should attentional control (mindfulness) training help? An information processing analysis. *Behaviour Research and Therapy, 33,* 25-39.

Wachtel, P. L. (1994). Cyclical processes in personality and psychopathology. *Journal of Abnormal Psychology, 103,* 51-66.

Wachtel, P. L. (1997). *Psychoanalysis, behavior therapy, and the relational world.* Washington, DC: American Psychological Association.

Watkins, E., & Teasdale, J. D. (2001). Rumination and overgeneral memory in depression: Effects of self-focus and analytic thinking. *Journal of Abnormal Psychology, 110,* 353-357.

Watkins, P. C. (2002). Implicit memory bias in depression. *Cognition and Emotion, 16,* 381-402.

Weingartner, M., Miller, H., & Murphy, D. L. (1977). Mood-state-dependent retrieval of verbal associations. *Journal of Abnormal Psychology, 86,* 276-284.

Weiss, E. L., Longhurst, J. G., & Mazure, C. M. (1999). Childhood sexual abuse as a risk for depression in women: Psychological and neurobiological correlates. *American Journal of Psychiatry, 156,* 816-828.

Wessel, I., Meeren, M., Peeters, F., Arntz, A., & Merckelbach, H. (2001). Correlates of autobiographical memory specificity: The role of depression, anxiety and childhood trauma. *Behaviour Research and Therapy, 39,* 409-421.

Wilhelm, S., McNally, R. J., Baer, L., & Florin, I. (1997). Autobiographical memory in obsessive-compulsive disorder. *British Journal of Clinical Psychology, 36,* 21-31.

Williams, J. M. G. (1992). *The psychological treatment of depression: A guide to the theory and practice of cognitive behaviour therapy.* London: Routledge.

Williams, J. M. G. (1996). Depression and the specificity of autobiographical memory. In D. C. Rubin (Ed.), *Remembering our past. Studies in autobiographical memory* (pp. 244-267). Cambridge, NY: Cambridge University Press.

Williams, J. M. G., & Broadbent, K. (1986). Autobiographical memory in suicide attempters. *Journal of Abnormal Psychology, 95,* 144-149.

Williams, J. M. G., & Dritschel, B. H. (1988). Emotional disturbance and the specificity of autobiographical memory. *Cognition and Emotion, 2,* 221-234.

Williams, J. M. G., Ellis, N. C., Tyers, C., Healy, H., Rose, G., & MacLeod, A. K. (1996). Specificity of autobiographical memory and imageability of the future. *Memory and Cognition, 24,* 116-125.

Williams, J. M. G., & Scott, J. (1988). Autobiographical memory in depression. *Psychological Medicine, 18,* 689-695.

Williams, J. M. G., Teasdale, J. D., Segal, Z. V., & Soulsby, J. (2000). Mindfulness-based cognitive therapy reduces overgeneral autobiographical memory in formerly depressed patients. *Journal of Abnormal Psychology, 109,* 150-155.

Williams, J. M. G., Watts, F., MacLeod, C., & Mathews, A. (1997). *Cognitive psychology and emotional disorders* (2nd ed.). Chichester: John Wiley & Sons.

Chapter 3

The Convergence Among Psychodynamic and Cognitive-

Behavioral Theories of Depression: Theoretical Overview

Patrick Luyten, Sidney J. Blatt, & Jozef Corveleyn

Over the last decades, there has been a growing trend towards integration among psychodynamic and cognitive-behavioral theories (Jones & Pulos, 1993; Milton, 2001; Ryle, 1995; Wachtel, 1997; Westen, 2000), specifically concerning the conceptualization and treatment of depression (Clark & Beck, 1999; Blatt, 2004; Blatt & Maroudas, 1992). In general, two related factors are responsible for this trend. First, as mentioned in the introduction of this volume, findings on the natural course of depression have changed our view of this disorder in important ways. Research has shown that depression tends to be a recurrent and even chronic disorder (e.g., Costello et al., 2002; see also Chapter 1, this volume), which has a high comorbidity with personality disorders (Klein & Hayden, 2000; Mulder, 2002). Second, so-called "evidence-based" brief treatments of depression, such as "traditional" cognitive-behavioral treatments and interpersonal therapy, have limited effects (Luyten, Lowyck, & Corveleyn, 2003; Shea et al., 1992; Westen & Morrison, 2001; Westen, Novotny, & Thompson-Brenner, 2004). These findings have not only led to a renewed interest in theories and techniques that are based on long-term treatments of depression, such as psychodynamic theories (Blatt, 2004; Jones & Pulos, 1993; Kwon, 1999), in which considerations concerning personality and particularly personality organization often play a central role (Westen, 2000), but also in the relationship between personality and depression in general (Klein, Durbin, Shankman, & Santiago, 2002; Klein, Kupfer, & Shea, 1993; Gunderson et al., 1999).

In this chapter, we focus on a very specific move towards the integration between psychodynamic and cognitive-behavioral formulations concerning the conceptualization and treatment of depression (Blatt, 2004; Robins, 1993; Sabbe, 2002). More specifically, we will focus on four groups of authors that have proposed similar personality dimensions as vulnerability factors for both clinical and non-clinical forms of depression and dysphoria. Blatt (1974, 1998, 2004; Blatt & Zuroff, 1992), from an object-relational and cognitive-developmental perspective, has described *dependency* and *self-critical perfectionism*[1] as vulnerability factors for depression, resulting in a dependent (or anaclitic) versus a self-critical/perfectionistic (or introjective) type of depression, as well as possible mixed forms of dependent and self-critical depression. Anaclitic depression is characterized by feelings of helplessness, loneliness, weakness, and intense and often chronic fears of being abandoned. Introjective depression, in contrast, is characterized by self-criticism and feelings of guilt, inferiority, failure, and a chronic fear of being disapproved and criticized.

Beck (1983, 1991, 1999; Clark & Beck, 1999) has made a similar distinction from a cognitive-behavioral perspective between *sociotropy* and *autonomy* as cognitive-affective personality styles that confer a vulnerability for depression, which at a descriptive level shows many similarities with Blatt's concepts of dependency and self-critical perfectionism respectively. Bowlby (1980, 1988) has distinguished from a psychodynamic/ethological perspective between *anxious* and *compulsive self-reliant attachment styles* predisposing to depression. Arieti and Bemporad (Arieti & Bemporad, 1978; Bemporad, 1992), finally, distinguish from an interpersonal psychodynamic perspective between *dominant other* and *dominant goal* personality structures predisposing to depression.

However, most research has concentrated on Blatt's and Beck's formulations of dependency/sociotropy and self-critical perfectionism/autonomy (e.g., see Blatt, 1998, 2004; Clark & Beck, 1999). Despite almost three decades of empirical research, this area of research is often little known, even among those who have specialized in mood disorders research or treatment (Luyten et al., 2003). In this chapter, we therefore present an overview of the main theoretical assumptions of these models. Because both Blatt's and Beck's views of depression are part of a more general theory of normal and pathological personality development, we first outline these general views briefly. Next, we focus specifically on Blatt's and Beck's conceptualizations concerning depression, including their views of the treatment of depression. Relevant empirical research is reviewed in the next chapter. Despite the fact that these theories offer important avenues towards integration concerning the conceptualization and treatment of depression, we also believe that there are some important barriers that limit further integration among

---

[1] Blatt (e.g., Blatt, 1974) originally used the term "self-criticism" to refer to this second personality dimension. However, in keeping with his more recent views (see Chapter 5, this volume) and given the fact that self-criticism is only one characteristic of this personality dimension, we prefer the notion "self-critical perfectionism" to refer to this personality dimension as a whole.

these theories. These barriers are discussed in a separate section. In a final section, we discuss more general issues concerning these theories and their potential for further integration in research and treatment of depression.

Blatt's and Beck's Theory of Normal and Pathological Personality Development

Blatt's Theory of Normal and Psychopathological Personality Development

According to Blatt (e.g., Blass & Blatt, 1996; Blatt, 1995a; Blatt & Blass, 1990; Blatt & Shichman, 1983; Guisinger & Blatt, 1994), personality development can be conceptualized as a dialectical interaction between two fundamental developmental lines, namely (1) an *anaclitic* or *relatedness* line that normally leads to increasingly mature, complex, and mutually satisfying interpersonal relations, and (2) an *introjective* or *self-definitional* line that normally leads to the development of a stable, realistic, and essentially positive self and identity. In "normal" development, these two developmental lines are in constant reciprocal or dialectic interaction. Thus, an increasingly stable and differentiated self-definition leads to more differentiated and complex interpersonal relationships and vice versa. Hence, in the case of "optimal" development, high levels of identity and autonomy go together with the capacity to form and maintain complex, differentiated and satisfying interpersonal relationships, and vice versa. One is at the same time able to relate to others in complex, reciprocal ways, without losing one's sense of self and identity. Such differentiated and reciprocal relationships in turn contribute to the development of even more integrated and positive feelings of identity and autonomy.

Based on this theory of normal personality development, psychopathology can be conceptualized as an *overemphasis* on or an *exaggeration* of one of these two developmental lines and the *neglect* or *defensive avoidance* of the other line (e.g., Blatt, 1991a, 1991b; Blatt & Maroudas, 1992; Blatt & Shichman, 1983). Thus, following this view, psychopathology is characterized by a disruption of the dialectical interaction of these two developmental lines – by a rigid, one-sided overemphasis of one line (e.g., interpersonal relationships), and the neglect and/or defensive avoidance of the other line (e.g., feelings of identity and autonomy). Whereas in "normal" development anaclitic and introjective developmental lines interact synergistically, and thus are in constant dialectical interaction, psychopathology is characterized by a rigid overemphasis of one developmental line at the expense of the other. Thus two *clusters* or *configurations of psychopathology* can be distinguished, depending on which developmental line *predominates* and which developmental line is *neglected* or *defended* against, i.e., an *anaclitic* and an *introjective cluster*. Blatt distinguishes several symptom ("Axis I") and personality ("Axis II") disorders in each developmental line on three structural levels, i.e., the psychotic, borderline, and neurotic level, which can be seen as different rigid exaggerations of one developmental line and the neglect or defensive avoidance of the other (see below; Blatt & Shichman, 1983). To distinguish between adaptive and maladaptive dimensions on each developmental line, Blatt has introduced the terms *relatedness* versus *dependency* or *neediness*, and *efficacy* versus *self-criticism* or *self-critical perfectionism* respectively (Blatt, 2004; Zuroff, Mongrain, & Santor, 2004; see also Chapter 5, this volume).

Thus, the name of these two developmental lines not only refers to the central dominant developmental theme in each line, but also to the central problem in case of disturbance (Blatt, 1974; Blatt & Shichman, 1983). The notion "anaclitic" refers to the development of interpersonal relations that prototypically find their origin in the relation with the first significant other, mostly the mother. Disturbances in this developmental line can give rise to anaclitic psychopathology, which is primarily characterized by problems concerning relatedness, such as intimacy, caring, and sexuality. These concerns can range from desires and conflicts concerning primitive, dyadic relationships, in which (primitive) symbiotic desires are central, as in nonparanoid schizophrenia (psychotic level) and, on somewhat higher levels, in hysteroid borderline personality disorder, histrionic (borderline level) and dependent personalities (low neurotic level). At the higher neurotic level, desires and conflicts concern more triadic, oedipal relationships, as in hysteria. According to Blatt (Blatt & Levy, 1998), the DSM-IV Axis II dependent, histrionic, passive-aggressive and borderline personality disorders belong to the anaclitic cluster (Blatt & Levy, 1998; Shahar, Blatt, & Ford, 2003).

The notion "introjective" in turn refers to the development of a stable, differentiated and integrated self by means of identification or introjection. Introjective pathology is according to Blatt primarily characterized by a focus on issues such as self-control, guilt, identity, and autonomy (Blatt & Shichman, 1983). Again, this focus can range from very primitive desires for autonomy, for instance in striving for isolation and defensive separation, such as in paranoid schizophrenia (psychotic level) and to a lesser extent in more "ideational" borderlines (borderline level), and in paranoid personalities, to a rigid control over impulses, as in obsessive-compulsive neurosis, and to an exaggerated focus on self-worth, power and identity in introjective depression and phallic narcissism (or narcissistic personality disorder) (neurotic level). The DSM-IV Axis II schizoid, schizotypic, paranoid, narcissistic, antisocial, avoidant, self-defeating, and obsessive-compulsive personality disorders belong in this cluster according to Blatt (Blatt & Levy, 1998; Shahar et al., 2003).

In general, introjective patients are expected to be more ideational than anaclitic patients and more concerned with identity and autonomy than with interpersonal relations and affects (Blatt & Shichman, 1983). Moreover, introjective patients are assumed to have a more sequential cognitive style that focuses on details, responsibility, and cause-effect relationships, whereas the cognitive style of anaclitic patients is expected to be more impressionistic and global. Conflicts or problems with anger and aggression dominate the clinical picture in introjective patients, while libidinal issues predominate in anaclitic patients.

Finally, Blatt (e.g., Blatt & Maroudas, 1992; Blatt & Shichman, 1983) hypothesizes that there are important gender differences in the emphasis on these two developmental lines and thus perhaps also in the two clusters of psychopathology. First, several psychological theories suggest that the primary identification figure throughout female development is typically the mother, whereas the male child has to switch in development from the mother to the father figure (Chodorow, 1978; Baker Miller, 1976). Thus, the male child is typically forced to de-identify with the mother and thus to de-emphasize relationships to attain a stable identity and autonomy, whereas there is much more continuity in the emphasis on relationships in the female child. In addition, at least in our western society there (still) is on average more emphasis on relatedness for females and achievement and autonomy for males (Chevron, Quinlan, & Blatt, 1978; Gilligan, 1982). Accordingly, one could expect that anaclitic psychopathology is more prevalent in women and introjective psychopathology in men. However, according to Blatt (e.g., Blatt, Quinlan, Chevron, McDonald, & Zuroff, 1982), gender incongruence might also play an important role. That is, for men high dependency and for women high self-critical perfectionism might be associated with an increased risk for psychopathology.

Possible limitations of this model of normal and pathological personality development include the fact that personality development is perhaps conceptualized in a too linear-causal way. However, Blatt (1974; Blatt & Shichman, 1983) explicitly refers to the fact that on each line progression and regression is possible. Thus, on each line, patients will tend to show – especially in stressful situations – a mix of different forms and levels of psychopathology that are typical for that developmental line. Moreover, the theoretical model also leaves room for the role of deferred action (*Nachträglichkeit*) (Blatt, 1974). A second possible limitation concerns the assumption in Blatt's original formulations (Blatt, 1991a; Blatt & Shichman, 1983) that individuals "choose" early in life between the two developmental lines. However, even Blatt's original formulations did not suggest a rigid dichotomy between anaclitic and introjective (Zuroff et al., 2004), but included the possibility that patients show both anaclitic and introjective features. Furthermore, it is a common misunderstanding to interpret the distinction between anaclitic and introjective as a *qualitative* or even *dichotomous* distinction, instead as one of *relative emphasis*. Blatt's theory emphasizes that the distinction between anaclitic and introjective should be made on the basis of which developmental line predominates and which line is *relatively* neglected or defended against. In addition, according to Blatt (e.g., Blatt & Shichman, 1983), "normality" is precisely defined by a *synergistic dialectic interaction* between these two developmental lines (although this does not mean that also within the "normal" range individuals can differ in relative emphasis on both lines), whereas psychopathology is characterized by a *rigid* emphasis on one line and the *neglect* or *defensive* avoidance of the other. For both reasons, anaclitic and introjective characteristics should not be considered to be mutually exclusive. Yet, notwithstanding these

71

important nuances, there has been a dearth of theoretical and especially empirical research on so-called "mixed anaclitic-introjective" patients. Recent theoretical developments and empirical research that addresses these issues are discussed in detail by Blatt and Shahar in Chapter 5 (see also Zuroff et al., 2004; Shahar, Blatt, & Ford, 2003).

Beck's Theory of Normal and Psychopathological Personality Development

Over the last two decades, Beck's views have evolved from a fairly simple schema theory towards a psychoevolutionary theory that conceptualizes pathological personality development, as does Blatt, as an exaggerated or distorted form of normal personality development (Beck, 1991, 1999; Beck & Freeman, 1990).

According to Beck (1999), psychological disorders can be seen as basic patterns of behavior that once had survival value, but that have often become maladaptive in our current modern society (the so-called "evolutionary friction rub"). For instance, depression according to Beck (1999) is a reaction to a loss that reactivates an "innate program consisting of giving up and withdrawal (in other words, depression) [which] would serve to reduce the individual's "needs" until new resources were developed" (Beck, 1999, p. 413). This innate program once clearly had survival value, because in the wild the loss of a partner, for instance, could mean that one had to survive for a considerable amount of time with limited resources. However, in our society, this is no longer the case and thus such innate programs often become maladaptive. Hence, such innate programs should largely be seen as "anachronistic symbols inherited from the past" (Beck, 1999, p. 413).

Beck (Beck, 1999; Beck & Freeman, 1990) has proposed that such *patterns* or *strategies* make up *normal personality* development. A certain "harmony" with and adaptation to the environment characterizes, according to Beck, "normal" or "functional personality". However, in an *exaggerated form* these patterns or strategies give rise to different forms of *psychopathology*. Thus, psychopathology arises when these strategies are used *excessively*, *compulsively* and/or *inappropriately* (Beck, 1999). Moreover, Beck proposes that these strategies are associated with specific beliefs, attitudes, and assumptions (Beck, 1999). These strategies and accompanying core beliefs form the basis of Beck's classification of personality disorders summarized in Table 1.

Furthermore, Beck's (1983, 1999) most recent views clearly exemplify the so-called "psychoanalytic drift" (Power, 1991; Milton, 2001) in cognitive psychology. Under the influence of psychodynamic formulations, Beck (1983, 1999) now distinguishes between two basic "self-concepts": on the one hand the self-concept "I am helpless", which according to Beck refers to survival; on the other hand, a self-concept centered around the core belief "I am unlovable", which refers to relatedness and attachment. Beck (1983, 1999) also calls these two basic self-concepts *sociotropic* and *autonomous personality dimensions* or "modes". Sociotropic individuals according to Beck are fundamentally oriented toward interpersonal relationships. Their self-esteem is mainly dependent on receiving love, care and acceptance from others. Autonomous individuals on the other hand, are predominantly oriented toward autonomy, control, and independence, and thus their self-esteem is mainly dependent on the achievement of goals and control. Although some important differences have been identified, sociotropy and autonomy resemble in important respects, at least at a descriptive level, Blatt's concepts of relatedness and self-definition (Blatt & Maroudas, 1992; Clark & Beck, 1999; Zuroff et al., 2004).

Moreover, like Blatt (Blatt & Levy, 1998; Blatt & Shichman, 1983), Beck (1999) has proposed that in an exaggerated form, these two personality dimensions give rise to *two clusters of psychopathology* that match in general Blatt's categorization of personality disorders into anaclitic and introjective clusters. According to Beck (1999) the dependent, histrionic, avoidant, passive-aggressive and borderline[2] personality disorder belong to the *sociotropic* cluster, whereas the schizoid, paranoid, narcissistic, antisocial, and obsessive-compulsive personality disorders make up the *autonomous* cluster.

TABLE 1
Strategies and core beliefs in personality disorders (Based on Beck, 1999)

Strategy	Core belief	Personality disorder
Predatory	People are there to be taken	Antisocial
Help-eliciting	I am helpless	Dependent
Competitive	I am special	Narcissistic
Exhibitionistic	I need to impress	Histrionic
Autonomous	I need plenty of space	Schizoid
Defensive	People are potential adversaries	Paranoid
Withdrawal	I may get hurt	Avoidant
Ritualistic	Errors are bad	Compulsive

Like Blatt, Beck's theoretical formulations have some important limitations (see Blatt & Maroudas, 1992). First, Beck's assumption of a link between evolutionary inherited strategies and Axis I and Axis II disorders is very speculative. Moreover, we believe that Beck's conceptualization of depression as an "anachronistic symbol inherited from the past" (Beck, 1999, p. 413) is not only speculative, but is also based on an overly rationalistic human anthropology which assumes that loss (e.g., loss of a partner, of a job, etc.) in our contemporary society should in fact not be associated with feelings of sadness and depression. However, we believe that such feelings are part and parcel of the human condition precisely because human beings possess the capacity to emotionally invest in what they value. Thus, feelings of sadness and depression after loss appear to be the other side of the coin of the human capacity for caring. Third, it has been repeatedly pointed out that Beck's terminology is often imprecise and vague (Clark & Beck, 1999). For instance, the relationship between concepts such as schemas, beliefs, automatic thoughts,

---

[2] Note that the borderline personality disorder is not included in Table 1. For a discussion, see below.

personality dimensions, and "modes" is often not clear. Fourth, Beck's theory only refers to content, but not to the structural level of psychopathology (e.g., psychotic, borderline, neurotic). This lack of a structural perspective on personality development and organization appears to be an important shortcoming of Beck's views (see also Westen, 2000). This becomes clear, for example, when Beck describes the reasons why the borderline personality disorder is not included in his views about the relationships between evolutionary inherited strategies and beliefs. According to Beck, this is due to the fact that patients with borderline personality disorder not only combine several "core beliefs", but also "are uniquely characterised by 'ego defects' in impulse control, affect stability, and reality testing rather than by a specific content" (Beck, 1999, p.422), a description which is heavily loaded with concepts that refer to a (psychodynamic) structural perspective on psychopathology.

Advantages over the DSM Approach

Despite these possible limitations, both Blatt's and Beck's views offer some important advantages over the atheoretical approach of DSM (Blatt, 2004; Blatt & Levy, 1998). It is well known that precisely because of its symptomatic and atheoretical approach, patients diagnosed with major depressive disorder (and other mood disorders) according to the DSM show considerable heterogeneity in terms of etiology, pathogenesis, prognosis, and treatment responsivity (Blatt, 2004; Van Praag, 1998; Westen et al., 2004). Moreover, the DSM is clearly inspired by a disease model, which assumes that a disease is either present or absent based on a counting of symptoms. However, research tends to favor a more continuous view of depression, going from mild dysphoria to full-blown depression (Judd et al., 1998; Kendler & Gardner, 1998; see also Chapter 1, this volume). Thus, in sum, a DSM diagnosis gives little information concerning theoretically and clinically important variables. In addition, the reification of the construct of depression by DSM, as if it were a disease entity that is either present or absent and that has its own specific etiology, pathogenesis, and treatment, hampers further research.

Blatt's and Beck's approach, in contrast, is clearly theoretical and geared towards providing the clinician (and researcher) with clinically important information. Blatt as well as Beck propose that psychopathology can be seen as an exaggerated form of normal personality development, thus linking the field of "normal" and "abnormal", "clinical" and "positive" psychology, and the study of psychopathology and developmental psychopathology (see also Chapter 7, this volume). In particular, their views imply that depression should not be seen as a distinct disease entity, for which only some people are vulnerable. To the contrary, depression is situated within a broader model of normal and pathological personality development: it can range from mild dysphoria to clinical depression. Moreover, clinical depression is not seen as a distinct *disease*, but as one possible *disorder* among many other *related* disorders. Thus, as we will show in detail later in this chapter, Blatt's and Beck's view that depression is related to personality development and structure has immediate implications for theoretically and clinically important information, such as etiology, pathogenesis, and treatment responsivity. This opens up several new perspectives from a research as well as from a clinical perspective.

Dependency/Sociotropy, Self-Critical Perfectionism/Autonomy, and Depression

Introduction

Blatt's and Beck's views about depression share two basic assumptions which are often misunderstood (Zuroff et al., 2004). A first assumption is that both dependency/sociotropy and self-critical perfectionism/autonomy are continuous dimensions. Thus, individuals can show all combinations of dependency/sociotropy and self-critical perfectionism/autonomy. However, Blatt's and Beck's views are often interpreted as attempts to distinguish between two *types* of depression, i.e., an anaclitic/sociotropic versus a perfectionistic/autonomous type of depression. The fact that both Blatt and Beck often present their views, mainly for didactical purposes, in a way that suggests a typology, has considerably added to this misunderstanding (Zuroff et al., 2004). However, both authors clearly hold the view that all combinations of dependent and perfectionistic features are possible and that only at the extreme ends of the continuum do relatively "pure" cases of anaclitic and perfectionistic depression exist. We will return to this issue at the end of this chapter.

A second assumption concerns the fact that Blatt and Beck also advocate a continuum view of depression (Blatt, 1974; Clark & Beck, 1999). This view holds that there is a continuum going from "normal" or mild forms of dysphoria to clinical, diagnosable depression, differing only in the severity (and perhaps also the persistence) of symptoms. A discontinuity or categorical view of depression on the other hand argues that there are not only quantitative, but also qualitative differences between feelings of dysphoria and diagnosable depression (e.g., see Vredenburg, Flett, & Krames, 1993 for a review). Although most research evidence seems to support a continuum view, the debate on this issue is far from settled (e.g., Clark & Beck, 1999). However, if diagnosable depression is qualitatively different from dysphoria, then studies investigating Blatt's and Beck's views in nonclinical samples might not generalize to clinical samples (Coyne & Whiffen, 1995; Flett, Hewitt, Endler, & Bagby, 1995; Ingram & Hamilton, 1999). In the next chapter, where we will review empirical research concerning Blatt's and Beck's view, we will return to this issue.

Taking these remarks into account, we will in the remainder of this chapter outline the main aspects of recent psychodynamic and cognitive-behavioral theories of depression. Because Blatt's model is the most encompassing, it will form the basis of our overview. However, we will also discuss important differences between Blatt's views and those of Beck, Arieti and Bemporad, and Bowlby. In short, Blatt (Blatt, 1974, 1998, 2004; Blatt & Shichman, 1983) proposes that general predisposing factors (genetic, biological and environmental), in interaction with specific environmental factors, can lead to disturbances in the anaclitic and/or introjective developmental line, resulting in two personality dimensions or structures that confer a specific vulnerability for depression. Moreover, both Blatt (e.g., Blatt & Zuroff, 1992) and Beck (1983, 1999) have proposed that dependent/sociotropic and self-critical/autonomous individuals are particularly vulnerable for life events that match their personal vulnerability. This hypothesis, which has been termed the personality-event congruency hypothesis (Robins, 1995), suggests that dependent/sociotropic individuals are more likely to become dysphoric/depressed following negative interpersonal events, such as rejection or loss, whereas selfcritical/autonomous individuals are more likely to become depressed following negative achievement-related events, such as failure at work or school. Both personality dimensions are also hypothesized to be associated with a specific relational style that enhances the risk for depression. Finally, when depressed, both personality dimensions are expected to influence the clinical presentation of depression. In what follows, we will for didactical reasons describe these features in relatively "pure" types, keeping in mind that patients may show "mixed" characteristics.

Anaclitic/Sociotropic Depression

Clinical presentation. The clinical presentation of dependent depressed patients is characterized by feelings of loneliness, helplessness, weakness, and fears of abandonment (Blatt, 1974). Often, these patients seek refuge in the use of alcohol, drugs, or excessive eating ("oral traits") (Blatt et al., 1982). Anxiety and agitation would often color the clinical picture ("anxious depression"). Depression would also often be masked by or show itself in somatic complaints (Blatt & Shichman, 1983). Suicide attempts would be less violent or more "passive" than in perfectionistic patients (e.g., overdose of medication) (Beck, 1983; Blatt et al., 1982). In addition, Beck (1983) has proposed that the mood of these patients would be more reactive to both positive and negative events (e.g., a new relationship ameliorates symptoms). They are also expected to be very sensitive to even minor frustrations. However, aggression would be denied or inhibited for fear of losing the care and love of others on whom one is dependent (Blatt & Shichman, 1983). In other respects, dependent depressed patients according to Blatt (1974) are characterized by marked impulsivity and problematic impulse control, and/or a

76

hypomanic mood, which can result in "intense seeking and clinging to objects" (Blatt, 1974, p. 118; Blatt & Shichman, 1983). They would also readily ask for (professional) help, although often in a clinging and claiming way (Blatt & Levy, 1998). Finally, Beck (1983) argues that these patients are often overly optimistic about treatment, resulting in a significant (but often temporary) relief of symptoms (see also Blatt & Maroudas, 1992).

Personality structure. According to Blatt (e.g., Blatt & Shichman, 1983), anaclitic depression is situated at the lower neurotic level. At this level, individuals in whom anaclitic needs predominate show a number of specific personality characteristics, which also differentiate them from individuals functioning predominantly on higher (e.g., hysterical) or lower (e.g., hysteroid borderline) anaclitic levels. First, they are overly dependent on others for their self-esteem. They have a tendency to idealize significant others and prefer symbiotic-like relationships, reminiscent of what Kohut and Wolf (1978) have called "merger-hungry" or "ideal-hungry" persons. When depressed, Arieti and Bemporad (1978) describe their depression in terms of a *dominant other* or *claiming* type of depression, because these patients typically are overly dependent on one or more "dominant others". Sometimes their exaggerated needs for dependency are expressed in what Bowlby (1980) has described as "compulsive caregiving". Compulsive caregivers typically feel guilty and anxious about leaving home, while simultaneously feeling resentful at being forced to stay at home, mostly to care for a disturbed or sick parent. However, they are highly dependent on the person(s) they care for and/or on the caring as such in that they care for others in the way they would like to be cared for (Blatt et al., 1982; Blatt & Maroudas, 1992).

Second, concerning ego functioning, dependent individuals heavily rely on denial, especially of aggression towards significant others. They are very sensitive to experiences of loss and abandonment (Blatt, 1974; Blatt & Shichman, 1983) and attempt to deny the importance of such painful experiences by frenetic activity. This denial would sometimes lead to hypomanic episodes, compulsive caregiving, somatic complaints, eating disturbances, alcohol or drug abuse or the frantic search for substitutes, which can result in hypersexual and/or promiscuous behavior. In addition, these patients show a tendency to externalize their problems, often accompanied by feelings of entitlement (see Kernberg, 1975). These feelings of entitlement show up not only in a claiming attitude, but also in an often "silent" rebellion against authority and rules ("passive-aggressive"). For instance, in therapy these patients demand extra therapeutic sessions or try to violate time limits of sessions (Blatt, 1974; Beck, 1983). Finally, from a drive perspective, libidinal issues and conflict dominate the clinical picture in dependent individuals (Blatt & Shichman, 1983).

Characteristic interpersonal style. Relationships of dependent individuals would be predominantly dyadic in nature, with little differentiation (Blatt, 1974; Blatt & Zuroff, 1992). Others are primarily valued only for (immediate) need gratification ("self-objects"), and not as separate individuals with their own needs and desires. They often have a strong need for immediate, visual contact with others (e.g., the importance of "touching", "hugging"), resulting in a claiming relational style, with much difficulty in tolerating delay and postponement. According to Blatt (1974), self-representations and object-representations in these individuals are predominantly on a sensorimotor level. This level refers to a stage in development where others are only valued for direct, immediate need gratification. Internalization of the object is incomplete, and thus there is much need for the real and immediate physical presence of the object (Blatt, 1974).

Dependent individuals would also often have excessive fears of abandonment and of object loss in general (Blatt & Shichman, 1983). Typically, aggression towards significant others is denied or displaced, for fear of losing these significant others ("rage threatens the very hand that feeds"). In addition, others are often put in a domineering position in that dependency "pulls" for dominance from others. Paradoxically, despite the fact that dependent individuals seek stability in relationships, this stability is mostly not found. According to Blatt (e.g., Blatt & Zuroff, 1992), the claiming, demanding, consuming relational style of these individuals tends to evoke irritation and dissatisfaction in others, and therefore often rejection and abandonment. Arieti and Bemporad (1978), in contrast, maintain that these individuals often have long and stable, but overly dependent relationships with one or more dominant others (e.g., parent, partner).

Proximal precipitating factors: The interaction with life events. It is well established that there is a modest, though important, relationship between negative life events and depression (Kessler, 1997; Tennant, 2002). Blatt and Beck take this finding one step further in that they propose that dependent and perfectionistic individuals are particularly vulnerable for life events that match their specific personal vulnerability ("personality-event congruency hypothesis") (Blatt & Zuroff, 1992; Clark & Beck, 1999; Robins, 1995). Thus, dependent individuals are expected to be particularly vulnerable for "interpersonal" life events, such as separation, divorce, or death of a significant other. However, dependent individuals are not considered to be mere passive recipients of their environment (Blatt & Zuroff, 1992; Zuroff, 1992). First, congruent with their underlying fear of rejection and abandonment, they are expected to show a tendency to interpret life events in terms of rejection or abandonment. Second, dependent individuals are also expected to *enhance* the risk of congruent life events (Blatt & Zuroff, 1992; Zuroff et al., 2004). Because of their claiming, consuming relational style, dependent individuals are expected to invoke irritation and frustration in others, often leading to rejection and abandonment and thus "congruent" life events.

Distal precipitating factors. The four groups of authors differ the most in their descriptions of the distal antecedents of both personality dimensions. Beck (1983, 1999), consistent with his emphasis on the present, refers only in general terms to "early life experiences" influencing the development of personality. Among the psychodynamically oriented authors, there seems to be general agreement that dependency is associated with parental inconsistency, neglect, or abandonment and/or overprotection, resulting in (defensive) excessive dependency on others and fear of rejection and abandonment. Beyond this point, there is much disagreement. Blatt (1974) links the origin of dependency to disturbances in preoedipal phases, i.e., issues related to the early separation-individuation phases. Bowlby (1980) emphasizes that as a child, these individuals are made to feel guilty and/or neglected by their parents, resulting in guilt over separation, excessive need for love, and fear of rejection. Whereas Blatt and Bowlby propose that dependency and self-critical perfectionism are associated with different parental styles, Arieti and Bemporad (1978) maintain that both personality dimensions have their origin in similar parenting styles. According to Arieti and Bemporad (1978), initially the mother is appropriately responsive and often even too responsive to the child's needs, resulting in a strong, often symbiotic-like relationship. However, with the advent of the child's desires for autonomy and independence towards the second year of life, the mother's (and later on father's) attitude to the child drastically changes. From then on, love and care are given only conditionally and the child is forced to conform to parental expectations in order to receive love. Depending on the specific circumstances, the child then can either be forced to remain in a dependent, submissive position, resulting in a clinging, dependent personality style, or is forced to conform to parental expectations concerning achievement, resulting in a dominant goal (or self-critical) type of personality.

Introjective/Autonomous Depression

Clinical presentation. When depressed, perfectionistic/autonomous individuals typically show self-criticism, guilt, shame, worthlessness, and often a chronic fear of being criticized or disapproved. There is constant self-scrutiny, often together with a feeling of having failed to live up to expectations (Beck, 1983; Blatt, 1974). They often have the feeling that they are constantly being watched and criticized. Self-criticism and guilt can become psychotic (e.g., delusions of poverty, feelings of immortal sin, etc.). Instead of feeling unloved, a feeling that dominates anaclitic/sociotropic depression, they would rather feel unlovable (Blatt, 1974). Obsessive-compulsive and paranoid-like symptoms can be present (e.g., distrust, a feeling of being constantly evaluated, delusions of punishment, etc.) (Arieti & Bemporad, 1978; Blatt, 1995b; Blatt & Shichman, 1983). Suicide would be more active and violent in these individuals (e.g., use of firearms) (Beck, 1983; Blatt et al., 1982).

According to Beck (1983), when depressed, these individuals withdraw from personal contact, seek isolation, and are less likely to seek (professional) help. Moreover, they are expected to be more pessimistic about being helped (e.g., about psychotherapy), despite the fact that they often have a good capacity for introspection (Beck, 1983; Blatt & Maroudas, 1992). Their depressed mood is according to Beck (1983) also less reactive to positive and negative events and immediate precipitating events can often not be identified. Instead, depression is caused more by internal factors (e.g., the feeling of having not lived up to one's own high standards). Hence, not surprisingly, Beck (1983) has proposed that his distinction between a sociotropic and autonomous depression matches the "classical" distinction between a reactive and an endogenous type of depression (e.g., see Gillespie, 1929; Kiloh & Garside, 1963). Indeed, the differences between autonomous and sociotropic depression in terms of symptomatology, reactivity of mood, and presence or absence of proximal precipitating events overlaps with the distinguishing features of endogenous and reactive depression. Blatt (1991a, 1998; Blatt, Schaffer, Bers, & Quinlan, 1992), however, maintains that distinctions between types of depression based on symptoms are unproductive because they are unlikely to lead to significant advances in our understanding of depression.

Personality structure. According to Blatt (e.g., Blatt & Shichman, 1983), the personality structure of introjectively depressed individuals is situated at a higher neurotic level. First, they typically have high and often rigid personal standards, in combination with strong self-criticism. In psychodynamic terms this means that they possess an overly harsh and rigid superego, in combination with an ego ideal that is characterized by strivings for perfectionism and control (Blatt & Shichman, 1983; Blatt, 1995b). Interestingly, Beck (1983) emphasizes in his theoretical descriptions more the control and independence component, while Blatt (1974) emphasizes more the high achievement standards and self-critical perfectionism of these individuals. Arieti and Bemporad (1978) coined the notion of a *dominant goal* personality. This dominant goal most often concerns professional issues (e.g., being successful in business), but according to Arieti and Bemporad (1978) it can also manifest itself in relationships. Relationships are then not so much valued for the interpersonal aspect as such, but rather for fulfilling certain role expectations or being "successful" in relations (e.g., the ideal of being a perfect husband, father and lover).

A second characteristic personality feature of these indidivuals is their high level of premorbid functioning (Arieti & Bemporad, 1978; Beck, 1983; Blatt, 1995b). Before becoming depressed, they are often very successful and praised by their environment for their achievements. However, equally characteristic is that they often have little lasting satisfaction (Arieti & Bemporad, 1978; Blatt, 1974). In addition, because of their "hypermorality", they frequently have the feeling of being superior to "ordinary" people, who they look down upon (Arieti & Bemporad, 1978). Thus, self-critical individuals remind us of what Nietzsche said about Christians: "They say that they have been redeemed, but then they should look more redeemed".

Traditionally, these individuals are expected to show a conflict over ambivalence in the strict sense of the term, i.e., aggression is repressed and thus absent on the manifest level (Freud, 1917/1957; Vergote, 1976). However, Blatt (1974; Blatt & Zuroff, 1992), as well as Arieti and Bemporad (1978), Beck (1983), and Bowlby (1980), maintain that these patients show a marked *manifest* ambivalence. Relationships of perfectionistic/autonomous individuals in particular would be characterized by much manifest ambivalence, and hence conflict and distance. However, in this regard there is a small, but important difference in the theoretical views of Beck, Bowlby, and Blatt. According to Beck (1983) and Bowlby (1980), autonomous individuals want to remain relatively distant and aloof from others ("defensive separation"), while Blatt (Blatt & Maroudas, 1992) maintains that introjective individuals do desire interpersonal contact and need others for appreciation and approval, but that they also simultaneously fear their disapproval and criticism.

The ego functioning of perfectionistic individuals is expected to be characterized by a tendency to assume blame and responsibility, and to attribute failures to oneself (Blatt & Shichman, 1983). This self-blaming, internalizing attitude is often combined with expectancies of punishment (Blatt, 1974). Not surprisingly, perfectionism in depression has traditionally been linked to pathological masochism (e.g., see Kernberg, 1992; Markson, 1993). From a drive perspective, aggression and its derivatives (e.g., competitiveness) are expected to dominate the personality structure of perfectionistic individuals.

Characteristic interpersonal style. As noted above, the interpersonal relationships of perfectionistic individuals are described as rather distant and cold (Blatt, 1974; Blatt & Zuroff, 1992). Beck (1983) and Bowlby (1980) maintain that autonomous individuals strive for independence and control, and thus avoid close interpersonal relationships, whereas Blatt (Blatt & Maroudas, 1992) stresses the conflictual and ambivalent nature of the relationships of perfectionistic individuals. On the one hand, they would desire interpersonal relations, especially for approval, while at the same time fearing disapproval and criticism from others.

Moreover, according to Blatt (Blatt & Shichman, 1983), relationships of introjective individuals are more triadic and thus more differentiated compared to anaclitic individuals. Object-representations and self-representations of introjective individuals are supposed to be at the developmentally more advanced perceptual and iconic levels (Blatt, 1974). This means that objects are recognized beyond their need-gratifying role, but that self-representations and object representations are still fragmented (i.e., based on part properties), contradictory and ambivalent. Negative part features of objects (such as criticism) and self (such as self-criticism) are exaggerated and not integrated with other features of self and others.

Proximal precipitating events. In line with the congruency hypothesis, both Blatt (Blatt & Zuroff, 1992) and Beck (1983) have proposed that perfectionistic/autonomous individuals are particularly vulnerable for life events that match their personal vulnerability. Thus, they are expected to be specifically vulnerable for life events related to achievement and control, such as missing a job promotion or failing at school or work. Again, however, Blatt (Blatt & Zuroff, 1992; Blatt et al., 2001) and Beck (1983; Clark & Beck, 1999) underline that introjective/autonomous individuals, in part, actively select, interpret and create their own environment. Hence, they are not only seen as particularly sensitive to failure, but they are also expected to enhance the risk of failure and thus congruent life events because of their often excessively high perfectionistic standards.

Distal precipitating factors. As for dependency/sociotropy, there is also disagreement among the four groups of authors concerning the developmental origins of perfectionism/autonomy. Whereas Beck's (1983) theory does not address the developmental origin of autonomy, Arieti and Bemporad (1978) emphasize high parental expectations concerning achievement. Bowlby (1980) has proposed that his anxious-avoidant type of attachment is associated with early loss and subsequent inadequate care and/or overcritical attachment figures, resulting in a tendency to be overly self-reliant and aloof. In a similar vein, Blatt (1974) suggests that self-critical perfectionism results from the identification with overcritical, hostile parental figures. In addition, reaction formation and overcompensation are used in reaction to supposed failures to live up to personal or parental standards. Like Arieti and Bemporad, Blatt (Blatt, 1974; Blatt & Homann, 1992) suggests that parents of future perfectionistic individuals link love too strongly to the attainment of parental standards and expectations, which prevents the development of real autonomy and results in the inhibition of "normal" impulsivity and creativity (Blatt & Homann, 1992). Finally, Blatt (1974) has proposed that the origin of self-critical perfectionism is situated at a higher developmental level than dependency, namely at the phallic and oedipal level, whereas Arieti and Bemporad (1978) maintain that for both dependency and self-critical perfectionism the reaction of the parents to the advent of strivings for autonomy around the age of two is crucial.

Clinical Implications: Do Different Kinds of Folks Need Different Kinds of Strokes?

All four groups of authors have outlined detailed treatment principles that are directly derived from their theoretical conceptualizations (see Blatt, 2004). Because most research has concentrated on Blatt's and Beck's formulations, we will restrict our discussion mainly to their views. In short, Blatt (e.g., Blatt & Felsen, 1993; Blatt, Shahar, & Zuroff, 2002) as well as Beck (1983) have argued that (predominantly) dependent/sociotropic and perfectionistic/autonomous individuals have very different needs and expectations about treatment and thus respond differently to (and often to different) treatment-related events (Blatt et al., 2002). Accordingly, both Blatt and Beck have suggested that these patients demand different therapeutic approaches and perhaps even different forms of psychotherapy. As Blatt puts it: "different folks may need different kinds of strokes" (Blatt & Felsen, 1993).

Especially in the early phases of psychotherapy, dependent/sociotropic and perfectionistic/autonomous patients are expected to show marked differences in the central transference and countertransference themes. Transference (and countertransference) themes in anaclitic/sociotropic patients are likely to center on libidinal issues, such as care, intimacy, loss, rejection, and abandonment; whereas in introjective/autonomous patients, issues such as aggression, power, control, autonomy, self-worth, criticism, self-criticism, and guilt are likely to be central. Thus, in the early phases, the therapeutic relationship is colored by "personality-congruent" themes, while themes from the "other" developmental line only emerge after some therapeutic work has been done.

Dependent/sociotropic and perfectionistic/autonomous patients are also expected to respond initially to different dimensions in the psychotherapeutic setting and thus to demand somewhat different therapeutic approaches (Beck, 1983; Blatt et al., 2002). According to Blatt (Behrends & Blatt, 1985; Blatt & Behrends, 1987), one can distinguish two general therapeutic factors in any form of psychotherapy, namely *insight* (explanation, interpretation) on the one hand and the *therapeutic relationship* on the other hand. In the initial phase of therapy, dependent/sociotropic patients are likely to be more responsive to the interpersonal and supportive dimension of psychotherapy and thus to the therapeutic relationship as such. Although explanations are readily accepted, it is not so much the concrete content or the correctness of these explanations that are important, but rather the fact that these explanations are interpreted in terms of empathy and support and thus strengthen the therapeutic relationship (Beck, 1983; Blatt & Maroudas, 1992). Self-critical/autonomous patients, on the other hand, because of their more "intellectual" style and their difficulties in relating to others, respond initially better to the interpretative aspects of psychotherapy (e.g., explanation, interpretation, insight), than to aspects related to the therapeutic relationship. The therapeutic relationship is initially likely to be colored by the ambivalence, need for control, and even somewhat distrustful, paranoid features that characterize these patients. Thus, self-critical/autonomous patients are expected to need more time to establish a safe and "good enough" therapeutic alliance (Blatt & Maroudas, 1992).

However, congruent with Blatt's theory of "normal" personality development and his characterization of psychopathology as a rigid overemphasis on one developmental line at the expense of the other, eventually both type of patients must deal with and thus work through issues of both developmental lines. Thus, during the therapeutic process, dependent/sociotropic patients eventually have to deal with introjective issues (such as self-definition, autonomy, and identity), whereas self-critical/autonomous patients eventually have to deal with interpersonal themes (such as intimacy, love, and care) (Blatt & Maroudas, 1992). If treatment goes well, discussion and working through of interpersonal issues in dependent/sociotropic patients leads to a working through of themes related to self-definition and autonomy. After some time, they come to realize that they have been overly dependent on one or more significant others and that their life has often been completely dominated by their tendency to please and comfort others. According to Arieti and Bemporad (1978), this is an important turning point in the psychotherapy of these patients. Moreover, this phase is often characterized by much anger (which previously was denied or displaced) towards significant others. Because of this anger, and because of the fact that the patient is changing and is becoming more assertive in general, significant others, such as the partner, often try to undermine the therapeutic process at this point. Thus, according to Arieti and Bemporad (1978), couple or family therapy should routinely be considered for these patients.

In self-critical/autonomous patients, the therapeutic relationship appears to form the vehicle for discussing and working through interpersonal themes, such as trust, love, and intimacy. The therapeutic situation thus can be seen in these patients as an "interpersonal laboratory", where they can "experiment" with relationships. In our view, benevolent neutrality, which counteracts these patients' fear of criticism and disapproval in combination with the interpretation of transference and counter-transference issues concerning relatedness once a good therapeutic alliance has been established, is vital in this context. However, it can take some time to establish such a good therapeutic alliance. And even then it might often not be simple to overcome these individuals' fear of criticism and sometimes even downward distrust of the good intentions of others, as well as their tendency to rationalize or intellectualize emotions and relationships.

In sum, Blatt has proposed that one can conceptualize the therapeutic process as a reinitiation of normal psychological development or the "reactivation of [a] disrupted developmental process" (Blatt & Shichman, 1983, p. 249), namely of a dialectical interaction between relatedness (anaclitic line) and separation-individuation (introjective line) towards more differentiated and integrated inter-personal relationships and self-definition. Conceptualizing the therapeutic process in this way clearly shows that these formulations are not limited to patients that can easily be categorized as predominantly anaclitic or introjective (i.e., relatively "pure" types), because issues of attachment/relatedness and separation/identity are important issues in all patients. In addition, these formulations are relevant for each psychotherapist, regardless of theoretical orientation and regardless of whether short-term or long-term treatment is considered (Blatt & Maroudas, 1992).

According to Blatt it is moreover likely that anaclitic and introjective patients need different kinds or forms of psychotherapy (Blatt & Felsen, 1993). In this context, Blatt refers to the fact that decades of psychotherapy research has not only identified few specific psychotherapeutic factors, but also few differences in the effectiveness of different forms of psychotherapy (the famous "Dodo bird verdict") (Blatt et al., 2002; Luborsky et al., 1993). In this respect, Blatt (Blatt & Felsen, 1993) argues that patient (and therapist) characteristics are potentially much more important than supposed differences between the various forms of psychotherapy and thus that one can expect patient-therapy interactions (see also Beutler, 1991; Beutler, Clarkin, & Bongar, 2000). For instance, anaclitic patients can be expected to respond better to more supportive, and possibly standardized forms of psychotherapy, in which the therapist is more active, supportive, and directive. Introjective patients are expected to benefit more from long-term, interpretative forms of psychotherapy, in which insight plays a central role and the autonomy and control, so important for these patients, is not restricted by the directive stance of the therapist or by the arbitrary amount of sessions fixed in advance, as is characteristic in short-term, standardized forms of treatments.

However, it is important to underline that we are not proposing here that because dependent patients might respond well to short-term psychotherapy, which is often more supportive, that they should not be referred to long-term psychotherapy, and vice versa for introjective patients. While short-term treatment of depression may result in symptom reduction and sometimes also in lasting changes in personality structure, many, if not most, patients do not show significant changes in personality structure after short-term psychotherapy. This is not mere speculation. In fact, research has shown that short-term treatment has limited effects, even in terms of symptom reduction (Westen et al., 2004). As noted in the introduction to this volume, on average only about 50% of patients show a substantial reduction in symptoms after brief psychotherapy. Moreover, studies concerning the long-term effects of short-term psychotherapy are largely lacking and the few studies that do exist show relapse rates around 70% after two years (Westen & Morrison, 2001). Congruent with these findings, we believe that for many patients, short-term psychotherapy does not result in lasting changes in personality structure, which could partly explain high relapse rates after such treatments. Thus, not only perfectionistic, but many dependent patients may also need long-term psychotherapy to work through both anaclitic and introjective issues (Luyten et al., 2003). This issue will be discussed in more detail in the next chapter, in which we will review relevant empirical research.

Barriers to Integration between Cognitive and Psychodynamic Theories of Depression

The literature reviewed in this chapter clearly indicates a clear trend towards integration between psychodynamic and cognitive thinking concerning depression. However, it should be underlined that up to this point we mainly emphasized the similarities between the theories of Blatt, Beck, Arieti and Bemporad, and Bowlby. However, differences between these theories have been identified (e.g., Blatt & Maroudas, 1992), as well as between psychodynamic and cognitive-behavioral formulations in general (Millon, 2001; Westen, 2000). These differences might pose important barriers towards further integration.

We believe that such differences are of two types. First, there are what we refer to as *minor differences* between these theories which concern concrete hypotheses at low levels of theorizing. In our view, these minor differences do not constitute a real barrier towards further integration because they can be easily translated into research hypotheses, and thus can subsequently lead to changes in theoretical assumptions. For instance, the four groups of authors discussed in this chapter differ in their conceptualization of the developmental origins of dependency and perfectionism. Future research could investigate these various hypotheses and then the four groups of authors could subsequently modify their views depending on the outcome of these studies. Another example of such a minor difference is the fact that Blatt and Beck differ with regard to the capacity for introspection of dependent individuals. According to Beck (1983), these individuals show a good capacity for introspection, whereas Blatt (1974) maintains that dependent individuals have very limited capacities for introspection.

Whereas these minor differences can be easily put to the test, other more fundamental or *substantial* differences are more difficult, if not impossible, to evaluate empirically. Moreover, these differences do form important barriers towards further integration. In this context, the views of Safran and Inck (1995) concerning integration between various psychotherapeutic orientations or "schools" are particularly interesting. Briefly, they have argued that the possibilities of integration between various theoretical orientations vary according to the level of theorizing. At lower levels of theoretical conceptualizations, often few differences are identifiable between various theoretical models, offering considerable possibilities for integration. This certainly seems to be true for Beck's and Blatt's models, which show many similarities at concrete or low levels of theorizing. On higher levels of theoretical reasoning, however, substantial differences often exist between different theoretical views, making integration much more difficult, if not impossible. Ultimately, on the highest level of theorizing, differences concern the concept of human nature and the worldview underlying a particular theoretical model or orientation (Safran & Inck, 1995). At this particular level, major differences exist between the psychodynamic views of Blatt (and Bowlby and Arieti and Bemporad) and Beck's cognitive-behavioral theories (see also Milton, 2001).

Whereas both Beck and Blatt conceptualize dependency/sociotropy and self-critical perfectionism/autonomy as central dimensions in personality development, their underlying concept of human nature is very different. These differences center particularly on Blatt's and Beck's ideas concerning the relationship between "normality" and psychopathology and their subsequent views on psychotherapy. In accordance with the cognitive-behavorial perspective, Beck (Beck & Freeman, 1990; Clark & Beck, 1999) sees human beings as rational scientists that can be dominated by (inherited or acquired) irrational schemas, which can be adjusted or "replaced" in short-term psychotherapy. Thus, both implicitly and explicitly, Beck assumes a more or less clear-cut difference between "normality" and psychopathology, and this despite the fact that Beck (like Blatt) proposes that psychopathology is in fact an exaggeration of normal personality development. Beck's view is intimately associated with a strong belief in reason and rationality and with a strong therapeutic optimism. From a cognitive-behavioral perspective, "we know what is wrong" or we will at least be able in the future to identify what is "wrong". For instance, we know when a particular depressed patient has a "maladaptive" belief. Put differently: we know what a "normal", "rational" or "adaptive" schema is and thus we can change or try to change "irrational" schemas. Although in recent years Beck's therapeutic optimism has been tempered somewhat (e.g., see Beck, 1999), his theory (e.g., Beck, 1991) – and the cognitive-behavioral literature in general – is still characterized by a strong belief in the possibilities of (short-term) cognitive behavioral therapy (for a good recent example of this optimism, see Hollon, 2003).

In contrast, and consistent with classic psychoanalytic thinking, Blatt's theory implies an essential continuity between normality and psychopathology. This means, in other words, that human beings are expected to be always troubled by conflict and frustration. Conflict is considered to be – to a certain extent – normal and thus is viewed as an intrinsic part of the human condition. A life without conflict and frustration is impossible and thus the possibility of psychopathology is present in everyone, and not just in some unhappy few who happen to have some special vulnerability or dysfunctional schemas. Moreover, for some (possibly for many), psychological problems we have no "rational", "normal" or "good" solutions. For instance, how should one deal with the death of a loved one? Is there a "rational", "adaptive", "normal" way to deal with this? Or, is there a "rational" way to deal with an overcritical parent? In addition, are some patients not correct in seeing themselves as, for instance, aloof, overcritical, and unlovable (Westen, 2000)?

This more "tragic" view of human nature (Westen, 2000) is associated with a completely different outlook on treatment. To begin with, in the therapeutic process there is not only an emphasis on reason and rationality (insight), but also on what since Alexander and French (1946) has come to be known as (corrective) emotional experience. Congruent with this view, Blatt (e.g., Blatt & Behrends, 1987; Blatt & Maroudas, 1992) describes the therapeutic process as a series of gratifying involvements at a succession of different developmental levels of relatedness and self-definition, leading to the internalization of these experiences. Thus, the therapeutic process enables the patient to reenact and subsequently renegotiate these issues. In addition, ultimately, the goal of psychodynamic psychotherapy is not only to obtain symptomatic improvement or to teach patients more adaptive modes of dealing with their current life circumstances, but to produce a significant change in personality structure, thus reducing vulnerability to relapse. While this is also the ultimate goal of cognitive-behavioral therapy (e.g., Beck & Freeman, 1990), studies of cognitive-behavioral therapy have generally tended to focus on short-term symptom improvement and not on changes in long-term reduction in vulnerability (Westen & Morrison, 2001). Moreover, from a psychodynamic point of view, even changing vulnerability does not imply a "total cure", whatever one may understand by that term, since vulnerability to psychopathology is part and parcel of the human condition. Stated otherwise, as Freud (1895/1953, p. 305) once said, psychotherapy can be nothing but transforming misery into common human unhappiness. Thus, this view implies a more pessimistic – or should we perhaps say realistic – view of therapeutic success.

These substantial differences are bound to limit the possibility of further integration on a *theoretical* level (Arkowitz, 1997; Messer, 1986; Westen, 2000) and this despite the fact that there is an increasing tendency towards *technical* integration (i.e., the use of cognitive-behavioral techniques in psychodynamic psychotherapy and vice versa, e.g., see Jones & Pulos, 1993) and an emphasis on *common factors* (such as the therapeutic relationship, e.g., see Waddington, 2002).

Conclusions and Future Perspectives for Integration

Psychodynamic and cognitive-behavioral theories of depression have proposed similar personality dimensions, i.e., interpersonal dependency/sociotropy and self-critical perfectionism/autonomy, as vulnerability factors for clinical and nonclinical forms of depression. Moreover, these theories are embedded in more general theoretical frameworks concerning normal and disrupted personality development. Having their origin in clinical experience as well as in empirical research, these theoretical perspectives provide both the researcher and the clinician with a rich heuristic theoretical framework.

Though these theories have a remarkable synthetic and heuristic power, it is clear that they also have a number of limitations. First, despite the fact that both Blatt and Beck have conceptualized dependency/sociotropy and perfectionism/autonomy as continuous dimensions, there is an urgent need for more theoretical and empirical research concerning "mixed" types (Coyne & Whiffen, 1995; Flett et al., 1995).

One likely candidate for such a "mixed" type of depression seems to be the so-called depressive-masochistic personality (e.g., Kernberg, 1992). Traditional descriptions suggest that these individuals are characterized by a severe superego, marked dependency, and difficulties in the expression of aggression, thus combining important aspects of both perfectionism and dependency. The issue of mixed types is further discussed in Chapter 5.

Second, because of their focus on broad personality dimensions, the dynamics involved in depression are somewhat less emphasized by these theories. In classical psychodynamic theorizing, for instance, depression is conceptualized as an active and basic psychobiological reaction to loss (e.g., see Bibring, 1953; Engel, 1962; Sandler & Joffe, 1965; Spitz, 1946). This implies that depression is not just a passive state, but an active and to a certain extent adaptive reaction to loss. In addition, classic psychodynamic descriptions of depression have emphasized the dynamics involved in discrepancies between ego and ego ideal (Bleichmar, 1996; Lax, 1989; Miller, 1979; Milrod, 1988; Morrison, 1989; Vergote, 1976). Because Blatt and Beck focus on the role of personality dimensions in depression, they place less emphasis on these detailed dynamic formulations. Future theoretical and empirical research should therefore concentrate more on the dynamics involved in dependency/sociotropy and perfectionism/autonomy. For instance, psychodynamic formulations suggest that both dependent/sociotropic and self-critical/autonomous individuals have much difficulty in abandoning unattainable goals or formulating more realistic goals, even in the face of repeated failures and/or frustrations. Future studies could focus on the dynamics (e.g., defensive processes, underlying narcissistic fantasies, etc.) involved in this inability to relinquish unattainable goals.

Despite these limitations, these theories emphasize the importance of considering personality factors in depression. Thus, they see depression not as an isolated disease entity, but as the result of distortions of normal development. As we said earlier, this view opens up several interesting perspectives for the integration between various psychological and biological approaches to depression (Blatt & Maroudas, 1992). First, concerning the integration between psychological theories of depression, this view makes integration possible between various domains in psychological research that have often developed in relative isolation, such as the relationships between "normal" and "psychopathological" development, between life-span developmental theory and developmental psychopathology, and between "clinical" and "positive" psychology. Second, concerning the integration between psychological and biological approaches, research has made increasingly clear that biological, social, and psychological processes are intimately interwoven in both normal and pathological personality development (Rutter et al., 1997). Research on depression could therefore benefit from being embedded in a more encompassing *biopsychosocial theoretical framework* concerning normal and pathological personality development, such as the one proposed by Blatt and Beck (Abramson, Alloy, Hankin, Haeffel, MacCoon, & Gibb, 2002). For instance, recent studies have lent considerable evidence for passive and active person-environment correlations and interactions (see Rutter et al., 1997, for an overview), linking temperamental and personality characteristics to neurobiological and genetic factors on the one hand and environmental factors on the other hand. These views are congruent with both Blatt's (Blatt & Zuroff, 1992) and Beck's (1983) emphasis on the active influence of anaclitic/sociotropic and self-critical/autonomous individuals on their environment. Moreover, Blatt's (Blatt, Cornell, & Eshkol, 1993; Blatt & Maroudas, 1992) and Beck's (1983) formulations explicitly refer to the (neuro)biological underpinnings of personality. Blatt has hypothesized that both dependency and self-critical perfectionism may have genetic roots (Blatt & Shichman, 1981) and are related to biological processes involved in neoplastic and cardiovascular disease, respectively (Blatt, Cornell, & Eshkol, 1993). In addition, Blatt (Blatt & Maroudas, 1992) has proposed that dependent individuals may initially show a positive placebo effect to antidepressant treatment, because of their optimism regarding treatment, especially when this treatment can be experienced by the patient as "being cared for and fed" by a physician. Self-critical patients, on the contrary, are expected to show a negative placebo effect, because of their pessimism regarding treatment and because they would feel unworthy of treatment. Beck (1983), in turn, has hypothesized that the autonomous type of depression is similar to the concept of endogenous depression and hence is more biological in origin. Thus, autonomous patients are expected to show a better response to antidepressant treatment than sociotropic patients.

Moreover, Blatt's and Beck's formulations are also congruent with recent studies showing that early life stress (ranging from severe trauma or neglect to low quality of parental care) is associated with biopsychosocial vulnerability to current life stress (e.g., Davidson, Pizzagalli, & Nitschke, 2002; Gunnar, 1998; see also Chapter 8, this volume). In this context, an increasing number of studies show that early adversity and later life stress have a profound impact on the hypothalamic-pituitary-adrenocortical (HPA) axis (Kandel, 1999; Gunnar, 1998; Tsigos & Chrousos, 2002), which has been linked to depression (Raison & Miller, 2003). Blatt's theory is also compatible with studies on "kindling" and "scarring" (see Chapter 1, this volume) since it emphasizes the recursive, cyclical interaction between personality, environment, and depression (Zuroff et al., 2004). In sum, we believe these findings and formulations clearly emphasize the urgent need for more integrative biopsychosocial theoretical frameworks regarding normal and pathological personality development (see also Chapters 1 and 8 in this volume). Research concerning such integrative theories could not only improve our insight into mood and other disorders, but is also likely to have important therapeutic implications. We will return to these issues in the Epilogue of this volume.

However, the conceptualization of depression, not as an isolated disorder, but as a distortion of normal personality development that can range from mild dysphoric reactions to full-blown clinical depression, may also constitute a main obstacle to the further integration between these theories and mainstream research on depression. Currently dominant theories of depression, in line with the DSM, view various forms of depression and other disorders as categorically distinct disease entities. Moreover, the DSM explicitly avoids any etiological considerations in the classification of mental disorders. Despite the fact that many of the key assumptions underlying DSM have been invalidated and thus hamper further research (Blatt & Levy, 1998; Westen & Shedler, 1999; Wampold, 1997), including the search for genetic and other biological factors involved in depression (e.g., Van Praag, 1998), the DSM remains the gold standard in mainstream depression research. Until this tension between descriptive and etiological viewpoints is solved, integration among the views of Blatt, Beck, Arieti and Bemporad and Bowlby with DSM-inspired research on mood and other disorders will be difficult.

References

Abramson, L. Y., Alloy, L. B., Hankin, B. L., Haeffel, G. J., MacCoon, D. G., & Gibb, B. E. (2002). Cognitive-vulnerability-stress models of depression in a self-regulatory and psychobiological context. In I. H. Gotlib & C. L. Hammen (Eds.), *Handbook of depression* (pp. 268-294). New York/London: The Guilford Press.

Alexander, F., & French, T. M. (1946). *Psychoanalytic therapy. Principles and application.* New York: The Ronals Press Company.

Arieti, S., & Bemporad, J. (1978). *Psychotherapy of severe and mild depression.* Northvale/London: Jason Aronson.

Arkowitz, H. (1997). Integrative theories of therapy. In P. Wachtel & S. Messer (Eds.), *Theories of psychotherapy: Origins and evolution* (pp. 227-288). Washington, DC: American Psychological Association Press.

Baker Miller, J. (1976). *Toward a new psychology of women.* London: Penguin Books.

Beck, A. T. (1983). Cognitive therapy of depression: New perspectives. In P. J. Clayton & J. E. Barrett (Eds.), *Treatment of depression: Old contro-versies and new approaches* (pp. 265-290). New York: Raven Press.

Beck, A. T. (1991). Cognitive therapy: A 30-year retrospective. *American Psychologist, 46,* 368-375.

Beck, A. T. (1999). Cognitive aspects of personality disorders and their relation to syndromal disorders: A psychoevolutionary approach. In C. R. Cloninger (Ed.), *Personality and psychopathology* (pp. 411-429). Washington, DC/London: American Psychiatric Press.

Beck, A. T., & Freeman, A. (1990). *Cognitive therapy of personality disorders.* New York: Guilford Press.

Behrends, R. S., & Blatt, S. J. (1985). Internalization and psychological development throughout the life cycle. *Psychoanalytic Study of the Child, 40,* 11-39.

Bemporad, J. R. (1992). Psychoanalytically orientated psychotherapy. In E. S. Paykel (Ed.), *Handbook of affective disorders* (2nd ed.) (pp. 465-473). Edinburgh: Churchill Livingstone.

Beutler, L. E. (1991). Have all won and must all have prizes? Revisiting Luborsky et al.'s verdict. *Journal of Consulting and Clinical Psychology, 59,* 226-232.

Beutler, L. E., Clarkin, J. F., & Bongar, B. (2000). *Guidelines for the systematic treatment of the depressed patient.* New York/Oxford: Oxford University Press.

Bibring, E. (1953). The mechanism of depression. In P. Greenacre (Ed.), *Affective disorders. Psychoanalytic contribution to their study* (pp. 13-48). New York: International Universities Press.

Blass, R. B., & Blatt, S. J. (1996). Attachment and separateness in the experience of symbiotic relatedness. *Psychoanalytic Quarterly, 65,* 711-746.

Blatt, S. (1974). Levels of object representation in anaclitic and introjective depression. *The Psychoanalytic Study of the Child, 29,* 107-157.

Blatt, S. J. (1991a). A cognitive morphology of psychopathology. *Journal of Nervous and Mental Disease, 179,* 449-458.

Blatt, S. J. (1991b). Depression and destructive risk-taking behavior in adolescence. In L. P. Lipsitt & L. L. Mitnick (Eds.), *Self-regulatory behavior and risk-taking: Causes and consequences* (pp. 285-309). Norwood, NJ: Ablex Press.

Blatt, S. J. (1995a). Representational structures in psychopathology. In D. Cicchetti & S. L. Toth (Eds.), *Emotion, cognition, and representation (Rochester Symposium on developmenal psychopathology Vol. 6)* (pp. 1-33). New York: University of Rochester Press.

Blatt, S. J. (1995b). The destructiveness of perfectionism. Implications for the treatment of depression. *American Psychologist, 50,* 1003-1020.

Blatt, S. J. (1998). Contributions of psychoanalysis to the understanding and treatment of depression. *Journal of the American Psychoanalytic Association, 46*, 722-752.

Blatt, S. J. (2004). *Experiences of depression: Theoretical, clinical and research perspectives.* Washington, DC: American Psychological Association.

Blatt, S. J., & Behrends, R. S. (1987). Internalization, separation-individuation, and the nature of therapeutic action. *International Journal of Psycho-Analysis, 68*, 279-297.

Blatt, S. J., & Blass, R. B. (1990). Attachment and separateness. A dialectic model of the products and processes of development throughout the life cycle. *Psychoanalytic Study of the Child, 45*, 107-127.

Blatt, S. J., Cornell, C. E., & Eshkol, E. (1993). Personality style, differential vulnerability and clinical course in immunological and cardiovascular disease. *Clinical Psychology Review, 13*, 421-450.

Blatt, S. J., & Felsen, I. (1993). Different kinds of folks may need different kinds of strokes: The effect of patients' characteristics on therapeutic process and outcome. *Psychotherapy Research, 3*, 245-259.

Blatt, S. J., & Levy, K. N. (1998). A psychodynamic approach to the diagnosis of psychopathology. In J. W. Baron (Ed.), *Making diagnosis meaningful. Enhancing evaluation and treatment of psychological disorders* (pp. 73-109). Washington, DC: American Psychological Association.

Blatt, S. J., & Maroudas, C. (1992). Convergence among psychoanalytic and cognitive-behavioral theories of depression. *Psychoanalytic Psychology, 9*, 157-190.

Blatt, S. J., Quinlan, D. M., Chevron, E. S., McDonald, C., & Zuroff, D. (1982). Dependency and self-criticism: Psychological dimensions of depression. *Journal of Consulting and Clinical Psychology, 50*, 113-124.

Blatt, S. J., Schaffer, C. E., Bers, S. A., & Quinlan, D. M. (1992). Psychometric properties of the Depressive Experiences Questionnaire for adolescents. *Journal of Personality Assessment, 59*, 82-98.

Blatt, S. J., Shahar, G., & Zuroff, D. C. (2002). Anaclitic/Sociotropic and Introjective/Autonomous dimensions. In J. C. Norcross (Ed.), *Psychotherapy relationships that work. Therapist contributions and responsiveness to patients* (pp. 315-333). Oxford: Oxford University Press.

Blatt, S. J., & Shichman, S. (1983). Two primary configurations of psychopathology. *Psychoanalysis and Contemporary Thought, 6*, 187-254.

Blatt, S. J., & Zuroff, D. C. (1992). Interpersonal relatedness and self-definition: Two prototypes for depression. *Clinical Psychology Review, 12*, 527-562.

Bleichmar, H. B. (1996). Some subtypes of depression and their implications for psychoanalytic treatment. *International Journal of Psycho-Analysis, 77*, 935-961.

Bowlby, J. (1980). *Attachment and loss Vol. 3 Loss: Sadness and depression.* London: The Hogarth Press.

Bowlby, J. (1988). *A secure base: Clinical applications of attachment theory.* London: Routledge.

Chevron, E. S., Quinlan, D. M., & Blatt, S. J. (1978). Sex roles and gender differences in the experience of depression. *Journal of Abnormal Psychology, 87*, 680-683.

Chodorow, N. (1978). *The reproduction of mothering. Psychoanalysis and the sociology of gender.* Berkeley: University of California Press.

Clark, D. A., & Beck, A. T. (1999). *Scientific foundations of cognitive theory and therapy of depression.* New York: John Wiley & Sons.

Costello, E. J., Pine, D. S., Hammen, C., March, J. S., Plotsky, P. M., Weissman, M. M., Biederman, J., Goldsmith, H. H., Kaufman, J., Lewinsohn, P. M., Hellander, M., Hoagwood, K., Koretz, D. S., Nelson, C. A., & Leckman, J. F. (2002). Development and natural history of mood disorders. *Biological Psychiatry, 52*, 529-542.

Coyne, J. C., & Whiffen, V. E. (1995). Issues in personality as diathesis for depression: The case of sociotropy-dependency and autonomy-self-criticism. *Psychological Bulletin, 118*, 358-378.

Davidson, R. J., Pizzagalli, D., & Nitschke, J. B. (2002). The representation and regulation of emotion in depression: Perspectives from affective neuroscience. In I. H. Gotlib & C. L. Hammen (Eds.), *Handbook of depression* (pp. 219-244). New York/London: The Guilford Press.

Engel, G. L. (1962). Anxiety and depression-withdrawal: The primary affects of unpleasure. *International Journal of Psycho-Analysis, 43*, 89-97.

Flett, G. L., Hewitt, P. L., Endler, N. S., & Bagby, R. M. (1995). Conceptualization and assessment of personality factors in depression. *European Journal of Personality, 9*, 309-350.

Freud, S. (1953). Studies on Hysteria. In J. Strachey (Ed. & Transl.), *The standard edition of the complete psychological works of Sigmund Freud* (Vol. 2). London: Hogarth Press. (Original work published 1895).

Freud, S. (1957). Mourning and melancholia. In J. Strachey (Ed. & Transl.), *The standard edition of the complete psychological works of Sigmund Freud* (Vol. 14, pp. 243-258). London: Hogarth Press.

91

(Original work published 1917).

Gillespie, R. D. (1929). The clinical differentiation of types of depression. *Guy's Hospital Reports, 9,* 306-344.

Gilligan, C. (1982). *In a different voice. Psychological theory and women's development.* Cambridge/London: Harvard University Press.

Guisinger, S., & Blatt, S. J. (1994). Individuality and relatedness. *American Psychologist, 49,* 104-111.

Gunderson, J. G., Triebwasser, J., Philips, K. A., & Sullivan, C. N. (1999). Personality and vulnerability to affective disorders. In C. R. Cloninger (Ed.), *Personality and psychopathology* (pp. 3-32). Washington, DC/London: American Psychiatric Press.

Gunnar, M. E. (1998). Quality of early care and buffering of neuroendocrine stress reactions: Potential effects on the developing human brain. *Preventive Medicine, 27,* 208-211.

Hollon, S. D. (2003). Does cognitive therapy have an enduring effect? *Cognitive Therapy and Research, 27,* 71-75.

Ingram, R. E., & Hamilton, N. A. (1999). Evaluating precision in the social psychological assessment of depression: Methodological considerations, issues, and recommendations. *Journal of Social and Clinical Psychology, 18,* 160-180.

Jones, E. E., & Pulos, S. M. (1993). Comparing the process of psychodynamic and cognitive-behavioral therapies. *Journal of Consulting and Clinical Psychology, 61,* 306-316.

Judd, L. J., Akiskal, H. S., Maser, J. D., Zeller, P. J., Endicott, J., Coryell, W., Paulus, M. P., Kunovac, J. L., Leon, A. C., Mueller, T. I., Rice, J. A., & Keller, M. B. (1998). A prospective 12-year study of subsyndromal and syndromal depressive symptoms in unipolar major depressive disorders. *Archives of General Psychiatry, 55,* 694-700.

Kandel, E. R. (1999). Biology and the future of psychoanalysis: A new intellectual framework for psychiatry revisited. *American Journal of Psychiatry, 156,* 505-524.

Kendler, K. S., & Gardner, C. O. (1998). Boundaries of major depression: An evaluation of DSM-IV criteria. *American Journal of Psychiatry, 155,* 172-177.

Kernberg, O. F. (1975). *Borderline conditions and pathological narcissism.* New York: Jason Aronson.

Kernberg, O. F. (1992). *Aggression in personality disorders and perversions.* New Haven/London: Yale University Press.

Kessler, R. C. (1997). The effects of stressful life events on depression. *Annual Review of Psychology, 48,* 191-214.

Kiloh, L. G., & Garside, R. F. (1963). The independence of neurotic depression and endogenous depression. *British Journal of Psychiatry, 109,* 451-463.

Klein, D. N., Durbin, E., Shankman, S. A., & Santiago, N. J. (2002). Depression and personality. In I. H. Gotlib & C. L. Hammen (Eds.), *Handbook of depression* (pp. 115-140). New York/London: The Guilford Press.

Klein, D. N., & Hayden, E. P. (2000). Dysthymic disorder: Current status and future directions. *Current Opinion in Psychiatry, 13,* 171-177.

Klein, M. H., Kupfer, D. J., & Shea, M. T. (1993). *Personality and depression. A current view.* New York/London: The Guilford Press.

Kohut, H., & Wolf, E. S. (1978). The disorders of the self and their treatment: An outline. *International Journal of Psycho-Analysis, 59,* 413-425.

Kwon, P. (1999). Attributional style and psychodynamic defense mechanisms: Toward an integrative model of depression. *Journal of Personality, 67,* 645-658.

Lax, R. F. (1989). The narcissistic investment in pathological character traits and the narcissistic depression: Some implications for treatment. *International Journal of Psycho-Analysis, 70,* 81-90.

Luborsky, L., Diguer, L., Luborsky, E., Singer, B., Dickter, D., & Schmidt, K. A. (1993). The efficacy of dynamic psychotherapies: Is it true that "Everyone has won and all must have prizes"? In N. E. Miller, L. Luborsky, J. P. Barber & J. P. Docherty (Eds.), *Psychodynamic treatment research. A Handbook for clinical practice* (pp. 497-516). New York: Basic Books.

Luyten, P., Lowyck, B., & Corveleyn, J. (2003). Teoria y tratamiento de la depression: Hacia su integracion? [Theory and treatment of depression: Towards integration?]. *Persona, 6,* 81-97.

Markson, E. R. (1993). Depression and moral masochism. *International Journal of Psycho-Analysis, 74,* 931-940.

Messer, S. (1986). Behavioral and psychoanalytic perspectives at therapeutic choice points. *American Psychologist, 41,* 1261-1272.

Miller, A. (1979). Depression and grandiosity as related forms of narcissistic disturbances. *International Review of Psycho-Analysis, 6,* 61-76.

Milrod, D. (1988). A current view of the psychoanalytic theory of depression. With notes on the role of identification, orality, and anxiety. *The Psychoanalytic Study of the Child, 43*, 83-99.

Milton, J. (2001). Psychoanalysis and cognitive behaviour therapy. Rival paradigms or common ground? *International Journal of Psychoanalysis, 82*, 431-447.

Morrison, A. P. (1989). *Shame. The underside of narcissism*. Hillsdale, NJ: The Analytic Press.

Mulder, R. T. (2002). Personality pathology and treatment outcome in major depression: A review. *American Journal of Psychiatry, 159*, 359-371.

National Institute of Mental Health (2003). *Breaking ground, breaking through: The Strategic Plan for Mood Disorders Research*. Retrieved September 3, 2004, from http://www.nimh.nih.gov/strategic/mooddisorders.pdf

Power, M. (1991). Cognitive science and behavioural psychotherapy: Where behaviour was, there shall cognition be? *Behavioural Psychotherapy, 19*, 20-41.

Raison, C. L., & Miller, A. H. (2003). When not enough is too much: The role of insufficient glucocorticoid signaling in the pathophysiology of stress-related disorders. *American Journal of Psychiatry, 160*, 1554-1565.

Robins, C. J. (1993). Implications of research in the psychopathology of depression for psychotherapy integration. *Journal of Psychotherapy Integration, 3*, 313-330.

Robins, C. J. (1995). Personality-event interaction models of depression. *European Journal of Personality, 9*, 367-378.

Rutter, M., Dunn, J., Plomin, R., Simonoff, E., Pickles, A., Maughan, B., Ormel, J., Meyer, J., & Eaves, L. (1997). Integrating nature and nurture: Implications of person-environment correlations and interactions for developmental psychopathology. *Development and Psychopathology, 9*, 335-364.

Ryle, A. (Ed.). (1995). *Cognitive Analytic Therapy: Developments in theory and practice*. New York: Wiley.

Sabbe, B. G. C. (2002). Psychotherapie bij depressie: Integratie? [Psychotherapy for depression: Integration?] In W. Trijsburg, S. Colijn, E. Collumbien & G. Lietaer (Eds.), *Handboek voor integratieve psychotherapie [Handbook of integrative psychotherapy]* (VI, 5.1-32). Leusden, The Netherlands: De Tijdstroom.

Safran, J. D., & Inck, T. A. (1995). Psychotherapy integration: Implications for the treatment of depression. In E. E. Beckham & W. R. Leber (Eds.), *Handbook of depression* (2nd ed.) (pp. 425-434). New York/London: The Guilford Press.

Sandler, J., & Joffe, W. G. (1965). Notes on childhood depression. *International Journal of Psycho-Analysis, 46*, 88-96.

Shahar, G., Blatt, S. J., & Ford, R. Q. (2003). Mixed anaclitic-introjective psychopathology in treatment-resistant inpatients undergoing psychoanalytic psychotherapy. *Psychoanalytic Psychology, 20*, 84-102.

Shea, M. T., Elkin, I., Imber, S. D., Sotsky, S. M., Watkins, J. T., Collins, J. F., Pilkonis, P. A., Beckham, E., Glass, D. R., & Dolan, R. T. (1992). Course of depressive symptoms over follow-up. Findings from the NIMH treatment of depression collaborative research program. *Archives of General Psychiatry, 49*, 782-787.

Spitz, R. A. (1946). Anaclitic depression. *The Psychoanalytic Study of the Child, 2*, 313-342.

Tennant, C. (2002). Life events, stress and depression: A review of recent findings. *Australian and New Zealand Journal of Psychiatry, 36*, 173-182.

Tsigos, C., & Chrousos, G. P. (2002). Hypothalamic-pituitary-adrenal axis, neuroendocrine factors and stress. *Journal of Psychosomatic Research, 53*, 865-871.

Van Praag, H. M. (1998). Inflationary tendencies in judging the yield of depression research. *Neuropsychobiology, 37*, 130-141.

Vergote, A. (1976). Névrose depressive [Depressive neurosis]. *Topique, 17*, 97-126.

Vredenburg, K., Flett, G. L., & Krames, L. (1993). Analogue versus clinical depression: A critical reappraisal. *Psychological Bulletin, 113*, 327-344.

Wachtel, P. L. (1997). *Psychoanalysis, behavior therapy, and the relational world*. Washington, DC: American Psychological Association Press.

Waddington, L. (2002). The therapy relationship in cognitive therapy: A review. *Behavioural and Cognitive Psychotherapy, 30*, 179-191.

Wampold, B. E. (1997). Methodological problems in identifying efficacious psychotherapies. *Psychotherapy Research, 7*, 21-43.

Westen, D. (2000). Integrative psychotherapy: Integrating psychodynamic and cognitive-behavioral theory and technique. In C. R. Snyder & R. E. Ingram (Eds.), *Handbook of psychological change* (pp. 217-242). New York: Wiley.

93

Westen, D., & Morrison, K. (2001). A multidimensional meta-analysis of treatments for depression, panic, and generalized anxiety disorder: An empirical examination of the status of empirically supported therapies. *Journal of Consulting and Clinical Psychology, 69,* 875-899.

Westen, D., & Shedler, J. (1999). Revising and assessing Axis II, Part I: Developing a clinically and empirically valid assessment method. *American Journal of Psychiatry, 156,* 258-272.

Westen, D., Novotny, C. M., & Thompson-Brenner, H. (2004). The empirical status of empirically supported psychotherapies: Assumptions, findings, and reporting in controlled clinical trials. *Psychological Bulletin, 130,* 631-663.

Zuroff, D. C. (1992). New directions for cognitive models of depression. *Psychological Inquiry, 3,* 274-277.

Zuroff, D. C., Mongrain, M., & Santor, D. (2004). Conceptualizing and measuring personality vulnerability to depression: Comment on Coyne and Whiffen (1995). *Psychological Bulletin, 130,* 489-511.

Chapter 4

The Convergence among Psychodynamic

and Cognitive-Behavioral Theories of Depression:

A Critical Review of Empirical Research

Patrick Luyten, Jozef Corveleyn, & Sidney J. Blatt

The previous chapter presented a theoretical overview of the growing integration among psychodynamic and cognitive-behavioral theories of depression. This chapter reviews empirical research relevant to the theoretical formulations of Sidney Blatt and Aaron Beck about the psychological dimensions of depression. First, we discuss the assessment of Dependency/Sociotropy and Self-Critical Perfectionism/Autonomy and then consider the three most central tenets of Blatt's and Beck's theories: (1) the relationship between Dependency/Sociotropy and Self-Critical Perfectionism/Autonomy and depression, (2) the relationship of these dimensions to stressful life events, and (3) the characteristic interpersonal styles and attitudes associated with these personality dimensions. We close this chapter with a review of research on the clinical implications of these formulations and some conclusions.

Despite a growing literature that employs other research methods, such as experiments and interviews, most research on the psychological dimensions of depression has relied on self-report instruments to assess dependent/sociotropic and self-critical perfectonistic/autonomous personality dimensions. Four such instruments are currently used to assess these dimensions: the Depressive Experiences Questionnaire (DEQ), developed by Blatt and his colleagues (Blatt, D'Afflitti, & Quinlan, 1976),[1] two instruments developed to assess Beck's cognitive-behavioral views, namely the Sociotropy-Autonomy Scale (SAS; Beck, Epstein, Harrison, & Emery, 1983) and the Dysfunctional Attitude Scale (DAS; Cane, Olinger, Gotlib, & Kuiper, 1986), and finally the Personal Style Inventory (PSI; Robins et al., 1994), which was developed to integrate both Blatt's and Beck's constructs.

Notwithstanding the fact that these instruments have produced interesting results, theoretical and/or psychometrical problems have been identified with each of these instruments (e.g., Blatt, 2004; Luyten, Fontaine, Soenens, Meganck et al., 2004). For instance, although the internal factor structure of the DEQ has been replicated in several cultures in nonclinical samples, it has not always been fully replicated in clinical samples (e.g., Bagby, Parker, Joffe, & Buis, 1994). The subscales of the DAS are highly correlated (Blaney & Kutcher, 1991; Blatt, Shahar, & Zuroff, 2002), suggesting that the two DAS subscales have substantial overlap. One of the most important assessment problems centers on the assessment of Beck's autonomy concept. It has repeatedly been shown that the SAS Autonomy scale measures counterdependency rather than autonomy (Blaney & Kutcher, 1991; Rude & Burnham, 1993). Attempts to improve the construct validity of the SAS Autonomy subscale have only been partially successful (Bieling, Beck, & Brown, 2000; Clark & Beck, 1991; Clark, Steer, Beck, & Ross, 1995; Sato & McCann, 1997), and the PSI Autonomy subscale appears to suffer from similar problems as the SAS Autonomy subscale (Bagby, Parker, Joffe, Schuller, & Gilchrist, 1998; Hong & Lee, 2001; Kwon, Campbell, & Williams, 2001; Sato & McCann, 1997).[2]

In addition to these instruments, several other scales measure aspects of Dependency/Sociotropy and Self-Critical Perfectionism/Autonomy. The most well-known include the Interpersonal Dependency Inventory (IDI; Hirschfeld, et al., 1977) and two multidimensional measures of perfectionism, both entitled Multidimensional Perfectionism Scale (MPS), one developed by Frost, Marten, Lahart and Rosenblate (1990) (MPS-F), the other one (MPS-H) by Hewitt and Flett

---

[1] Blatt and his colleagues also developed a version of the DEQ for adolescents (DEQ-A; Blatt, Schaffer, Bers, & Quinlan, 1992).

[2] Although somewhat imprecise, for didactical reasons in our discussion we will consider these four instruments (DEQ, SAS, DAS, PSI) as equivalent measures of the constructs of Dependency/Sociotropy and Self-Critical Perfectionism/Autonomy, except when results differ depending upon the instrument used. For the same reason, we will in general not distinguish between Blatt's and Beck's constructs, unless this is important for a correct interpretation of results.

(1991). Factor analytic studies suggest that two dimensions underlie these two perfectionism scales, namely adaptive or "healthy" and maladaptive or "unhealthy" perfectionism (Enns, Cox, & Clara, 2002). Similarly, recent research suggests that interpersonal dependency also is multidimensional and has both adaptive and maladaptive aspects (Blatt; 2004; Bornstein, 1992; Pincus & Gurtman, 1995). Consistent with these findings, Blatt and his colleagues have recently distinguished between adaptive and maladaptive forms of self-definition and interpersonal relatedness. This chapter, however, concentrates mainly on research concerning maladaptive aspects of self-definition and relatedness. In the next chapter, Blatt and Shahar will focus on both adaptive and maladaptive aspects of these two dimensions. In addition, our review is mainly limited to research with the DEQ, SAS, DAS, and PSI for two reasons. First, we believe that it is vital to retain a clear distinction between results from studies that have employed instruments that explicitly assess Blatt's and Beck's views and instruments that were developed based on other theoretical frameworks.[3] Second, specifically concerning the MPS-F and MPS-H, we believe that further research is needed to investigate whether these instruments indeed contain two underlying dimensions that can be interpreted as adaptive versus maladaptive perfectionism.[4]

The Relationship Between Dependency/Sociotropy, Self-Critical Perfectionism/Autonomy, and Depression

Cross-sectional Studies

Severity of depression. Over the past decades, cross-sectional studies in various nonclinical populations (adolescents, students, adults, elderly) and in inpatient and outpatient clinical populations have in general shown a consistent relationship between Dependency/Sociotropy, Self-Critical Perfectionism/Autonomy, and self-

---

[3] For instance, recent research shows that the DEQ and the DAS Perfectionism subscales both capture and thus confound Hewitt and Flett's socially prescribed and self-oriented perfectionism (Enns & Cox, 1999; Hewitt & Flett, 1993; Hewitt, Flett, Besser, Sherry, & McGee, 2003), which makes it difficult to compare results obtained with the Hewitt and Flett scales and results from scales that have been developed from Blatt's and Beck's theories.

[4] In fact, several studies have found that "adaptive" perfectionism scales are related to measures of distress and psychopathology (e.g., Bieling, Israeli, & Antoni, 2004; Enns, Cox, Sareen, & Freeman, 2001) as well as somatic complaints and Chronic Fatigue Syndrome (Luyten, Van Houdenhove, Cosyns, & Vandenbroucke, 2004; Saboonchi & Lundh, 2003). Thus, we believe that caution should be exercised in calling these scales "adaptive". It appears that these so-called adaptive scales represent *less pathological* forms of perfectionism. Second, although some forms or aspects of perfectionism (e.g., high personal standards) might be adaptive temporarily (e.g., when one has to finish a project in time) or in some circumstances (e.g., during an exam period), in the long term they might be quite detrimental for one's psychical and physical health and/or for others (Blatt, 1995; Shafran & Mansell, 2001).

report and interview-based measures of the severity of depression (for overviews, see Blatt, 2004; Clark & Beck, 1999; Nietzel & Harris, 1990). A typical finding in this respect is that Self-Critical Perfectionism shows a stronger relation to severity of depression than Dependency/Sociotropy. Nietzel & Harris (1990), for instance, in a meta-analysis of cross-sectional studies, found a mean effect size of $r = .28$ for Dependency/Sociotropy and $r = .49$ for Self-Critical Perfectionism/Autonomy in their association with measures of depression. No differences were found, however, in association with severity of depression between Autonomy and Dependency/ Sociotropy in studies using the SAS. This finding, consistent with findings from a number of other studies, again points to psychometric problems with the SAS Autonomy scale (Clark & Beck, 1999). While the relationship between measures of depression and Dependency/Sociotropy is typically smaller than for Self-Critical Perfectionism/Autonomy, in some studies Dependency/ Sociotropy is even unrelated to severity of depression (e.g., Fichman, Koestner, & Zuroff, 1996; Ouimette & Klein, 1993; Overholser & Freiheit, 1994; Santor & Zuroff, 1997). One possible explanation for this finding is that traditional measures of the severity of depression are more heavily weighted with symptoms typical for self-criticism, leading to an underdiagnosis of anaclitic depression, which is more concerned with loneliness, abandonment, and somatic complaints than with self-criticism and guilt (Blatt, 1998; Blatt, Quinlan, Chevron, McDonald, & Zuroff, 1982).

Consistent with Blatt's and Beck's predictions, females generally have higher levels of Dependency/Sociotropy than males, but gender differences are usually not found on Self-Critical Perfectionism/Autonomy (Blatt, 2004). Some evidence indicates that gender incongruence (high Dependency/Sociotropy in males and high Self-Critical Perfectionism/Autonomy in females) is associated with a higher risk for depression (Mongrain & Zuroff, 1994; Sanathara, Gardner, Prescott, & Kendler, 2003; Smith, O'Keeffe, & Jenkins, 1988) and a greater number of negative life events (Mongrain & Zuroff, 1994; Fichman, Koestner, & Zuroff, 1994; Little & Garber, 2000; Smith et al., 1988).

Diagnosis of depression. Several cross-sectional studies have shown that both Dependency/Sociotropy and Self-Critical Perfectionism/Autonomy are consistently associated with *current major depression* (e.g., Cox, McWilliams, Enns, & Clara, 2004; Mazure, Bruce, Maciejewski, & Jacobs, 2000; Mazure & Maciejewski, 2003; Mazure, Maciejewski, Jacobs, & Bruce, 2002; Nelson, Hammen, Daley, Burge, & Davila, 2001; Raghavan, Le, & Berenbaum, 2002). Also, case-control studies, comparing clinical and control groups, have consistently found that depressed patients exhibit higher levels of both Dependency/Sociotropy and Self-Critical Perfectionism/Autonomy than nonclinical groups of students and adults (Bagby, Schuller, Parker, Levitt, Joffe, & Shafir, 1994; Bieling & Alden, 2001; Blatt et al., 1982; Fairbrother & Moretti, 1998; Franche & Dobson, 1992; Gudleski & Shean, 2000; Klein, Harding, Taylor, & Dickstein, 1988; Lehman et al., 1997; Mazure, Bruce, Maciejewski, & Jacobs, 2000; Mazure, Maciejewski, Jacobs, & Bruce, 2002; Mazure, Raghavan, Maciejewski, Jacobs, & Bruce, 2001; Moore & Blackburn, 1996; Robins et al., 1994; Rosenfarb, Becker, Kahn, & Mintz, 1998; Sahin, Ulusoy, & Sahin, 1993).[5] In addition, Lehman et al. (1997) found that depressed inpatients scored higher on both dimensions than depressed outpatients (see also Morse, Robins, & Gittes-Fox, 2002). One study comparing depressed and mixed psychiatric patients (Luyten, 2002) found that depressed inpatients exhibited significantly higher scores on Dependency/Sociotropy than mixed psychiatric inpatients, but no difference was found for Self-Critical Perfectionism/Autonomy, suggesting that Self-Critical Perfectionism/Autonomy is a more general vulnerability factor than Dependency/Sociotropy.

Ouimette, Klein, Clark and Margolis (1992) found that only Self-Critical Perfectionism/Autonomy was related to *life time major depression* as well as to interview assessed depressive personality (see also Zuroff & Blatt, 2002). Other studies have found that both Dependency/Sociotropy and Self-Critical Perfectionism/Autonomy are associated with life time major depression (Cox et al., 2004; Nordahl & Stiles, 2000; Ouimette, Klein, & Pepper, 1996; Sakado et al., 1999; Sanathara et al., 2003). Sanathara et al. (2003), for instance, reported that Interpersonal Sensitivity, as assessed by the IDI (Hirschfeld et al., 1977), which is closely related to the construct of Dependency/Sociotropy, was strongly associated with life time major depression as assessed by the Structured Clinical Interview for DSM-III-R in the Virginia Twin Registry population-based sample of 7,174 twins. Cox et al. (2004) reported that both personality dimensions were associated with life time major depression as assessed by the Composite International Diagnostic Interview in the National Comorbidity Survey (NCS), a study of a population based representative sample (*N*=5,877).

Dependency/Sociotropy and Self-Critical Perfectionism/Autonomy have also been related to *dysthymic disorder* (Goldberg, Segal, Vella, & Shaw, 1989; Ouimette et al., 1996). Moreover, Klein, Taylor, Dickstein and Harding (1988) reported that patients with early-onset Dysthymic Disorder had higher scores on Self-Critical Perfectionism/Autonomy, but not Dependency/Sociotropy, compared to patients with major depressive disorder.

Finally, some studies have investigated the stability of both personality dimensions using cross-sectional designs by comparing currently depressed and recovered patients. Results of these studies have been somewhat mixed (Fairbrother & Moretti, 1998; Hartlage, Arduino, & Alloy, 1998; Klein, Harding et al., 1988; Rosenfarb et al., 1998; Zuroff, Blatt, Sanislow, Bondi, & Pilkonis, 1999). Recovered depressed patients, however, have consistently been found to exhibit higher levels of both Dependency/Sociotropy and Self-Critical Perfectionism/Autonomy than never depressed controls (Solomon, Haaga, Brody, Kirk, & Friedman, 1998; Solomon, Arnow, Gotlib, & Wind, 2003). Thus, while depression may influence levels of Dependency/Sociotropy and Self-Critical Perfectionism/Autonomy (state effect), recovered depressed patients still show higher levels of both personality dimensions compared to normal controls, which is congruent with a

---

[5] It should be noted that four studies did not find a significant difference in levels of Autonomy between depressed patients and normals controls (Mazure, Maciejewski, Jacobs, & Bruce, 2002; Moore & Blackburn, 1996; Sahin, Ulusoy, & Sahin, 1993; Vogel, Stiles, & Nordahl, 2000). However, all these studies employed the SAS Autonomy subscale which, as we noted, has serious psychometric limitations. In fact, recent research indicates that the SAS Autonomy scale also contains both adaptive and maladaptive dimensions (Blatt, 2004).

vulnerability model. Family studies have also investigated the vulnerability status of Dependency/Sociotropy and Self-Critical Perfectionism/Autonomy because it is well known that biological offspring of depressed patients are at high risk for affective disorders. However, Ouimette et al. (1992) found no differences in levels of both personality dimensions between a high risk group (offspring of patients with affective disorders) and normal controls. While these findings may contradict the vulnerability hypotheses, Self-Critical Perfectionism/Autonomy in the total sample was associated with lifetime major depression and depressive personality. In another study, Ouimette et al. (1996) found evidence for a scar effect in that relatives of depressed patients with a history of affective disorders had higher levels of both Dependency/Sociotropy and Self-Critical Perfectionism/Autonomy compared to those relatives without a history of affective disorders.

Though cross-sectional studies clearly suggest that Dependency/Sociotropy and Self-Critical Perfectionism/Autonomy are possible etiological or pathogenetic factors associated with both severity of depression and depression diagnosis, these studies are limited in the investigation of these dimensions as possible causal antecedents or vulnerability factors in depression (Barnett & Gottlib, 1988). Simple cross-sectional studies, for example, cannot rule out that these personality dimensions are mere concomitants or consequences ("scar-hypothesis", see Chapter 1, this volume) of depression. Likewise, cross-sectional case control studies that compare remitted and currently depressed patients as well as family studies of offspring of depressed patients are also limited in drawing causal conclusions. Even though state effects may influence personality, this does not eliminate the possibility of a vulnerability component. In fact, Blatt and Beck do not imply absolute stability of Dependency/Sociotropy and Self-Critical Perfectionism/Autonomy. Rather, their theoretical views imply both state and trait effects, thus environmental stressors can intensify dependent/sociotropic or self-critical/autonomous needs and conflicts (Zuroff, 1992). Conversely, pharmacological or psychotherapeutic treatment may deactivate or modify these personality dimensions. Moreover, Blatt's formulations (e.g., Blatt & Shichman, 1983) also imply the possibility of regression as well as progression on each of these dimensions. Hence, only longitudinal studies can definitely test the stability and temporal antecedence of these personality dimensions.

Longitudinal Research

Stability. Evidence for the stability of both personality dimensions comes from several studies that have shown good test-retest reliability of the DEQ, SAS, PSI, and DAS in both clinical and nonclinical samples over periods ranging from three weeks to up to three years (Brewin & Firth-Cozens, 1997; Hammen, Marks, deMayo, & Mayol, 1985; Hammen, Ellicott, & Gitlin, 1989; Kasch, Klein, & Lara, 2001; Ouimette & Klein, 1993; Overholser & Freiheit, 1994; Segal, Shaw, Vella, &

Katz, 1992; Voyer & Cappeliez, 2002; Zuroff, Moskowitz, Wielgus, Powers, & Franko, 1983; Zuroff, Igreja, & Mongrain, 1990; Zuroff et al., 1999). In addition, Koestner, Zuroff and Powers (1991) reported considerable stability of self-criticism as measured by a specially constructed scale in adolescent and young adult females, but not in males. Self-criticism in males at age 12, however, predicted inhibition of aggressive impulses at age 31.

Follow-up studies. Follow-up studies of depressed patients have shown that levels of both Dependency/Sociotropy and Self-Critical Perfectionism/Autonomy remain elevated in remitted depressed patients compared to normal controls, even after brief pharmacological and/or psychotherapeutic treatment (Bagby, Schuller et al., 1994; Bagby et al., 2001; Enns, Cox, & Pidlubny, 2002; Frank et al., 1997; Kasch et al., 2001; Mazure et al., 2000; Moore & Blackburn, 1996; Ouimette & Klein, 1993; Segal et al., 1992; Solomon et al., 2003; Voyer & Cappeliez, 2002; Zuroff et al., 1999). Moreover, Zuroff et al. (1999) showed in a re-analysis of data from the National Institute of Mental Health Treatment of Depression Collaborative Research Program (TDCRP) that changes over time in mean scores that are found in some studies (e.g., Enns, Cox, & Pidlubny, 2002; Moore & Blackburn, 1996; Ouimette et al., 1996; Rector, Bagby, Segal, Joffe, & Levitt, 2000; Rosenfarb et al., 1998) do not necessarily imply that Dependency/Sociotropy and Self-Critical Perfectionism/Autonomy are mere concomitants of depression. Using Structural Equation Modeling (SEM), these investigators found that a model that included both state and trait effects better fitted the data than a pure state or pure trait model. Both during, but particularly after treatment, both personality dimensions showed remarkable stability. These findings have been replicated since in two other studies (Cox & Enns, 2003; Shahar, Blatt, Zuroff, Kuperminc, & Leadbeater, 2004). Consistent with formulations by Blatt and Beck, these findings suggest that the measurement of Dependency/Sociotropy and Self-Critical Perfectionism/Autonomy in both clinical and non-clinical samples includes both state and trait components, with trait components accounting for most of the variance.

Prospective studies. While some studies found that neither Dependency/Sociotropy nor Self-Critical Perfectionism/Autonomy predict *severity of depression* over time (Mazure et al., 2000; Overholser & Freiheit, 1994; Voyer & Cappeliez, 2002), most studies found that both personality dimensions predict severity of depression over time (Brewin & Firth-Cozens, 1997; Fresco, Sampson, Craighead, & Koons, 2001; Lakey & Ross, 1994; Mongrain, Lubbers, & Struthers, 2004; Mongrain & Zuroff, 1994; Priel & Shahar, 2000; Robins, Hayes, Block, Kramer, & Villena, 1995; Shahar, Joiner, Zuroff, & Blatt, 2004; Shahar & Priel, 2003; Zuroff, Stotland, Sweetman, Craig, & Koestner, 1995; Zuroff et al., 1999). Two other studies reported that only Self-Critical Perfectionism/Autonomy (Shahar, Blatt, Zuroff, Kuperminc, & Leadbeater, 2004) or Dependency/Sociotropy (Alford & Gerrity, 1995) predicted depression severity. One likely explanation for these mixed findings is that all negative studies (with the exception of Shahar, Blatt et al., 2004) are based on very small samples (*N*'s ranging between 41-75 in negative studies and between 48-603 in positive studies), most probably resulting in inadequate statistical power to detect significant effects (Cohen, 1988). Of particular importance is a study by Brewin and Firth-Cozens (1997), which reported that both Dependency/Sociotropy and Self-Critical Perfectionism/Autonomy predicted severity of depression, especially in males, after 2 and 10 years, even after controlling for initial symptoms and workload in a sample of medical students. To address the issue of scar effects, Shahar, Blatt, Zuroff, Kuperminc and Leadbeater (2004), investigating a pure vulnerability, a pure scar, and a reciprocal model (including both vulnerability and scar effects) of the relationship between Dependency/Sociotropy and Self-Critical Perfectionism/Autonomy and severity of depression in a one-year longitudinal study of 452 adolescents, found a reciprocal relationship between Self-Critical Perfectionism/Autonomy, but not Dependency/ Sociotropy, and depressive symptoms. However, the scar effect was small compared to the vulnerability effect and was only found in girls. In addition, pure vulnerability and pure scar models provided a significantly poorer fit to the data than a reciprocal model.

Both Dependency/Sociotropy and Self-Critical Perfectionism/Autonomy have also been shown to predict several variables related to the *course of depression*, including severity of depression and worse global functioning at a 6-month follow-up (Klein, 1989), increased time to recovery (Kasch et al., 2001), non-recovery (Bothwell & Scott, 1997), and relapse (Lam, Green, Power, & Checkley, 1996; Wilhelm, Boyce, & Brownhill, 2004).

Longitudinal studies of the relationship between Dependency/Sociotropy and Self-Critical Perfectionism/Autonomy and the *onset of depression* are scant, mainly because of their high cost and effort. Wilhelm et al. (2004) found that Separation Anxiety, a core component of Dependency/Sociotropy, predicted repeated episodes of major depression in a 5-year follow-up study of 156 community participants. Spasojevic and Alloy (2001) found that both Dependency/Sociotropy and Self-Critical Perfectionism/Autonomy predicted the number of future episodes of major depression in 137 students who were followed for 2.5 years. In a 6-year prospective study in a sample of first-degree relatives of patients with affective disorders, Hirschfeld et al. (1989) reported that Dependency/Sociotropy, as measured by the IDI, predicted first onset of depression among older subjects (aged 31-41), but not among younger (aged 17-30). The study by Sanathara et al. (2003), discussed earlier, evaluated vulnerability, state, and scar models of the relationship between Dependency/Sociotropy as assessed by the IDI, and major depression as measured by the SCID, in a one-year prospective study in a community-based sample of 7,174 twins. Sanathara et al. (2003) reported, congruent with a vulnerability model, that pre-morbid Dependency/Sociotropy predicted future onset of major depression among those that had no prior depressive episodes (N=1,328). Congruent with the state model, they also found that levels of Dependency/Sociotropy were influenced by current depression. However, in contrast with the scar model, Dependency/ Sociotropy scores were not significantly elevated by a history of depression. Interestingly, they also reported that Dependency/Sociotropy scores showed a trend towards elevation during and after experiencing a major depressive episode. Fitting a regression line to the change observed in Dependency/Sociotropy scores as a function of time, they showed that Dependency/Sociotropy scores would return to baseline in approximately 6 months after a depressive episode.

Conclusions

Existing research clearly suggests that Dependency/Sociotropy and Self-Critical Perfectionism/Autonomy are relatively stable factors influencing the onset and course of depression as well as the severity of depression. In particular, the relationship between these personality dimensions and depression appears to be best described by a trait/state/scar model, with trait effects accounting for most variance. Although state and "scar" effects are not negligible, they appear to be small. Moreover, "scar" effects seem to "wear off" over time.

However, more well designed prospective studies of the relationship between these personality dimensions and the onset and course of several forms of clinical depression are needed to further validate these conclusions. For instance, whereas both personality dimensions might predict onset of major depression, Dependency/Sociotropy might actually be a protective factor against post-partum depression (Franche, 2001; Franche & Mikail, 1999; Priel & Besser, 1999, 2000; however, see Boyce, Parker, Barnett, Cooney, & Smith, 1991). Future studies should also consider the possibility of age and cohort effects because the meaning and thus effect of Dependency/Sociotropy and Self-Critical Perfectionism/Autonomy might change over time and with age. For instance, Hirschfeld et al. (1989) reported that Dependency/Sociotropy predicted first onset of depression in subjects aged 31-41, but not in young adults. Mazure and Maciejewski (2003) in turn found in a sample of 170 subjects aged 20-91 years that the risk for clinical depression was quite uniform across age for Dependency/Sociotropy, whereas the effect for Self-Critical Perfectionism/Autonomy was strongest in younger adulthood and declined with age.

Finally, it should be pointed out that the studies reviewed in this section only provide a partial test of Blatt's and Beck's hypothesis that Dependency/Sociotropy and Self-Critical Perfectionism/Autonomy are antecedent vulnerability factors of depression because they only consider the diathesis (i.e., personality) component. However, as noted in the previous chapter, Blatt's and Beck's views imply in fact a diathesis-stress model in which these personality dimensions confer a vulnerability (diathesis) to depression either alone or in interaction with (congruent) stressors (stress). In the next section, we review studies concerning this congruency hypothesis.

Proximal Precipitating Factors: The Congruency Hypothesis

The relationship between (severe) negative life events and the onset and course of depression is well documented (Kessler, 1997; Tennant, 2002). Blatt as well as Beck extend traditional theories of the relationship between life events and depression in two ways. First, a key assumption of Blatt's and Beck's views is that Dependency/Sociotropy and Self-Critical Perfectionism/Autonomy are expected to interact with congruent or matching events to predict depression (e.g., interpersonal events vs. achievement events) (Blatt & Zuroff, 1992). This "key-and-lock" hypothesis has also been called the congruency hypothesis (Robins, 1995). A second extension of research on the relationship between life events and depression involves the view that personality, depression, and life stressors are not independent, but dynamically interact with each other. This view implies that dependent/sociotropic and self-critical/autonomous individuals, in part, generate their own (congruent) life stressors. Thus, dependent/sociotropic subjects are expected to generate interpersonal stress events (e.g., dissolution of relationships, family quarrels), while self-critical/autonomous subjects are expected to cause more achievement related events (e.g., failure to obtain a job promotion). Moreover, (congruent) life stressors may increase levels of Dependency/Sociotropy and Self-Critical Perfectionism/Autonomy (Zuroff, 1992). For instance, dependent individuals' fear of rejection might be increased by frequently experiencing rejection by significant others, whereas the fear of failure and disapproval of self-critical individuals increases their vulnerability to experiencing failure. Finally, depression may influence both personality ("scar-effect") as well as life events (see also Hammen, 1991).

Unfortunately, most research concerning the congruency hypothesis has not investigated this *dynamic interactionism perspective*, but has rather adopted a *mechanistic interactionism* view (Zuroff, 1992). That is, most studies have treated personality and environment as distinct, static, independent entities. Life events are thus often conceptualized as moderators (Baron & Kenny, 1986), whereas Blatt's and Beck's views imply in fact that life events act as mediators in the relationship between personality and depression. First, we review studies that have either implicitly or explicitly adopted a mechanistic view of Dependency/Sociotropy and Self-Critical Perfectionism/Autonomy and their interaction with life events. Next, research concerning the dynamic interactionism hypothesis is examined.

Mechanistic interactionism. More than 40 empirical studies have investigated the "mechanistic" congruency hypothesis. A considerable number of these studies found evidence for the congruency hypothesis for both personality dimensions (Blaney, 2002; Brown, Hammen, Craske, & Wickens, 1995; Dunkley, Zuroff, & Blankstein, 2003; Fichman, Koestner, & Zuroff, 1997; Giordana, Wood, & Michela, 2000; Gruen, Silva, Ehrlich, Schweitzer, & Friedhoff, 1997; Hammen & Goodman-Brown, 1990; Hammen, Marks, Mayol, & deMayo, 1985; Hammen, Ellicott & Gitlin, 1989; Hammen, Ellicott, Gitlin, & Jamison, 1989; Lam et al., 1996; Mazure & Maciejewski, 2003; Mazure et al., 2002; Mongrain & Zuroff, 1994; Robins, 1990, Study 2; Segal et al., 1992), other studies only found evidence for Dependency/Sociotropy (Allen, Horne, & Trinder, 1996; Bartelstone & Trull, 1995; Clark, Beck, & Brown, 1992; Dozois & Backs-Dermott, 2000; Ewart, Jorgensen, & Kolodner, 1998; Hammen, Ellicott, & Gitlin, 1992; Lakey & Ross, 1994; Priel & Shahar, 2000; Raghavan et al., 2002; Robins, 1990, Study 1; Robins & Block, 1988; Rude & Burnham, 1993; Segal, Shaw, & Vella, 1989; Shahar, Joiner, Zuroff, & Blatt, 2004; Solomon et al., 1998; Voyer & Cappeliez, 2002; Whiffen & Aube, 1999; Zuroff & Mongrain, 1987), while in one study there was only evidence for a specific interaction between Self-Critical Perfectionism/Autonomy and congruent life events (Clark & Oates, 1995). In addition, some studies have found no evidence for the congruency hypothesis for neither Dependency/ Sociotropy nor Self-Critical Perfectionism/Autonomy (Burgess, Lorah, Haaga, & Chrousos, 1996; Flett, Hewitt, Garshowitz, & Martin, 1997; Fresco et al., 2001; Kwon & Whisman, 1998; Mazure et al., 2000; Robins et al., 1995; Santor & Zuroff, 1997; Santor, Pringle, & Israeli, 2000; Shahar & Priel, 2003; Smith et al., 1988; Zuroff et al., 1990). [6]

Studies concerning the interaction between Dependency/Sociotropy and Self-Critical Perfectionism/Autonomy and specific types of daily hassles have yielded more mixed results, with some studies finding support for the congruency hypothesis (Sherry, Hewitt, Flett, & Harvey, 2003; Dunkley, Zuroff, & Blankstein, 2003), others only in depressed patients, but not in mixed psychiatric patients (Hewitt & Flett, 1993), and still others finding none or only limited evidence for a congruency effect (Clark & Oates, 1995; Santor & Patterson, 2003).

In sum, support for the mechanistic congruency hypothesis has been fairly consistent for Dependency/Sociotropy, but more mixed for Self-Critical Perfectionism/Autonomy (Blatt, 2004; Coyne & Whiffen, 1995; Nietzel & Harris, 1990; Robins, 1995), and is mainly limited to negative life events, but not daily hassles. It is noteworthy, however, that the evidence for a congruency effect for both dimensions is most clear when one considers the qualitatively best studies (i.e., using a prospective design, interview-based measures of life events and clinical depression and/or standardized measures of the severity of depression). For example, Hammen, Ellicott, Gitlin and Jamison (1989) found that both Dependency/Sociotropy and Self-Critical Perfectionism/Autonomy in interaction with interview-assessed congruent life events predicted both the onset of major depressive episodes and the severity of depressive symptoms in a sample of unipolar depressed patients during a 6 month follow-up.

Studies on the congruency hypothesis also lend further support for the status of Dependency/Sociotropy and Self-Critical Perfectionism/Autonomy as vulnerability factors for depression. Not only do both personality dimensions directly and independently predict depression, but most studies have found that the interaction between these two personality dimensions and life events is not only statistically significant, but also accounts for a substantial, and thus clinically relevant, amount of additional variance in predicting depression. Mazure et al. (2002), for instance, reported that whereas a clinical diagnosis of major depression was 0.5 to 3 times more likely when subjects had high levels of Dependency/Sociotropy and Self-Critical Perfectionism/Autonomy, the interaction between these personality dimensions and congruent life events made clinical depression 6 to 11 times more likely (for similar results, see Raghavan et al., 2002).

---

[6] Only two studies investigated the congruency hypothesis in bipolar patients. In a 6-month follow-up study of bipolar patients, Hammen, Ellicott, Gitlin and Jamison (1989) did not find evidence for neither Dependency/Sociotropy nor Self-Critical Perfectionism/Autonomy, while Hammen, Ellicott and Gitlin (1992) reported that the interaction between Dependency/Sociotropy and interpersonal events predicted symptom severity, but not onset of symptoms, in an 18-month follow-up study of bipolar patients. For Self-Critical Perfectionism/Autonomy, no evidence for the congruency hypothesis was found.

Dynamic interactionism. Early studies of the effect of Dependency/Sociotropy and Self-Critical Perfectionism/Autonomy on the occurrence of life events have yielded remarkably inconsistent results, most likely because of small samples sizes (Connor-Smith & Compas, 2002; Hammen, Marks, deMayo, & Mayol, 1985; Mongrain & Zuroff, 1989, 1994; Robins & Block, 1988). In what is probably the most sophisticated study of the dynamic interactionism theory to date, Simons, Angell, Monroe and Thase (1993) investigated the influence of Dependency/Sociotropy and Self-Critical Perfectionism/Autonomy on the definition, rating, and generation of life events as measured by both self-report and interview in a sample of 55 depressed patients. Self-Critical Perfectionism/Autonomy predicted the total number as well as severity of self-reported achievement, but not interpersonal, events. Dependency/Sociotropy was unrelated to the total number and severity of self-reported interpersonal as well as achievement events. Thus, Self-Critical Perfectionism, but not Dependency/Sociotropy, was related to a tendency to overreport and overrate the importance of congruent, but not incongruent, life events (see also Gruen et al., 1997). Moreover, Simons et al. (1993) found that both Dependency/Sociotropy and Self-Critical Perfectionism/Autonomy predicted the generation of fateful (i.e., self-generated) congruent, but not incongruent, life events, particularly in patients with no prior history of depression. Importantly, both personality dimensions were unrelated to independent (not self-generated) events. Daley and colleagues (1997) reported in a 2-year follow-up study of 134 late adolescent women that Self-Critical Perfectionism/Autonomy, and to a lesser extent Dependency/Sociotropy, predicted fateful, but not independent, life events. Interestingly, both Dependency/Sociotropy and Self-Critical Perfectionism/Autonomy predicted interpersonal conflict stress (see also Flett et al., 1997). Unfortunately, Daley and colleagues (1997) did not investigate whether these personality dimensions also predicted achievement stress. In addition, in line with the dynamic interactionism model, Daley et al. (1997) also found that depression predicted fateful, but not independent, events. However, these fateful events occurred mainly outside depressive episodes. Similarly, Lakey and Ross (1994) reported that dysphoria predicted severity of depression and both interpersonal and achievement life events in a sample of 133 students. However, controlled for initial levels of dysphoria, Dependency/Sociotropy still interacted only with congruent events, whereas Self-Critical Perfectionism/Autonomy interacted with both congruent and incongruent events. In line with these findings, several studies have reported that levels of distress do not predict subsequent life events when controlled for Dependency/Sociotropy and Self-Critical Perfectionism/Autonomy (Priel & Shahar, 2000; Shahar & Priel, 2003; Shahar, Blatt, Zuroff, Krupnick, & Sotsky, 2004). These results are consistent with the notion that the generation of stress mostly occurs outside depressive episodes, and that relatively stable personality features, such as Dependency/Sociotropy and Self-Critical Perfectionism/Autonomy, rather than depressed mood, are responsible for stress generation (see also Daley et al., 1997).

Recent studies by Shahar and colleagues suggest important differences between Dependency/Sociotropy and Self-Critical Perfectionism/Autonomy and responsivity to and generation of stress. Priel & Shahar (2000) reported that only Self-

Critical Perfectionism/Autonomy, but not Dependency/Sociotropy, was related to life stress in a 9-week prospective study of 182 young adults. In line with these results, they reported that a moderating model best described the relationship between Dependency/Sociotropy, negative life events, and dysphoria, whereas a mediating model represented the best fit to the data for the relationship between Self-Critical Perfectionism/Autonomy, negative life events, and dysphoria. Moreover, Dependency/Sociotropy was associated with higher levels of perceived social support, which in turned was associated with lower levels of distress. Self-Critical Perfectionism/Autonomy on the contrary predicted decreased social support over time, which in turn predicted elevated distress.

Hence, self-critical, but not dependent, individuals seemed to generate their own negative life events and further "degenerate" levels of social support. These results were replicated in a 5-week longitudinal study of 198 university students (Shahar, Joiner, Zuroff, & Blatt, 2004). Moreover, whereas Dependency/Sociotropy interacted with congruent stressors related to family and friends, Self-Critical Perfectionism/Autonomy predicted the generation of both congruent (e.g., friends-related) and incongruent stress (e.g., school stress). In a 16-week longitudinal study, Shahar and Priel (2003) found that both personality dimensions predicted the generation of negative life events. One possible explanation of these divergent findings for the effect of Dependency/Sociotropy is that the stress generation effect of Dependency/Sociotropy may be smaller, and thus is perhaps harder to detect. Interestingly, Shahar and Priel (2003) also reported that Dependency/Sociotropy predicted the experience of positive events over time, which suppressed the negative effect of Dependency/Sociotropy, whereas Self-Critical Perfectionism/Autonomy, in contrast, was negatively associated with positive events, which in turn predicted increased levels of distress. Hence, while both Dependency/Sociotropy and Self-Critical Perfectionism/Autonomy were associated with the generation of negative life events, Dependency/Sociotropy also increased the number of positive experiences, whereas Self-Critical Perfectionism/Autonomy decreased the number of positive events.

In summary, the vulnerability associated with Dependency/Sociotropy appears to be somewhat more passive-reactive. The fact that Dependency/Sociotropy is, at best, only weakly related with the generation of life stress could be explained by the tendency of dependent/sociotropic individuals to avoid conflicts, especially in interpersonal relationships, and to generate, at least temporarily, social support (Blatt & Zuroff, 1992). Alternatively, because of this tendency to avoid conflicts, they may underreport interpersonal conflicts. Evidence is more clear in suggesting that their vulnerability for life stress is specific, in that dependent/sociotropic individuals show increased vulnerability for depression in reaction to particular classes (i.e., congruent) of stressors. Moreover, Dependency/Sociotropy is also associated with the generation of protective factors such as positive life events and perceived social support. Thus, Dependency/Sociotropy appears to include aspects of vulnerability as well as resilience (Blatt, 2004; Bornstein, 1992; Shahar, Joiner et al., 2004).[7] This conclusion is further substantiated by research showing that

---

[7] This might also explain its weaker relationship with distress compared to Self-Critical Perfectionism (Shahar & Priel, 2003).

faced with stress, dependent/sociotropic individuals tend to use both adaptive (i.e., active, approach) (Besser & Priel, 2003; Fichman, Koestner, Zuroff, & Gordon, 1999) as well as maladaptive coping styles such as venting or consumption-based self-indulgence (Fichman et al., 1999, Haaga, Fine, Terrill, Stewart, & Beck, 1995).

Vulnerability to life stress associated with Self-Critical Perfectionism/Autonomy, in contrast, appears to be more proactive but less specific. Self-critical/autonomous individuals seem to generate a wide range of stressors. In addition, unlike dependent/sociotropic individuals, they fail to generate positive, protective environmental factors such as positive events or social support. Moreover, they also tend to consistently use maladaptive (e.g., emotional, passive) coping strategies (Chang, 2000; Chang & Rand, 2000; Connor-Smith & Compas, 2002; Besser & Priel, 2003; Dunkley & Blankstein, 2000; Dunkley, Blankstein, Halsall, Williams, & Winkworth, 2000; Haring, Hewitt, & Flett, 2003; O'Connor & O'Connor, 2003). Faced with stress, they tend to withdraw and isolate themselves (Fichman et al., 1999). In all likelihood, this gives rise to a self-perpetuating cycle characterized by rumination, self-criticism, further withdrawal, and thus fewer opportunities to receive social support and to have positive experiences (Daley et al., 1997; Kasch et al., 2001). Finally, results from studies on the dynamic interactionism hypothesis may explain why evidence for the "mechanistic" congruency hypothesis is less equivocal for Dependency/Sociotropy than for Self-Critical Perfectionism/Autonomy. First, a moderating model, which is implied by a mechanistic view, seems to best describe the relationship between Dependency/Sociotropy and life events, whereas a mediating model best describes this relationship for Self-Critical Perfectionism/Autonomy. Moreover, Self-Critical-Perfectionism/Autonomy appears to be associated with a broader vulnerability to life stress than Dependency/Sociotropy.

Limitations of existing research. The above conclusions await further research because of several methodological and theoretical caveats, especially in studies that have adopted a mechanistic interpretation of the congruency hypothesis (see also Coyne & Whiffen, 1995). From a *methodological* point of view, findings concerning Self-Critical Perfectionism/Autonomy may be influenced by the fact that several studies of the congruency hypothesis have employed the SAS (Beck et al., 1983). Because the SAS Autonomy scale is often unrelated to depression, it should come as no surprise that some studies have found no interaction between SAS Autonomy and (congruent) life events (Bieling et al., 2000). Second, research concerning the congruency hypothesis should be better informed by current life stress research. For instance, most studies have relied on subjective, questionnaire-based measures of life stress rather than objective, interview-based measures of stress. Yet, studies have consistently shown that questionnaire-based measures of life stress tend to overestimate both the frequency and severity of life stress compared with interview-based measures (Monroe & Hadjiyannakis, 2002), possibly leading to an inflation of life events and their impact. Furthermore, interview-based assessment of life events also allows distinguishing between fateful and independent life events, which is crucial in investigating the dynamic interactionism hypothesis. In addition, many studies have typically employed small samples. In combination with the low incidence of depression and the fact that the ability to detect (personality-event) interactions typically requires a larger number of subjects than does the detection of main effects (McClelland & Judd, 1993), many studies in this domain suffer from inadequate statistical power. Also, often very short time frames (i.e., often only a few days or weeks) have been used in longitudinal studies of the congruency hypothesis. However, it is well known that the average person will experience very few severe negative life events in such short time spans (Tennant, 2002). Finally, it is well documented that the role of life stressors in the onset of depression decreases as the number of previous episodes increases, such that depression tends to run a more autonomous course, whereas those without a history of depression may be more responsive to stressors (see also Chapter 1 and Chapter 8 in this volume). The number of previous depressive episodes, however, is rarely taken into account in research concerning the congruency hypothesis. Hence, future studies should differentiate between pathways toward initial and subsequent episodes of depression.

Many existing studies in this domain also show important *theoretical limitations.* To begin with, the categorization of life events as either relevant for Dependency/Sociotropy or Self-Critical Perfectionism/Autonomy is not only difficult, but also to a certain extent arbitrary because dependent/sociotropic and self-critical/autonomous individuals may interpret the same life event in different ways (Blatt & Zuroff, 1992; Coyne & Whiffen, 1995). A dimensional approach, in which individuals rate life events in terms of the degree of relevance for Dependency/Sociotropy and Self-Critical Perfectionism/Autonomy is needed (Hammen, Ellicott, & Gitlin, 1989). In addition, a more idiographic assessment, which takes into account the meaning of a life stressor, rather than using general classes of life events (e.g., interpersonal versus achievement), may provide a better test of the congruency hypothesis. Assessment methods such as in vivo thought sampling or priming techniques are likely to yield more ecologically valid tests of the congruency hypothesis (Dozois & Backs-Dermott, 2000). Second, research suggests that most important negative life events are in the interpersonal domain, which could make it very hard to find a specific interaction between Self-Critical Perfectionism/Autonomy and achievement events (Coyne & Whiffen, 1995; Hammen, 1991; Zuroff et al., 1987). Third, some authors have argued that depression in self-critical/autonomous subjects may not require environmental activation, but primarily results from internal factors, such as continuous self-criticism and/or biological factors (Mongrain & Zuroff, 1994). In this context, it is important to note that Beck (1983) links his autonomous type of depression to endogenous depression. Fourth, very little research has explored cohort and age differences in the relationship between Dependency/Sociotropy and Self-Critical Perfectionism/Autonomy and life stress. In the only study addressing this issue, Mazure and Maciejewski (2003) reported that the impact of the interaction between Self-Critical Perfectionism/Autonomy and achievement events as a risk factor for clinical depression was strongest in young adulthood (increasing the likelihood of clinical depression more than 20 (!) times at age 25) and declined with age, whereas the reverse was found for the interaction between Dependency/Sociotropy and interpersonal events. Hence, these results suggest important age (and perhaps also gender and cohort) differences in that self-critical/

autonomous individuals are particularly at risk for depression in young adulthood when confronted with congruent stressors, whereas with age the likelihood of depression increases for dependent/sociotropic individuals if they experience congruent stressors.

Future research should focus more on the dynamic processes involved in the relationship between personality and life stress. As Hewitt and Flett (2002) have argued, personality dimensions such as Dependency/Sociotropy and Self-Critical Perfectionism/Autonomy are likely to influence not only the perception and generation of stress, but also the anticipation, enhancement, and perpetuation of stress. In addition, as research on gene- and person-environment correlations and interactions in other domains has shown (Rutter et al., 1997), a dynamic, reciprocal model of vulnerability to depression might also play an important role in the integration of biological and psychosocial factors in depression. Already, several studies have shown that not only subjective, but psychophysiological and biochemical stress as well might be contingent on the "fit" between personality and the nature of the stressor (Allen et al., 1996; Ewart et al., 1998; Gruen et al., 1997; Sauro et al., 2001). Gruen et al. (1997), for instance, found that Self-Critical Perfectionism/Autonomy, but not Dependency/Sociotropy, was associated with changes in plasma homovanillic acid (HVA), the primary dopamine metabolite in humans, during exposure to an induced failure-stressor. Hence, studies concerning the congruency hypothesis might play an important role in bridging the gap between psychological and biological approaches in research and treatment of depression.

Characteristic Interpersonal Style

Empirical research, especially on couples, has provided strong support for Blatt's and Beck's descriptions of the characteristic interpersonal style associated with Dependency/Sociotropy and Self-Critical Perfectionism/Autonomy. In addition, these studies also provide further support for the dynamic interactionism model proposed by Blatt and Zuroff (1992). Based on Buss (1987), Blatt and Zuroff (1992) proposed that dependent/sociotropic and self-critical/autonomous individuals select, evoke, and transform (manipulate) their social environment. *Selection* refers to the ways individuals choose different environments, *evocation* to the fact that individuals tend to elicit different environments, and *transformation* to the tendency of individuals to transform (or manipulate) their environment. We review evidence for each of these interactive processes in turn.

Selection. Research findings clearly indicate that dependent/sociotropic and self-critical/autonomous individuals prefer different (social) environments. Dependent/ sociotropic individuals are fundamentally oriented towards others in order to receive love and support, whereas self-critical/autonomous individuals are ambivalent and distant towards others and mainly value achievement and success (Blatt

& Zuroff, 1992; Zuroff & DeLorimier, 1989; Zuroff et al., 1995). Studies have consistently shown that Self-Critical Perfectionism/Autonomy is associated with a cold, distant relational style that is characterized by manifest hostility in relationships, even in intimate relationships such as with romantic partners (Alden & Bieling, 1996; Fichman et al., 1994; Vettese & Mongrain, 2000; Whisman & Friedman 1998; Zuroff & Duncan, 1999). In addition, Self-Critical Perfectionism/Autonomy is associated with dissatisfaction in relationships in general, including those with partner and children (Dimitrovsky, Levy-Schiff, & Schattner-Zanany, 2002; Haring et al., 2003; Lynch, Robins, & Morse, 2001; Zuroff & Duncan, 1999; Vettese & Mongrain, 2000; Whiffen, Aubé, Thompson, & Campbell, 2000; Zuroff, Koestner, & Powers, 1994), and with dissatisfaction concerning sexuality in particular (Morrison, Urquiza, & Goodlin-Jones, 1998). Self-Critical Perfectionism/Autonomy has also been associated with feelings of social isolation and loneliness (Besser, Flett, & Davis, 2003; Clark et al., 1995; Schachter & Zlotogorski, 1995; Wiseman, 1997). For self-critical/autonomous individuals, their worth often appears to be equated with their work. In line with theoretical expectations, they also tend to evaluate others negatively (Shapiro, 1988a, 1988b), show low levels of social acuity (Aube & Whiffen, 1996), are less likely to ask help from others when confronted with problems (Mongrain, 1998), and tend to experience various interpersonal problems. More specifically, studies have shown that self-critical/autonomous individuals have difficulty in connecting to people and have the feeling that they are too controlling in relationships (e.g., Fichman et al., 1994; Morrison et al., 1998).

Dependent/sociotropic individuals, in contrast, are more open towards others, report fewer problems with intimacy, and are more likely to ask for help from others, including medical assistance (Bornstein, 1992; Mongrain, 1998). However, studies have also shown that they consider themselves as non-assertive and submissive, but at the same time as demanding and as overly responsible in relationships (Alden & Bieling, 1996; Bornstein, 1992; Ewart et al., 1998; Lynch et al., 2003; Morrison et al., 1998; Whisman & Friedman, 1998). In addition, Dependency/Sociotropy, as expected, is associated with the inhibition of aggression in intimate relationships (Alden & Bieling, 1996; Mongrain et al., 2004; Mongrain & Zuroff, 1994; Mongrain, Vettese, Shuster, & Kendal, 1998; Vettese & Mongrain, 2000; Zuroff & Fitzpatrick, 1995; Zuroff et al., 1983), with difficulty in disclosing true feelings (Ewart et al., 1998; Mongrain & Zuroff, 1994; Zuroff et al., 1983), and with difficulties leaving relationships (Ewart et al., 1998; Kurdek, 2000).

In sum, contrary to some theories that conceptualize Dependency/Sociotropy as a maladaptive trait, but consistent with findings reviewed earlier on the relationship between Dependency/Sociotropy and life stress, Dependency/Sociotropy has adaptive (e.g., more openness, fewer problems with intimacy) as well as maladaptive (e.g., submissive, demanding) aspects. Similarly, Bornstein (1992) emphasizes that dependency should not be equated with passivity. As we will show below, dependency is often associated with very active and even manipulative behaviors to obtain the needed care, love and support. Self-Critical Perfectionism/Autonomy, in contrast, again emerges as a more "pure" vulnerability factor, in that self-critical/autonomous individuals tend to have ambivalent, distant, and cold

111

relationships, and tend to experience much conflict and dissatisfaction in their relationships, even in close, intimate relationships (Blatt, 1995, 2004).

Studies investigating the relationship between Dependency/Sociotropy and Self-Critical Perfectionism/Autonomy and attachment styles further add to this picture, but at the same time also highlight important differences between Blatt's and Beck's conceptualizations (Morrison et al., 1998; Murphy & Bates, 1997; Reis & Grenyer, 2002; Zuroff & Fitzpatrick, 1995). Both Dependency and Sociotropy are most closely associated with a preoccupied attachment style, characterized by a combination of desires for love, but also fear for loss of love. Blatt's concept of Self-Critical Perfectionism is more closely related to a fearful-avoidant attachment style, characterized by a longing for approval, together with fear for dependency and closeness, dissatisfaction and distrust of others. Thus, Self-Critical Perfectionism appears to be associated with an approach-avoidance conflict in relationships. Beck's (1983) Autonomy concept, however, is more closely related to a dismissive attachment style, characterized by the (defensive) avoidance of relationships. This is in keeping with Beck's (1983) emphasis on the strong needs for independence, solitude, and control of autonomous individuals, resulting in a defensive separation and even downright insensitivity to the needs of others (Clark et al., 1995).

Evocation. Dependent/sociotropic and self-critical/autonomous individuals also tend to elicit different reactions and thus environments. Moreover, they also tend to show marked differences in their perceptions of their social environment. In this context, research on the relationship between Dependency/Sociotropy and Self-Critical Perfectionism/Autonomy and social support is particularly interesting. Research has shown that low social support is an important antecedent of depression (Barnett & Gotlib, 1988). It is therefore generally accepted that positive social relationships and a good social integration buffer against depression, either directly or indirectly (Cohen & Wills, 1985). From this perspective, it should not be surprising that Dependency/Sociotropy in general shows a weaker relationship with depression than Self-Critical Perfectionism/Autonomy. Because of their fundamental orientation towards others, it could be argued that dependent/socio-tropic individuals tend to have larger social networks than self-critical/autonomous individuals and tend to have higher levels of perceived and/or actual social support (Mongrain, 1998). Moreover, dependent/sociotropic individuals might be less at risk for specific (congruent) life events (e.g., divorce, social isolation, etc.) known to be associated with depression (Brown & Harris, 1978). Conversely, it could also be argued that the often extreme neediness and claiming attitude of dependent/ sociotropic individuals leads to resentment in (significant) others, and finally in rejection, putting dependent/sociotropic individuals at *increased* risk for (con-gruent) life stress and thus depression (Mongrain, 1998). Self-critical individuals, in contrast, may have a more limited and less satisfying social network because of their cold, ambivalent relational style. The combination of this restricted and negative social network with their continuous self-criticism, places these individuals at greater risk for depression.

Studies in this area have again shown that while Dependency/Sociotropy contains elements of both vulnerability and resilience, Self-Critical Perfectionism/

Autonomy appears to be a more clear-cut vulnerability factor. Priel and Shahar (2000), for instance, found that Dependency/Sociotropy was associated with high levels of perceived social support, which buffer the effect of stress, while Self-Critical Perfectionism/Autonomy was associated with low levels of social support, which in turn predicted increased levels of distress (see also Shahar & Priel, 2003; Shahar, Henrich, Blatt, Ryan, & Little, 2003). Moreover, whereas Self-Critical Perfectionism/Autonomy has been consistently related to low levels of social support, evidence for Dependency/Sociotropy is more mixed, with some studies reporting a positive association (Mongrain, 1998; Priel & Besser, 1999; Priel & Shahar, 2000), others a negative association (Ewart et al., 1998), and still others no relationship (Reynolds & Gilbert, 1991). These mixed findings are consistent with the findings that the measures of Dependency/Sociotropy are often a complex mix of risk and resilience components (Blatt, 2004; Rude & Burnham, 1995). In addition, levels of social support may show strong fluctuations in dependent/ sociotropic individuals (e.g., disillusionment after initial idealization). Priel and Shahar (2000), for instance, found in a longitudinal study that Dependency/Socio-tropy was positively related to perceived social support at Time 1, but not nine weeks later. Such fluctuations may be especially pronounced when dependent/ sociotropic individuals experience stress. As noted in the previous section, faced with (interpersonal) stress, dependent/sociotropic individuals tend to seek help from others, but in an excessive, claiming way (Beck, Robbins, Taylor, & Baker, 2001; Shahar, Joiner et al., 2004), as well as using venting as a coping mechanism (Fichman et al., 1999), possibly leading to (further) resentment in others. In addition, several studies suggest that the good social integration and good quality of relationships of dependent/sociotropic individuals can be deceptive (Ewart et al., 1998; Flett et al., 1997; Mongrain, 1998; Whiffen & Aube, 1999; Whisman & Friedman, 1998; Zuroff et al., 1995). Zuroff et al. (1995), for instance, reported that although Dependency/Sociotropy was related to more frequent and more intimate relationships, it was also related to feelings of dissatisfaction and dysphoria in relationships. Thus, although relationships of dependent/sociotropic individuals may seem positive, they most likely are also characterized by underlying dissatisfaction and exaggerated fears of rejection.

Furthermore, all of these studies have focused on *perceived*, but not *actual* social support. This is noteworthy because several studies have shown that dependent/ sociotropic individuals perceive their relationships as positive, loving, and supporting, while others, including their partner, perceive these same relationships in less positive terms (Bieling & Alden, 1998; Lynch et al., 2003; Mongrain et al., 1998, 2004; Shapiro, 1988). Self-critical/autonomous individuals on the other hand not only report that they are more critical, hostile, and ambivalent towards others, but others, including their own partner, also perceive them as more critical and less loving and therefore tend to react more critical and hostile (Bieling & Alden, 1998; Lynch et al., 2003; Mongrain et al., 1998, 2004; Whiffen & Aube, 1999; Zuroff & Duncan, 1999). In addition, self-critical/autonomous individuals appear to exaggerate negative perceptions by others in that they think that others perceive them more negatively than is actually the case (Fichman et al., 1996, 1997). Thus, in sum, dependent/sociotropic individuals tend to show a positive, idealizing bias in their perceptions of their relationships, risking future disillusionment, while self-critical/autonomous individuals tend to show a negative bias in their perceptions of their relationships and in how they are perceived by others. These findings are congruent with Blatt's (Blatt & Shichman, 1983) proposition that Dependency is associated with the use of avoidant defense mechanisms, such as denial, whereas Self-Critical Perfectionism is characterized by a harsh, judgmental, internalizing stance.

Transformation. Empirical research has also yielded considerable support for Blatt's (Blatt & Zuroff, 1992) and Beck's (1983) prediction that dependent and perfectionistic subjects *actively influence and transform* their own environment. Santor and Zuroff (1997, 1998), for instance, found in two experimental studies that highly dependent/sociotropic women reacted to a situation threatening interpersonal relatedness by trying to maintain interpersonal contact, relinquishing control over the situation, and minimizing disagreement (e.g., praising friends even when they disagreed), whereas highly self-critical/autonomous women reacted to threats to status by actively trying to control the situation, even at the expense of a close friend. These results have been consistently replicated in other experimental studies in both nonclinical and clinical samples (Bieling & Alden, 1998, 2001; Santor et al., 2000; Vettese & Mongrain, 2000) and by research using self-report questionnaires. Dependent/sociotropic individuals value interpersonal goals at the expense of achievement goals, whereas self-critical/autonomous individuals mainly value achievement goals, at the expense of interpersonal goals (Ewart et al., 1998; Luyten, Fontaine, Soenens, Duriez, & Corveleyn, 2004; Rosenfarb et al., 1994; Mongrain & Zuroff, 1995; Zuroff & deLorimier, 1989; Zuroff, Moskowitz, & Côté, 1999; Zuroff et al., 1983). In addition, as noted earlier, others tend to react in critical, hostile ways to self-critical/autonomous individuals, whereas the clinging relational style of dependent/sociotropic individuals appears to eventually lead to irritation and resentment in others.

To summarize, both Dependency/Sociotropy and Self-Critical Perfectionism/Autonomy appear to be associated with *dysfunctional interpersonal transactional cycles* (Kiesler, 1983, see also Andrews, 1989; Safran, 1990; Wachtel, 1994). Such a cycle implies that one's interpersonal style leads to exactly these behaviors and reactions in others that one fears and attempts to avoid, which in turn confirms one's expectations. Whereas dependent/sociotropic individuals may be able to generate a positive social environment, at the same time they seem to elicit by their claiming, clinging relational style annoyance, resentment, and eventually rejection and abandonment, confirming their underlying fear for rejection and abandonment. Self-critical/autonomous individuals on the other hand are ambivalent, critical and distrustful in relationships because they constantly fear, as well as express, criticism and disapproval. Accordingly, they are perceived by others as cold and distant and are thus less liked by others. Thus, self-critical/autonomous individuals are likely to have not only few, but also very ambivalent relationships, confirming their conviction that others do not like them and criticize and disapprove of them. Moreover, they are unable to generate positive experiences and have also been found to continue to solicit social comparisons, particularly when these comparisons are unfavorable (Santor & Yazbek, 2003), which is likely to further confirm their negative self-views. In addition, as Whiffen and Aube (1999) have shown, complaints and criticism from others, especially from significant others, may lead to elevated levels of Dependency/Sociotropy and Self-Critical Perfectionism/Autonomy, further increasing the risk for the onset, exacerbation or relapse of depression.

The implications of these findings for clinical practice, and especially with regard to the nature of the therapeutic relationship, are readily apparent. As both Blatt (e.g., Blatt, 1974; Blatt et al., 2002) and Beck (1983) emphasize, dependent/sociotropic and self-critical/autonomous individuals not only bring very different needs and expectations into therapy, they will also perceive the therapeutic relationship differently. They construct the therapeutic relationship in congruent ways, so that their initial perceptions and experiences of the therapeutic relationship match their maladaptive beliefs and expectations. Hence, the therapeutic process should involve the identification, articulation and working through of these transference reactions. These and related issues are further discussed in the next section.

Clinical Implications

Impact of Dependency/Sociotropy and Self-Critical Perfectionism/Autonomy on Psychotherapy

Several studies have shown that Dependency/Sociotropy and Self-Critical Perfectionism/Autonomy influence the outcome of psychotherapy for depression. To begin with, Blatt and colleagues have reported several re-analyses of the extensive data from the well-known National Institute of Mental Health (NIMH)-sponsored Treatment of Depression Collaborative Research Program (TDCRP; Elkin, Parloff, Hadley, & Autry, 1985). In this elaborate and extensive randomized clinical trial, 239 depressed outpatients were randomly assigned to three brief treatments for depression, i.e., cognitive-behavioral therapy (CBT), interpersonal therapy (IPT), and medication (imipramine plus clinical management) (IMI-CM), and a placebo control plus clinical management (PLA-CM) condition. Initial analyses revealed few differences in the efficacy of these four treatments (Elkin et al., 1989). However, re-analyses by Blatt and his colleagues of these data showed that pre-treatment Self-Critical Perfectionism/Autonomy predicted poorer outcome in all four conditions on all primary outcome measures, including symptoms, general clinical functioning, and social adjustment, as rated by patients, therapists, and independent clinical evaluators, at termination (16 weeks), as well as at follow-up after 18 months (Blatt, Quinlan, Pilkonis, & Shea, 1995; Blatt, Zuroff, Bondi, Sanislow, & Pilkonis, 1998). Thus, these findings support Blatt's (e.g., Blatt &

Maroudas, 1992) contention that self-critical/autonomous patients do not respond well to short-term, standardized or manual directed therapy.

Further analyses showed that this negative effect of Self-Critical Perfectionism/Autonomy on outcome began to manifest itself primarily in the second half of the treatment (Blatt, Zuroff et al., 1998). Several explanations of this intriguing finding are possible. Self-critical/autonomous patients may in the second half of treatment begin to perceive the impending end of treatment as arbitrary and thus as impeding their sense of control and autonomy. Alternatively, because of their high standards, they may find their degree of therapeutic change insufficient. Yet another possibility is that self-critical/autonomous patients have difficulty in establishing a good therapeutic relationship and become disillusioned in their therapist and treatment in general. Congruent with this latter suggestion, further analyses of the TDCRP revealed that self-critical/autonomous patients showed smaller increases in the therapeutic alliance later in the treatment than other patients, regardless of treatment condition, which in turn predicted worse outcome (Blatt, Zuroff, Quinlan, & Pilkonis, 1996; Zuroff, Blatt, Sotsky, Krupnick, Martin, Sanislow, & Simmens, 2000). Additional analyses (Shahar, Blatt, Zuroff, Krupnick, & Sotsky, 2004) showed that Self-Critical Perfectionism/Autonomy also had a negative impact on social relationships outside treatment, which in turn predicted poorer outcome. Moreover, Self-Critical Perfectionism/Autonomy was also associated with increased vulnerability for (chronic) stress and stress-related increases in interview-assessed depressive symptoms during the 18-month follow-up period (Zuroff & Blatt, 2002). These findings are consistent with findings reviewed earlier concerning the distant, ambivalent interpersonal style of self-critical/autonomous individuals, which appears to further impair their social environment, thus placing them at increased risk for relapse/recurrence. In addition, Shahar, Blatt, Zuroff and Pilkonis (2003) showed that Self-Critical Perfectionism/Autonomy predicted negative outcome even controlled for personality disorders, which have been previously associated with worse outcome in the TDCRP (Shea et al., 1990). Moreover, Self-Critical Perfectionism/Autonomy also predicted poor therapeutic alliance and poor social relationship satisfaction outside treatment, whereas personality disorder features did not.

Blatt and colleagues also tried to identify factors that could mitigate the negative effects of Self-Critical Perfectionism/Autonomy in the TDCRP. They found that perfectionistic patients who had an early positive view of their therapist showed more therapeutic gain. However, this effect was only found for patients with moderate levels of perfectionism (Blatt, Zuroff, Quinlan, & Pilkonis, 1996). Furthermore, Blatt, Sanislow, Zuroff and Pilkonis (1996) reported that effective therapists, irrespective of the type of treatment they provided in the TDCRP, had a more psychological than biological orientation and used more psychotherapy than medical treatment for depression in their general clinical practice. Interestingly, more effective therapists also believed that change would take longer to manifest itself than less effective therapists. Finally, effective therapists also showed less variability in outcome, that is: they seemed to be able to work effectively with most of their patients. These findings are particularly impressive because they occurred in a relatively homogeneous group of highly experienced therapists in three manualized treatments.

Subsequent studies have consistently replicated the finding that Self-Critical Perfectionism/Autonomy negatively affects outcome of brief treatments. Rector, Zuroff and Segal (2000) found that Self-Critical Perfectionism/Autonomy negatively predicted outcome as measured by the Beck Depression Inventory (BDI; Beck & Steer, 1993) in a sample of 51 depressed outpatients treated with CBT. Enns, Cox and Pidlubny (2002) reported that Self-Critical Perfectionism/Autonomy negatively predicted outcome of brief group CBT in a sample of 65 patients with residual depression. Similarly, Enns, Cox and Inayatulla (2003) reported that Self-Critical Perfectionism/Autonomy negatively predicted outcome of inpatient treatment of 78 adolescent suicidal patients, even controlled for neuroticism. Cox, Walker, Enns and Karpinsky (2002), in turn, found that changes in levels of Self-Critical Perfectionism/Autonomy were significantly related to outcome in brief group CBT of 84 patients with generalized social phobia, even controlled for baseline severity of social phobia and depressive symptoms. Cox et al. (2002, p. 489) conclude from these findings that self-critical/autonomous patients "might benefit from treatment augmentation or tailoring".

This latter suggestion was partially addressed in the Riggs-Yale Project, a study of therapeutic change in a sample of 90 seriously disturbed, treatment-resistant psychiatric inpatients that received long-term, intensive psychoanalytically oriented treatment (4 to 5 times a week) (Blatt, Berman, Cook, & Ford, 1998; Blatt & Ford, 1994; Blatt, Ford, Berman, Cook, & Meyer, 1988). In general, it was found that after an average 15 months of intensive treatment, introjective patients demonstrated greater therapeutic gain than anaclitic patients. These findings are consistent with Blatt's suggestion that introjective patients typically need longer, insight-oriented treatment, whereas anaclitic patients may need more structured, supportive treatment. Moreover, both types of patients showed primarily changes in characteristics that were congruent with their dominant personality functioning. For instance, anaclitic patients showed primarily changes in the quality of interpersonal relationships, while introjective patients showed predominantly changes in cognitive functioning. Further evidence for patient-by-treatment interactions were found in re-analyses of another well-known psychotherapy study, the Menninger Psychotherapy Research Project, which compared the effect of psychoanalysis (5 times a week) and psychodynamic supportive-expressive psychotherapy (2-3 times a week). Although in general little differences in outcome were found in this study between psychoanalysis and psychodynamic psychotherapy, re-analyses showed that introjective patients had greater positive change in psychoanalysis than in psychodynamic therapy, while the reverse was found for anaclitic patients (Blatt, 1992; Blatt & Shahar, 2004).

Why would dependent/sociotropic patients benefit relatively more from supportive-expressive psychotherapy and self-critical/autonomous from insight-oriented psychotherapy? According to Blatt (e.g., Blatt & Ford, 1994; see also Beck, 1983), these findings are consistent with his suggestion that dependent/sociotropic might be particularly responsive to interpersonal factors in treatment, whereas self-critical/autonomous may benefit most from interpretation and insight.

117

Three studies have yielded supporting evidence for these assumptions. In another re-analysis of the Riggs-Yale Study, Fertuck, Bucci, Blatt and Ford (2004) found that the extent to which patients were able to articulate their feelings and thoughts predicted improvement in introjective patients, but was negatively associated with improvement in anaclitic patients. However, increased experiences of closeness predicted clinical improvement in anaclitic patients. Hence, anaclitic patients seem to be able to benefit from a good therapeutic alliance, rather than from exploration and insight, while introjective patients appeared to be especially responsive to interpretation and insight. Blatt and Shahar (2004), in turn, sought to identify factors that were responsible for the fact that introjective patients did better in psychoanalysis, while anaclitic patients showed more improvement in supportive-expressive psychotherapy in the Menninger Psychotherapy Research Project. They found that psychoanalysis was associated with increases in associational activity, whereas supportive-expressive psychotherapy led to decreased associational activity. Again, these findings suggest that introjective patients appear to benefit from insight, anaclitic patients from the therapeutic relationship. Piper, Joyce, McCallum, Azim and Ogrodniczuk (2001) reported similar findings. These investigators randomized 114 mixed psychiatric outpatients to either 20 weeks of manualized psychodynamically-oriented supportive or interpretive psychotherapy. Patients with higher quality of object relations fared better in interpretive therapy compared to those with lower levels of object relations. In addition, a relatively high frequency of transference interpretations predicted poorer outcome and a more negative therapeutic alliance in patients with low quality of object relations. These findings are consistent with Blatt's (1974) notion that patients with relatively high levels of object relations such as introjective patients fare better in interpretive psychotherapy, whereas those with lower quality of object relations such as anaclitic patients do not respond well to a highly interpretive approach, but benefit more from a supportive relationship. Together, these findings suggest that introjective patients, despite considerable problems in interpersonal relationships, are able to benefit from insight in the context of a therapeutic relationship that had sufficient time to develop. In contrast, anaclitic patients, perhaps because of the symbiotic-like quality of their relationships and the fact that they are less able to reflect on and articulate their feelings, might focus on the therapeutic relationship as such, and are therefore less capable to benefit from insight in psychotherapy. Hence, future research should investigate the relationship between the anaclitic-introjective distinction and the capacity for mentalization (Fonagy, Gergely, Jurist, & Target, 2002).

Research inspired by Beck's (1983) formulations adds further support for the influence of Dependency/Sociotropy and Self-Critical Perfectionism/Autonomy on psychosocial treatments. Zettle, Haflich and Reynolds (1992), for instance, reported that highly dependent/sociotropic depressed patients responded better to group CBT, while highly self-critical/autonomous patients showed more improvement in individual CBT, which is consistent with Blatt's and Beck's predictions that dependent/sociotropic patients benefit more from relational aspects (e.g., social support) and self-critical/autonomous patients from an individual, insight-oriented approach. Yet, in a similar study, Zettle and Herring (1995) found that depressed patients that received "matched" treatment (e.g., individual therapy for highly self-critical/autonomous patients) showed similar levels of severity of depression after treatment. However, at follow-up after two months, remission rates were significantly lower for "matched" patients. Kuyken, Kurzer, DeRubeis, Beck and Brown (2001), finally, reported that avoidant and paranoid beliefs (belonging to the introjective/autonomous cluster; Beck, 1999; Blatt & Shichman, 1983), but not dependent beliefs (that belong to the anaclitic/sociotropic cluster), negatively predicted outcome in CBT of 162 depressed outpatients.

In summary, self-critical/autonomous patients apparently require a substantial period of time and more intensive contact before they can establish an effective therapeutic relationship and can begin to change their harsh, overly self-critical views. In the long-term, however, these patients can make substantial therapeutic progress (Blatt & Ford, 1994; Blatt & Shahar, 2004). Dependent/sociotropic patients on the other hand, can more easily establish a therapeutic relationship and seem to benefit most, at least in the initial phases of treatment, but perhaps also during later stages of treatment, from interpersonal aspects of treatment and appear not to be as responsive to interpretation and insight.

Impact of Dependency/Sociotropy and Self-Critical Perfectionism/Autonomy on Pharmacotherapy of Depression

Few studies have systematically investigated the impact of Dependency/Sociotropy and Self-Critical Perfectionism/Autonomy on pharmacological treatment. In line with Beck's (1983) predictions, Peselow, Robins, Sanfilipo, Block and Fieve (1992) found in a study of 217 depressed outpatients that Dependency/Sociotropy negatively predicted outcome of antidepressant treatment, whereas Self-Critical Perfectionism/Autonomy was associated with good antidepressant response. In addition, highly self-critical/autonomous low dependent/sociotropic patients showed a significant better response to antidepressant drug treatment (74%) than placebo (25%) and than did highly dependent/sociotropic low self-critical/ autonomous patients (39%). Furthermore, this latter group showed no significant drug-placebo difference (39% versus 32%). In line with Beck's (1983) predictions, 91% of high self-critical/autonomous low dependent/sociotropic patients in their sample met Research Diagnostic Criteria (RDC; Spitzer, Endicott, & Robins, 1978) for endogenous depression as opposed to only 20% in the high dependent/ sociotropic low self-critical/autonomous group. Rector et al. (2000), however, found that Self-Critical Perfectionism/Autonomy was unrelated to pharmacothera-py outcome as measured by the BDI in a study of 58 depressed outpatients, while Blatt, Quinlan et al. (1995) found that pre-treatment Self-Critical Perfectionism/ Autonomy was a negative predictor of pharmacological treatment in the NIMH TDRCP.

There are a number of possible explanations for these divergent findings, including differences in the samples employed and/or different antidepressant

119

regimes. Interestingly, Scott (2001, cited in Flett & Hewitt, 2002) reported that Self-Critical Perfectionism/Autonomy was associated with several variables that predicted nonadherence to medication, which is consistent with Blatt's and Beck's views that these patients are pessimistic about professional help because of conscious and unconscious self-destructive tendencies (Blatt, 1995). Moreover, these patients might perceive the antidepressant treatment regime as undermining their need for personal control. Hence, their tendency for nonadherence could in part explain why Self-Critical Perfectionism/Autonomy could have a negative impact on outcome of pharmacological treatment (see also Demyttenaere, 1997). Thus, it is somewhat paradoxically that these patients respond well to pharmacotherapy as reported by Peselow et al. (1992).

Results for Dependency/Sociotropy have been somewhat more consistent. Bothwell and Scott (1997) reported that Dependency/Sociotropy predicted non-recovery in a 2-year follow-up study of depressed patients treated with antidepressant medication. Similarly, as Peselow et al. (1992), Frank, Kupfer, Jacob and Jarrett (1987) found that dependent patients were less responsive to pharmacotherapy. In line with these findings, several studies have found that Reward Dependency and Harm Avoidance, two dimensions in Cloninger's (Cloninger, Svrakic, & Przbybeck, 1993) psychobiological theory of temperament and personality, which are conceptually related to Blatt's and Beck's notions of Dependency/Sociotropy, negatively predicted pharmacological treatment, although some recent studies have failed to replicate these findings (Mulder, 2002).

Regarding the effect of pharmacotherapy on personality, in at least five studies of depressed patients it was found that brief pharmacological treatment did not significantly alter levels of both Dependency/Sociotropy and Self-Critical Perfectionism/Autonomy (Bagby et al., 1994, 2001; Franche & Dobson, 1992; Moore & Blackburn, 1996; Reda, Carpiniello, Secchariollo, & Blanco, 1985). Rector et al. (2000), however, reported that a 12-week antidepressant trial in a sample of 58 depressed outpatients led to significant decreases in levels of Dependency/Sociotropy and Self-Critical Perfectionism/Autonomy. Similarly, Hellerstein, Kocsis, Chapman, Stewart and Harrison (2000) reported that pharma-cological treatment resulted in a significant drop in levels of Harm Avoidance and Reward Dependence. As these two latter studies lack a control group of non-depressed and never-depressed individuals, these results are difficult to interpret. Moreover, as previously noted, one should be careful to draw any conclusions from such studies because measures of Dependency/Sociotropy and Self-Critical Perfectionism/Autonomy contain both state and trait elements (Zuroff et al., 1999). Moreover, whereas brief treatment may result in the (partial) deactivation of maladaptive cognitions and affects associated with these personality dimensions (e.g., Rector et al., 2000), as the data from the TDCRP (Zuroff et al., 1999) and priming studies (Segal & Ingram, 1994) suggest, Dependency/Sociotropy and Self-Critical Perfectionism/Autonomy may in fact show high levels of relative stability and may easily be re-activated. Hence, long-term follow-up is essential to measure the true efficacy of any treatment, pharmacological or psychosocial.

At the same time, it is clear that further research is needed concerning the relationship between these personality dimensions and pharmacological treatment.

On a theoretical note, these studies could play an important role in the integration of biological and psychological theories of depression. As noted in Chapter 3, both Blatt and Beck have speculated on the biological origins of Dependency/Sociotropy and Self-Critical Perfectionism/Autonomy (Beck, 1983; Blatt, Cornell, & Eshkol, 1993), and Cloninger et al. (1993) have proposed that Harm Avoidance and Reward Dependence are associated with serotonine and norepinephrine functioning respectively. From a clinical point of view, future studies exploring the relationship between personality and antidepressant response thus might also enable better matching of patients to specific pharmacological treatments (Mulder, 2002).

Treatment Implications

Several treatment strategies have been developed to treat Dependency/Socio-tropy and/or Self-Critical Perfectionism/Autonomy based on various theoretical perspectives, including behavioral and cognitive-behavioral (Beck, 1983; Di Bartolo, Frost, Dixon, & Almodovar, 2001; Ferguson & Rodway, 1994; Hirsch & Hayward, 1998), psychodynamic (Arieti & Bemporad, 1978; Blatt, 2004; Bowlby, 1980; Fredtoft, Poulsen, Bauer, & Malm, 1996), and integrative (Barrow & Moore, 1983; Halgin & Leahy, 1989) perspectives. Unfortunately, at present little is known about the efficacy of these specific treatments.

Studies so far suggest the following preliminary conclusions and guidelines. First, a growing research literature suggests that patient characteristics such as Dependency/Sociotropy and Self-Critical Perfectionism/Autonomy are important predictors of therapeutic outcome in the treatment of depression, regardless of therapeutic orientation, and should therefore be an important consideration in treatment planning. In addition, brief pharmacologic and psychotherapeutic treatments of depression appear to be relatively ineffective in altering both personality dimensions (Zuroff & Blatt, 2002). Self-Critical Perfectionism/ Autonomy appears to exert a particularly negative influence on outcome. This conclusion is further supported by the fact that pre-treatment Self-Critical Perfectionism/Autonomy in the NIMH TDCRP was associated with the opinion of independent clinical evaluators at termination and at follow-up that patients needed further treatment as well as with these patients's own dissatisfaction with their treatment (Blatt, Quinlan et al., 1995). Thus, treatments of depression that do not address personality issues might leave these vulnerabilities, which have both direct and indirect (e.g., through life stress) effects on depression, unaltered (Daley et al., 1998; Blatt & Zuroff, 2004).

Moreover, whereas dependent/sociotropic patients might initially respond better to brief (psychosocial) treatments, studies reviewed suggest that this initial response might be based more on positive transference feelings associated with these individuals tendency to feel relieved once they have the feeling that they are being helped, rather than by presumed neurobiological effects of antidepressants or specific psychotherapeutic techniques. This might also explain in part the high relapse rates after brief treatment of depression (Westen & Morrison, 2001). One possible explanation that deserves further investigation is that dependent/socio-tropic patients, in such brief treatments, establish a new and idealizing dependent relationship, which initially ameliorates their symptoms (e.g., see Arieti & Bemporad, 1978), what in psychoanalysis has been discussed as a transference cure. However, once this therapeutic relationship ends or becomes more negative (e.g., because of alliance ruptures), treatment effects may disappear. Future research should investigate this suggestion, and should moreover be aimed at identifying which patients benefit most from which forms of psychotherapy, or which aspects of the therapeutic process. For instance, future research should explore the possibility that dependent/sociotropic and self-critical/autonomous patients may benefit considerably from brief interventions that are specifically tailored to the needs and expectations of these patients. In fact, studies have found that although Self-Critical Perfectionism/Autonomy negatively predicts outcome in brief treatments, changes in Self-Critical Perfectionism/Autonomy predicted better outcome (Enns et al., 2002; Rector et al., 2000). In other words, the extent to which these brief treatments were able to modify levels of Self-Critical Perfectionism/ Autonomy was associated with better outcome. Similarly, future studies should identify depressed patients that typically need longer treatment. Another direction for future research is to examine how typical transference and countertransference issues associated with Dependency/Sociotropy and Self-Critical Perfectionism/ Autonomy emerge and are modified in the therapeutic relationship.

A second implication of the findings reviewed is that common factors such as therapist characteristics (e.g., empathy) and relationship factors (e.g., therapeutic alliance) are important predictors of therapeutic success in the treatment of depression, regardless of theoretical orientation (Blatt, Zuroff et al., 1996; Burns & Nolen-Hoeksema, 1992; Horvath & Symonds, 1991; Krupnick et al., 1996; Wampold, 1997). These are not isolated findings. In fact, Lambert and Barley (2002) estimated that specific techniques account for only approximately 15% in therapeutic outcome, whereas common factors explain about 30% in therapeutic change. Findings from the NIMH TDCRP are particularly informative in this context. While very few mode-specific effects were found for CBT and IPT, patient, therapist and interpersonal relationship factors did predict outcome, regardless of specific techniques (Blatt, Zuroff et al., 1996, 1998; Imber et al., 1990). In addition, as hypothesized by psychodynamic (e.g., Freud, 1912/1958), experiential (Rogers, 1957), and cognitive-behavioral (Beck, Rush, Shaw, & Emery, 1979) theorists, common factors such as a good therapeutic alliance appear to be an essential if not necessary condition for specific techniques to be effective across various forms of treatment (e.g., Division 29 Task Force on Empirically Supported Therapy Relationships, 2002; Gaston, Thompson, Gallagher, Cournoyer, & Gagnon, 1998; Rector et al., 1999). A "good-enough" therapeutic relationship seems to be the foundation on which specific techniques can exert their influence.

Thus, in our view it is time that patient and therapist characteristics are included in the assessment, treatment planning and actual treatment of depression. To those who are familiar with psychotherapy research, existing guidelines for the treatment of depression clearly underestimate, to say the least, the importance of patient and therapist factors, and overestimate the importance of specific techniques (Blatt & Zuroff, 2004). In addition, existing guidelines (e.g., American Psychiatric Association, 2000) incorrectly view patients in an undifferentiated way, expecting them to be uniformly responsive to different pharmacological and psychosocial treatments (Lambert & Ogles, 2004). Although the research literature just reviewed clearly has its limitations, the almost complete neglect of patient and therapist characteristics in these guidelines appears no longer warranted in the light of existing research (for similar opinions, see Beutler, Clarkin, & Bongar, 2000; Blatt & Zuroff, 2004; Division 29 Task Force on Empirically Supported Therapy Relationships, 2002; Lambert & Ogles, 2004; Lutz, 2002; Piper et al., 2001).

Conclusions and Directions for Future Research

Almost three decades of research have led to considerable integration among psychodynamic and cognitive-behavioral theories of depression and have found considerable support for these formulations. Both perspectives clearly have mutually influenced and enriched each other (Robins, 1993). Now, the time seems ripe to bridge the gap between these two psychosocial approaches and biological approaches of depression. In this chapter, we suggested several possibilities for such integration in various areas, including the biological determinants of temperament and personality (Cloninger et al., 1994; Woodside et al., 2002), the relationship between neurobiological responses to stress and personality (see also Chapter 8, this volume), and the influence of personality on the effects of pharmacotherapy.

To conclude, we are confident that the coming years will continue to see a growing number of studies concerning the role of Dependency/Sociotropy and Self-Critical Perfectionism/Autonomy in the etiology, pathogenesis, and treatment of depression. These studies will undoubtedly lead to modifications in both Blatt's and Beck's conceptualizations. These modifications are only natural, however, and are the essence of the development of scientific theories and investigations that enable us to achieve a greater understanding of depression that more closely matches the complexities of clinical reality.

References

Alden, L. E., & Bieling, P. J. (1996). Interpersonal convergence of personality constructs in dynamic and cognitive models of depression. *Journal of Research in Personality, 30,* 60-75.
Alford, B. A., & Gerrity, D. M. (1995). The specificity of sociotropy-autonomy personality dimensions to

depression vs. anxiety. *Journal of Clinical Psychology, 51*, 190-195.

Allen, N. B., Horne, D. J., & Trinder, J. (1996). Sociotropy, autonomy, and dysphoric emotional responses to specific classes of stress: A psychophysiological evaluation. *Journal of Abnormal Psychology, 105*, 25-33.

American Psychiatric Association (2000). *Practice guidelines for the treatment of patients with major depression.* Retrieved September 3, 2004, from
http://www.psych.org/psych_pract/treatg/pg/Depression2e.book.cfm

Andrews, J. D. W. (1989). Psychotherapy of depression: A self-confirmation model. *Psychological Review, 96*, 576-607.

Arieti, S., & Bemporad, J. (1978). *Psychotherapy of severe and mild depression.* Northvale/London: Jason Aronson.

Aube, J., & Whiffen, V. E. (1996). Depressive styles and social acuity: Further evidence for distinct interpersonal correlates of dependency and self-criticism. *Communication Research, 23*, 407-424.

Bagby, R. M., Gilchrist, E. J., Rector, N. A., Dickens, S. E., Joffe, R. T., Levitt, A., Levitan, R. D., & Kennedy, S. H. (2001). The stability and validity of the sociotropy and autonomy personality dimensions as measures by the Revised Personal Style Inventory. *Cognitive Therapy and Research, 25*, 765-779.

Bagby, R. M., Parker, J. D. A., Joffe, R. T., & Buis, T. (1994). Reconstruction and validation of the Depressive Experiences Questionnaire. *Assessment, 1*, 59-68.

Bagby, R. M., Parker, J. D. A., Joffe, R. T., Schuller, D., & Gilchrist, E. (1998). Confirmatory factor analysis of the revised Personal Style Inventory (PSI). *Assessment, 5*, 31-43.

Bagby, R. M., Schuller, D. R., Parker, J. D. A., Levitt, A., Joffe, R. T., & Shafir, M. S. (1994). Major depression and the self-criticism and dependency personality dimensions. *American Journal of Psychiatry, 151*, 597-599.

Barnett, P. A., & Gotlib, I. H. (1988). Psychosocial functioning and depression: Distinguishing among antecedents, concomitants, and consequences. *Psychological Bulletin, 104*, 97-126.

Baron, R. M., & Kenny, D. A. (1986). The moderator-mediator variable distinction in social psychological research: Conceptual, strategic, and statistical considerations. *Journal of Personality and Social Psychology, 41*, 1173-1182.

Barrow, J. C., & Moore, C. A. (1983). Group interventions with perfectionist thinking. *The Personnel and Guidance Journal, 61*, 612-615.

Bartelstone, J. H., & Trull, T. J. (1995). Personality, life events, and depression. *Journal of Personality Assessment, 64*, 279-294.

Beck, A. T. (1983). Cognitive therapy of depression: New perspectives. In P. J. Clayton & J. E. Barrett (Eds.), *Treatment of depression: Old controversies and new approaches* (pp. 265-290). New York: Raven Press.

Beck, A. T. (1999). Cognitive aspects of personality disorders and their relation to syndromal disorders: A psychoevolutionary approach. In C. R. Cloninger (Ed.), *Personality and psychopathology* (pp. 411-429). Washington, DC/London: American Psychiatric Press.

Beck, A. T., Epstein, N., Harrison, R. P., & Emery, G. (1983). *Development of the Sociotropy-Autonomy Scale: A measure of personality factors in psychopathology.* Unpublished manuscript, University of Pennsylvania, Philadelphia.

Beck, A. T., Rush, A. J., Shaw, B. F., & Emery, G. (1979). *Cognitive therapy of depression.* New York: The Guilford Press.

Beck, A. T., & Steer, R. A. (1993). *Beck Depression Inventory Manual.* San Antonio, TX: The Psychological Corporation.

Beck, R., Robbins, M., Taylor, C., & Baker, L. (2001). An examination of sociotropy and excessive reassurance seeking in the prediction of depression. *Journal of Psychopathology and Behavioral Assessment, 23*, 101-104.

Besser, A., Flett, G. L., & Davis, R. A. (2003). Self-Criticism, dependency, silencing the self, and loneliness: A test of a mediational model. *Personality and Individual Differences, 35*, 1735-1752.

Besser, A., & Priel, B. (2003). Trait vulnerability and coping strategies in the transition to motherhood. *Current Psychology: Developmental, Learning, Personality, Social, 22*, 57-72.

Beutler, L. E., Clarkin, J. F., & Bongar, B. (2000). *Guidelines for the systematic treatment of the depressed patient.* New York/Oxford: Oxford University Press.

Bieling, P. J., & Alden, L. E. (1998). Cognitive-interpersonal patterns in dysphoria: The impact of sociotropy and autonomy. *Cognitive Therapy and Research, 22*, 161-178.

124

Bieling, P. J., & Alden, L. E. (2001). Sociotropy, Autonomy, and the interpersonal model of depression: An integration. *Cognitive Therapy and Research*, *25*, 167-184.

Bieling, P. J., Beck, A. T., & Brown, G. K. (2000). The Sociotropy-Autonomy Scale: Structure and implications. *Cognitive Therapy and Research*, *24*, 763-780.

Bieling, P. J., Israeli, A. L., & Antony, M. M. (2004). Is perfectionism good, bad, or both? Examining models of the perfectionism construct. *Personality and Individual Differences*, *36*, 1373-1385.

Blaney, P. H. (2002). Stress and depression: A personality/situation interaction approach. In S. L. Johnson, A. M. Hayes, T. Field, P. McCabe, & N. Schneidermann (Eds.), *Stress, coping, and depression* (pp. 89-116). Mahwah, NJ: Erlbaum.

Blaney, P. H., & Kutcher, G. S. (1991). Measures of depressive dimensions: Are they interchangeable? *Journal of Personality Assessment*, *56*, 502-512.

Blatt, S. J. (1974). Levels of object representation in anaclitic and introjective depression. *The Psychoanalytic Study of the Child*, *29*, 107-157.

Blatt, S. J. (1992). The differential effect of psychotherapy and psychoanalysis with anaclitic and introjective patients: The Menninger psychotherapy research project revisited. *Journal of the American Psychoanalytic Association*, *40*, 691-724.

Blatt, S. J. (1995). The destructiveness of perfectionism. Implications for the treatment of depression. *American Psychologist*, *50*, 1003-1020.

Blatt, S. J. (1998). Contributions of psychoanalysis to the understanding and treatment of depression. *Journal of the American Psychoanalytic Association*, *46*, 722-752.

Blatt, S. J. (2004). *Experiences of depression: Theoretical, clinical and research perspectives*. Washington, DC: American Psychological Association.

Blatt, S. J., Berman, W. H., Cook, B. P., & Ford, R. Q. (1998). Effectiveness of long-term, intensive, inpatient treatment for seriously disturbed young adults: A reply to Bein. *Psychotherapy Research*, *8*, 42-53.

Blatt, S. J., Cornell, C. E., & Eshkol, E. (1993). Personality style, differential vulnerability and clinical course in immunological and cardiovascular disease. *Clinical Psychology Review*, *13*, 421-450.

Blatt, S. J., D'Afflitti, J. P., & Quinlan, D. M. (1976). Experiences of depression in normal young adults. *Journal of Abnormal Psychology*, *85*, 383-389.

Blatt, S. J., & Ford, R. Q. (1994). *Therapeutic change. An object relations perspective*. New York/London: Plenum Press.

Blatt, S. J., Ford, R. Q., Berman, W., Cook, B., & Meyer, R. (1988). The assessment of therapeutic change in schizophrenic and borderline young adults. *Psychoanalytic Psychology*, *5*, 127-158.

Blatt, S. J., & Maroudas, C. (1992). Convergence among psychoanalytic and cognitive-behavioral theories of depression. *Psychoanalytic Psychology*, *9*, 157-190.

Blatt, S. J., Quinlan, D. M., Chevron, E. S., McDonald, C., & Zuroff, D. (1982). Dependency and self-criticism: Psychological dimensions of depression. *Journal of Consulting and Clinical Psychology*, *50*, 113-124.

Blatt, S. J., Quinlan, D. M., Pilkonis, P. A., & Shea, M. T. (1995). Impact of perfectionism and need for approval on the brief treatment of depression: The National Institute of Mental Health Treatment of Depression Collaborative Research Program revisited. *Journal of Consulting and Clinical Psychology*, *63*, 125-132.

Blatt, S. J., Sanislow, C. A., Zuroff, D. C., & Pilkonis, P. A. (1996). Characteristics of effective therapists: Further analyses of data from the NIMH TDCRP. *Journal of Consulting and Clinical Psychology*, *63*, 125-132.

Blatt, S. J., Schaffer, C. E., Bers, S. A., & Quinlan, D. M. (1992). Psychometric properties of the Depressive Experiences Questionnaire for adolescents. *Journal of Personality Assessment*, *59*, 82-98.

Blatt, S. J., & Shahar, G. (2004). Psychoanalysis: With whom, for what, and how? Comparisons with psychotherapy. *Journal of the American Psychoanalytic Association*, *52*, 393-447.

Blatt, S. J., Shahar, G., & Zuroff, D. C. (2002). Anaclitic/Sociotropic and Introjective/Autonomous dimensions. In J. C. Norcross (Ed.), *Psychotherapy relationships that work. Therapist contributions and responsiveness to patients* (pp. 315-333). Oxford: Oxford University Press.

Blatt, S. J., & Shichman, S. (1983). Two primary configurations of psychopathology. *Psychoanalysis and Contemporary Thought*, *6*, 187-254.

Blatt, S. J., & Zuroff, D. C. (1992). Interpersonal relatedness and self-definition: Two prototypes for depression. *Clinical Psychology Review*, *12*, 527-562.

Blatt, S. J., & Zuroff, D. C. (2004). *Empirical evaluation of the assumptions in identifying evidence-based treatments in mental health*. Manuscript submitted for publication.

Blatt, S. J., Zuroff, D. C., Bondi, C. M., Sanislow, C. A., & Pilkonis, P. A. (1998). When and how perfectionism impedes the brief treatment of depression: Further analyses of The National Institute of Mental Health Treatment of Depression Collaborative Research Program. *Journal of Consulting and Clinical Psychology, 66*, 423-428.

Blatt, S. J., Zuroff, D. C., Quinlan, D. M., & Pilkonis, P. A. (1996). Interpersonal factors in brief treatment of depression: Further analyses of The National Institute of Mental Health Treatment of Depression Collaborative Research Program. *Journal of Consulting and Clinical Psychology, 64*, 162-171.

Bornstein, R. F. (1992). The dependent personality: Developmental, social, and clinical perspectives. *Psychological Bulletin, 112*, 3-23.

Bothwell, R., & Scott, J. (1997). The influence of cognitive variables on recovery in depressed inpatients. *Journal of Affective Disorders, 43*, 207-212.

Bowlby, J. (1980). *Attachment and loss Vol. 3 Loss: Sadness and depression*. London: The Hogarth Press.

Boyce, P., Parker, G., Barnett, S., Cooney, M., & Smith, F. (1991). Personality as a vulnerability factor to depression. *British Journal of Psychiatry, 159*, 106-114.

Brewin, C. R., & Firth-Cozens, J. (1997). Dependency and self-criticism as predictors of depression in young doctors. *Journal of Occupational Health Psychology, 2*, 242-246.

Brown, G. P., Hammen, C. L., Craske, M. G., & Wickens, T. D. (1995). Dimensions of dysfunctional attitudes as vulnerabilities to depressive symptoms. *Journal of Abnormal Psychology, 104*, 431-435.

Brown, G. W., & Harris, T. O. (1978). *Social origins of depression*. Routledge: London.

Burgess, E., Lorah, D., Haaga, D. A. F., & Chrousos, G. (1996). Sociotropy, Autonomy, stress, and depression in Cushing Syndrome. *Journal of Nervous and Mental Disease, 184*, 362-367.

Burns, D. D., & Nolen-Hoeksema, S. (1992). Therapeutic empathy and recovery from depression in cognitive-behavioral therapy: A structural equation model. *Journal of Consulting and Clinical Psychology, 60*, 441-449.

Buss, D. M. (1987). Selection, evocation, and manipulation. *Journal of Personality and Social Psychology, 53*, 1214-1221.

Cane, D. B., Olinger, L. J., Gotlib, I. H., & Kuiper, N. A. (1986). Factor stucture of the Dysfunctional Attitude Scale in a student population. *Journal of Clinical Psychology, 42*, 307-309.

Chang, E. C. (2000). Perfectionism as a predictor of positive and negative psychological outcomes: Examining a mediation model in younger and older adults. *Journal of Counseling Psychology, 47*, 18-26.

Chang, E. C., & Rand, K. L. (2000). Perfectionism as a predictor of subsequent adjustment: Evidence for a specific diathesis-stress mechanism among younger and older adults. *Journal of Counseling Psychology, 47*, 129-137.

Clark, D. A., & Beck, A. T. (1991). Personality factors in dysphoria: A psychometric refinement of Beck's Sociotropy-Autonomy Scale. *Journal of Psychopathology and Behavioral Assessment, 13*, 369-388.

Clark, D. A., & Beck, A. T. (1999). *Scientific foundations of cognitive theory and therapy of depression*. New York: John Wiley & Sons.

Clark, D. A., Beck, A. T., & Brown, G. K. (1992). Sociotropy, autonomy, and life event perceptions in dysphoric and nondysphoric individuals. *Cognitive Therapy and Research, 16*, 635-652.

Clark, D. A., & Oates, T. (1995). Dailey hassles, major and minor life events and their interaction with sociotropy and autonomy. *Behaviour Research and Therapy, 33*, 819-823.

Clark, D. A., Steer, R. A., Beck, A. T., & Ross, L. (1995). Psychometric properties of revised sociotropy and autonomy scales in college students. *Behaviour Research and Therapy, 33*, 325-334.

Cloninger, C. R., Svrakic, D. K., & Przbybeck, T. R. (1993). A psychobiological model of temperament and character. *Archives of General Psychiatry, 50*, 975-990.

Cohen, J. (1988). *Statistical power analysis for the behavioral sciences* (2nd ed.). Hillsdale, NJ: Erlbaum.

Cohen, S., & Wills, T. A. (1985). Stress, social support, and the buffering hypothesis. *Psychological Bulletin, 98*, 310-357.

Connor-Smith, J. K., & Compas, B. E. (2002). Vulnerability to social stress: Coping as a mediator or moderator of sociotropy and symptoms of anxiety and depression. *Cognitive Therapy and Research, 26*, 39-55.

Cox, B. J., & Enns, M. W. (2003). Relative stability of dimensions of perfectionism in depression. *Canadian Journal of Behavioural Science, 35*, 124-132.

Cox, B. J., McWilliams, L. A., Enns, M. W., & Clara, I. P. (2004). Broad and specific personality dimensions associated with major depression in a nationally representative sample. *Comprehensive*

Psychiatry, 45, 246-253.

Cox, B. J., Walker, J. R., Enns, M. W., & Karpinski, D. C. (2002). Self-criticism in generalized social phobia and response to cognitive-behavioral treatment. *Behavior Therapy, 33*, 479-491.

Coyne, J. C., & Whiffen, V. E. (1995). Issues in personality as diathesis for depression: The case of sociotropy-dependency and autonomy-self-criticism. *Psychological Bulletin, 118*, 358-378.

Daley, S. H., Hammen, C., Burge, D., Davila, J., Paley, B., Lundberg, N., & Herzberg, D. S. (1997). Predictors of the generation of episodic stress: A longitudinal study of late adolescent women. *Journal of Abnormal Psychology, 106*, 251-259.

Demyttenaere, K. (1997). Compliance during treatment with antidepressants. *Journal of Affective Disorders, 43*, 27-39.

Di Bartolo, P. M., Frost, R. O., Dixon, A., & Almodovar, S. (2001). Can cognitive restructuring reduce the disruption associated with perfectionistic concerns? *Behavior Therapy, 32*, 167-184.

Dimitrovsky, L., Levy-Schiff, R., & Schattner-Zanany, I. (2002). Dimensions of depression and perfectionism in pregnant and nonpregnant women: Their levels and interrelationsships and their relationship to marital satisfaction. *Journal of Psychology, 136*, 631-646.

Division 29 Task Force on Empirically Supported Therapy Relationships (2002). Conclusions and recommendations of the Division 29 Task Force. In J. C. Norcross (Ed.), *Psychotherapy relationships that work* (pp. 441-443). Oxford: Oxford University Press.

Dozois, D. J. A., & Backs-Dermott, B. J. (2000). Sociotropic personality and information processing following imaginal priming: A test of the congruency hypothesis. *Canadian Journal of Behavioural Science, 32*, 117-126.

Dunkley, D. M., & Blankstein, K. R. (2000). Self-critical perfectionism, coping, hassles, and current distress: A structural equation modeling approach. *Cognitive Therapy and Research, 24*, 713-730.

Dunkley, D. M., Blankstein, K. R., Halsall, J., Williams, M., & Winkworth, G. (2000). The relation between perfectionism and distress: Hassles, coping, and perceived social support as mediators and moderators. *Journal of Counseling Psychology, 47*, 437-453.

Dunkley, D. M., Zuroff, D. C., & Blankstein, K. R. (2003). Self-Critical perfectionism and daily affect: Dispositional and situational influences on stress and coping. *Journal of Personality and Social Psychology, 84*, 234-252.

Elkin, I., Parloff, M. B., Hadley, S. W., & Autry, J. H. (1985). NIMH Treatment of Depression Collaborative Research Program. *Archives of General Psychiatry, 42*, 305-316.

Elkin, I., Shea, M. T., Watkins, J. T., Imber, S. D., Sotsky, S. M., Collins, J. F., Glass, D. R., Pilkonis, P. A., Leber, W. R., Docherty, J. P., Fiester, S. J., & Parloff, M. B. (1989). NIMH treatment of depression collaborative research program: General effectiveness of treatments. *Archives of General Psychiatry, 46*, 971-983.

Enns, M. W., & Cox, B. J. (1999). Perfectionism and depression symptom severity in major depressive disorder. *Behaviour Research and Therapy, 37*, 783-794.

Enns, M. W., Cox, B. J., & Clara, I. (2002). Adaptive and maladaptive perfectionism: Developmental origins and association with depression proneness. *Personality and Individual Differences, 33*, 921-935.

Enns, M. W., Cox, B. J., & Inayatulla, M. (2003). Personality predictors of outcome for adolescents hospitalized for suicidal ideation. *Journal of the American Academy of Child & Adolescent Psychiatry, 42*, 720-727.

Enns, M. W., Cox, B. J., & Pidlubny, S. R. (2002). Group cognitive behaviour therapy for residual depression: Effectiveness and predictors of response. *Cognitive Behaviour Therapy, 31*, 31-40.

Enns, M. W., Cox, B. J., Sareen, J., & Freeman, P. (2001). Adaptive and maladaptive perfectionism in medical students: A longitudinal investigation. *Medical Education, 35*, 1034-1042.

Ewart, C. K., Jorgensen, R. S., & Kolodner, K. B. (1998). Sociotropic cognitions moderates blood pressure response to interpersonal stress in high-risk adolescent girls. *International Journal of Psychophysiology, 28*, 131-142.

Fairbrother, N., & Moretti, M. (1998). Sociotropy, autonomy, and self-discrepancy: Status in depressed, remitted depressed, and control participants. *Cognitive Therapy and Research, 22,* 279-296.

Ferguson, K. L., & Rodway, M. R. (1994). Cognitive behavioral treatment of perfectionism: Initial validation studies. *Research on Social Work & Practice, 4*, 283-308.

Fertuck, E. A., Bucci, W., Blatt, S. J., & Ford, R. Q. (2004). Verbal representation and therapeutic change in anaclitic and introjective patients. *Psychotherapy: Theory, Research, Practice, Training, 41*, 13-25.

Fichman, L., Koestner, R., & Zuroff, D. C. (1994). Depressive styles in adolescence: Assessment, relation to social functioning, and developmental trends. *Journal of Youth and Adolescence, 23*, 315-330.

Fichman, L., Koestner, R., & Zuroff, D. C. (1996). Dependency, self-criticism, and perceptions of inferiority at summer camp: I'm even worse than you think. *Journal of Youth and Adolescence, 25,* 113-126.

Fichman, L., Koestner, R., & Zuroff, D. C. (1997). Dependency and distress at summer camp. *Journal of Youth and Adolescence, 26,* 217-232.

Fichman, L., Koestner, R., Zuroff, D. C., & Gordon, L. (1999). Depressive styles and the regulation of negative affect: A daily experiences study. *Cognitive Therapy and Research, 23,* 483-495.

Flett, G. L., & Hewitt, P. L. (2002). Perfectionism and maladjustment: An overview of theoretical, definitional, and treatment issues. In G. L. Flett & P. L. Hewitt (Eds.), *Perfectionism. Theory, research, and treatment* (pp. 5-31). New York/London: Guilford Press.

Flett, G. L., Hewitt, P. L., Garshowitz, M., & Martin, T. R. (1997). Personality, negative social interactions, and depressive symptoms. *Canadian Journal of Behavioural Science, 29,* 28-37.

Fonagy, P., Gergely, G., Jurist, E, & Target, M. (2002*). Affect regulation, mentalization, and the development of the self.* New York: Other Press.

Franche, R.-L. (2001). Psychologic and obstetric predictors of couples' grief during pregnancy after miscarriage or perinatal death. *Obstetrics & Gynecology, 97,* 597-602.

Franche, R.-L., & Dobson, K. (1992). Self-criticism and interpersonal dependency as vulnerability factors to depression. *Cognitive Therapy and Research, 16* (4), 419-435.

Franche, R.-L., & Mikail, S. F. (1999). The impact of perinatal loss on adjustment to subsequent pregnancy. *Social Science & Medicine, 48,* 1613-1623.

Frank, E., Kupfer, D. J., Jacob, M., & Jarrett, D. (1987). Personality features and response to acute treatment in recurrent depression. *Journal of Personality Disorders, 1,* 14-26.

Frank, S. J., Van Egeren, L. A., Paul, J. S., Poorman, M. O., Sanford, K., Williams, O. B., & Field, D. T. (1997). Measuring self-critical and interpersonal preoccupations in an adolescent inpatient sample. *Psychological Assessment, 9,* 185-195.

Fredhoft, T., Poulsen, S., Bauer, M., & Malm, M. (1996). Dependency and perfectionism: Short term dynamic group psychotherapy for university students. *Psychodynamic Counselling, 24,* 476-497.

Fresco, D. M., Sampson, W. S., Craighead, L. W., & Koons, A. N. (2001). The relationship of sociotropy and autonomy to symptoms of depression and anxiety. *Journal of Cognitive Psychotherapy, 15,* 17-31.

Freud, S. (1958). The dynamics of transference. In J. Strachey (Ed.), *The standard edition of the complete psychological works of Sigmund Freud* (Vol. 12, pp. 99-108). London: Hogarth. (Original work published 1912)

Frost, R. O., Marten, P., Lahart, C. M., & Rosenblate, R. (1991). The dimensions of perfectionism. *Cognitive Therapy and Research, 14,* 449-468.

Gaston, L., Thompson, L., Gallagher, D., Cournoyer, L.-G., & Gagnon, R. (1998). Alliance, technique, and their interactions in predicting outcome of behavioral, cognitive, and brief dynamic therapy. *Psychotherapy Research, 8,* 190-209.

Giordani, C., Wood, J. V., & Michela, J. L. (2000). Depressive personality styles, dysphoria, and social comparisons in everyday life. *Journal of Personality and Social Psychology, 79,* 438-451.

Goldberg, J. O., Segal, Z. V., Vella, D. D., & Shaw, B. F. (1989). Depressive personality: Millon clinical multiaxial inventory profiles of sociotropic and autonomous subtypes. *Journal of Personality Disorders, 3,* 193-198.

Gruen, R. J., Silva, R., Ehrlich, J., Schweitzer, J. W., & Friedhoff, A. J. (1997). Vulnerability to stress: Self-Criticism and stress-induced changes in biochemistry. *Journal of Personality, 65,* 33-47.

Gudleski, G. D., & Shean, G. D. (2000). Depressed and nondepressed students: Differences in interpersonal perceptions. *The Journal of Psychology, 134,* 56-62.

Haaga, D. A. F., Fine, J. A., Terrill, D. R., Stewart, B. L., & Beck, A. T. (1995). Social problem solving deficits, dependency, and depressive symptoms. *Cognitive Therapy and Research, 16,* 409-418.

Halgin, R. P., & Leahy, P. M. (1989). Understanding and treating perfectionistic college students. *Journal of Counseling & Development, 68,* 222-225.

Hammen, C. (1991). Generation of stress in the course of unipolar depression. *Journal of Abnormal Psychology, 100,* 555-561.

Hammen, C., Ellicott, A., & Gitlin, M. (1989). Vulnerability to specific life events and prediction of course of disorder in unipolar depressed patients. *Canadian Journal of Behavioural Science, 21,* 377-388.

Hammen, C., Ellicott, A., & Gitlin, M. (1992). Stressors and sociotropy/autonomy: A longitudinal study of their relationship to the course of bipolar disorder. *Cognitive Therapy and Research, 16,* 409-418.

Hammen, C., Ellicott, A., Gitlin, M., & Jamison (1989). Sociotropy/autonomy and vulnerability to specific life events in patients with unipolar depression and bipolar disorders. *Journal of Abnormal Psychology*, *98*, 154-160.

Hammen, C., & Goodman-Brown, T. (1990). Self-schemas and vulnerability to specific life stress in children at risk for depression. *Cognitive Therapy and Research*, *14*, 215-227.

Hammen, C., Marks, T., deMayo, R., & Mayol, A. (1985). Self-schemas and risk for depression: A prospective study. *Journal of Personality and Social Psychology*, *49*, 1147-1159.

Hammen, C., Marks, T., Mayol, A., & deMayo, R. (1985). Depressive self-schemas, life stress, and vulnerability to depression. *Journal of Abnormal Psychology*, *94*, 308-319.

Haring, M., Hewitt, P. L., & Flett, G. L. (2003). Perfectionism, coping, and quality of intimate relationships. *Journal of Marriage and Family*, *65*, 143-158.

Hartlage, S., Arduino, K., & Alloy, L. B. (1998). Depressive personality characteristics: State dependent concomitants of depressive disorder and traits independent of current depression. *Journal of Abnormal Psychology*, *107*, 349-354.

Hellerstein, D. J., Kocsis, J. H., Chapman, D., Stewart, J. W., & Harrison, W. (2000). Double-blind comparision of sertraline, imipramine, and placebo in the treatment of dysthymia: Effects on personality. *American Journal of Psychiatry*, *157*, 1436-1444.

Hewitt, P. L., & Flett, G. L. (1991). Perfectionism in the self and social contexts: Conceptualization, assessment, and association with psychopathology. *Journal of Personality and Social Psychology*, *60*, 456-470.

Hewitt, P. L., & Flett, G. L. (1993). Dimensions of perfectionism, daily stress, and depression: A test of a specific vulnerability hypothesis. *Journal of Abnormal Psychology*, *102*, 58-65.

Hewitt, P. L., & Flett, G. L. (2002). Perfectionism and stress processes in psychopathology. In G. L. Flett & P. L. Hewitt (Eds.), *Perfectionism. Theory, research, and treatment* (pp. 255-284). New York/London: Guilford Press.

Hewitt, P. L., Flett, G. L., Besser, A., Sherry, S. B., & McGee, B. (2003). Perfectionism is multi-dimensional: A reply to Shafran, Cooper and Fairburn (2002). *Behaviour Research and Therapy*, *41*, 1221-1236.

Hirsch, C. R., & Hayward, P. (1998). The perfect patient: Cognitive behavioral therapy for perfectionism. *Behavioural and Cognitive Psychotherapy*, *26*, 359-364.

Hirschfeld, R. M. A., Klerman, G. L., Gough, H. G., Barrett, J., Korchin, S. J., & Chodoff, P. (1977). A measure of interpersonal dependency. *Journal of Personality Assessment*, *41*, 610-618.

Hirschfeld, R. M. A., Klerman, G. L., Lavori, P., Keller, M. B., Griffith, P., & Coryell, W. (1989). Premorbid personality assessment of first onset of major depression. *Archives of General Psychiatry*, *46*, 345-350.

Hong, S., & Lee, M. K. (2001). Hierarchical confirmatory factor analysis of the revised Personal Style Inventory: Evidence for the multidimensionality problem of perfectionism. *Educational and Psychological Measurement*, *61*, 421-432.

Horvath, A. O., & Symonds, B. D. (1991). Relation between working alliance and outcome in psychotherapy: A meta-analysis. *Journal of Counseling Psychology*, *38*, 139-149.

Imber, S. D., Pilkonis, P. A., Sotsky, S. M., Elkin, I., Watkins, J. T., Collins, J. F., Shea, M. T., Leber, W. R., & Glass, D. R. (1990). Mode-specific effects among three treatments for depression. *Journal of Consulting and Clinical Psychology*, *58*, 352-359.

Kash, K. L., Klein, D. N., & Lara, M. E. (2001). A construct validation study of the Response Styles Questionnaire Rumination Scale in participants with a recent-onset major depressive episode. *Psychological Assessment*, *13*, 375-383.

Kessler, R. C. (1997). The effects of stressful life events on depression. *Annual Review of Psychology*, *48*, 191-214.

Kiesler, D. J. (1983). The 1982 Interpersonal Circle: A taxonomy for complementarity in human transactions. *Psychological Review*, *90*, 185-214.

Klein, D. N. (1989). The Depressive Experiences Questionnaire: A further evaluation. *Journal of Personality Assessment*, *53*, 703-715.

Klein, D. N., Harding, K., Taylor, E. B., & Dickstein, S. (1988). Dependency and self-criticism in depression: Evaluation in a clinical population. *Journal of Abnormal Psychology*, *97*, 399-404.

Klein, D. N., Taylor, E. B., Dickstein, S., & Harding, K. (1988). Primary early-onset dysthymia: Comparison with primary nonbipolar nonchronic major depression on demographic, clinical, familial, personality, and socioenvironmental characteristics and short-term outcome. *Journal of Abnormal*

Psychology, 97, 387-398.

Koestner, R., Zuroff, D. C., & Powers, T. A. (1991). Family origins of adolescent criticism and its continuity into adulthood. *Journal of Abnormal Psychology, 100*, 191-197.

Krupnick, J. L., Sotsky, S. M., Simmens, S., Moyer, J., Elkin, I., Watkins, J. T., & Pilkonis, P. A. (1996). The role of therapeutic alliance in psychotherapy and pharmacotherapy outcome: Findings in the National Institute of Mental Health Treatment of Depression Collaborative Research Program. *Journal of Consulting and Clinical Psychology, 64*, 532-539.

Kurdek, L. A. (2000). The link between sociotropy/autonomy and dimensions of relationship commitment: Evidence from gay and lesbian couples. *Personal Relationships, 7*, 153-164.

Kuyken, W., Kurzer, N., DeRubeis, R. J., Beck, A. T., & Brown, G. K. (2001). Response to cognitive therapy in depression: The role of maladaptive beliefs and personality disorders. *Journal of Consulting and Clinical Psychology, 69*, 560-566.

Kwon, P., Campbell, D. G., Williams, M. G. (2001). Sociotropy and autonomy: Preliminary evidence for construct validity using TAT narratives. *Journal of Personality Assessment, 77*, 128-138.

Kwon, P., & Whisman, M. A. (1998). Sociotropy and autonomy as vulnerabilities to specific life events: Issues in life event categorization. *Cognitive Therapy and Research, 22*, 353-362.

Lakey, B., & Ross, L. T. (1994). Dependency and self-criticism as moderators of interpersonal and achievement stress: The role of initial dysphoria. *Cognitive Therapy and Research, 18*, 581-599.

Lam, D. H., Green, B., Power, M. J., & Checkley, S. (1996). Dependency, matching adversities, length of survival and relapse in major depression. *Journal of Affective Disorders, 37*, 81-90.

Lambert, M. J., & Barley, D. E. (2002). Research summary on the therapeutic relationship and psychotherapy outcome. In J. C. Norcross (Ed.), *Psychotherapy relationships that work* (pp. 17-32). Oxford: Oxford University Press.

Lambert, M. J., & Ogles, B. M. (2004). The efficacy and effectiveness of psychotherapy. In M. J. Lambert (Ed.), *Bergin and Garfield's handbook of psychotherapy and behavior change* (5th ed.) (pp. 139-193). New York: John Wiley & Sons.

Lehman, A. K., Ellis, B., Becker, J., Rosenfarb, I., Devine, R., Khan, A., & Reichler, R. (1997). Personality and depression: A validation study of the Depressive Experiences Questionnaire. *Journal of Personality Assessment, 68*, 197-210.

Little, S. A., & Garber, J. (2000). Interpersonal and achievement orientations and specific stressors predicting depressive and aggressive symptoms in children. *Cognitive Therapy and Research, 24*, 651-670.

Lutz, W. (2002). Patient-focused psychotherapy research and individual treatment progress as a scientific groundwork for an empirically based clinical practice. *Psychotherapy Research, 12*, 251-272.

Luyten, P. (2002). *Normbesef en depressie. Aanzet tot een integratief theoretisch kader en een empirisch onderzoek aan de hand van de depressietheorie van S. J. Blatt* [Personal standards and depression: A theoretical framework and an empirical investigation of S. J. Blatt's theory of depression]. Unpublished doctoral dissertation. University of Leuven, Leuven, Belgium.

Luyten, P., Fontaine, J. R. J., Soenens, B., Duriez, B., & Corveleyn, J. (2004). *What you risk reveals what you value. Depressive personality styles and value priorities.* Manuscript submitted for publication.

Luyten, P., Fontaine, J. R. J., Soenens, B., Meganck, S., Jansen, B., De Grave, C., Corveleyn, J., Maes, F., & Sabbe, B. (2004). *Factor structure, reliability, and content analysis of the Depressive Experiences Questionnaire (DEQ) in students, adults and psychiatric inpatients.* Manuscript submitted for publication.

Luyten, P., Van Houdenhove, B., Cosyns, N., & Vandenbroecke, A. (2004). *Are patients with Chronic Fatigue Syndrome perfectionistic – or were they? A case-control study.* Manuscript submitted for publication.

Lynch, T. R., Robins, C. J., & Morse, J. Q. (2001). Couple functioning in depression: The roles of sociotropy and autonomy. *Journal of Clinical Psychology, 57*, 93-103.

Mazure, C. M., Bruce, M. L., Maciejewski, P. K., & Jacobs, S. C. (2000). Adverse life events and cognitive-personality characteristics in the prediction of major depression and antidepressant response. *American Journal of Psychiatry, 157*, 896-903.

Mazure, C. M., & Maciejewski, P. K. (2003). A model of risk for major depression: Effects of life stress and cognitive style vary by age. *Depression and Anxiety, 17*, 26-33.

Mazure, C. M., Maciejewski, P. K., Jacobs, S. C., & Bruce, M. L. (2002). Stressful life events interacting with cognitive/personality styles to predict late-onset major depression. *American Journal of Geriatric Psychiatry, 10*, 297-304.

Mazure, C. M., Raghavan, C., Maciejewski, P. K., Jacobs, S. C., & Bruce, M. L. (2001). Cognitive personality characteristics as direct predictors of unipolar major depression. *Cognitive Therapy and Research, 25*, 215-225.

McClelland, G., & Judd, C. (1993). Statistical difficulties of detecting interaction and moderator effects. *Psychological Bulletin, 114*, 376-390.

Mongrain, M. (1998). Parental representations and support-seeking behaviors related to dependency and self-criticism. *Journal of Personality, 66*, 151-173.

Mongrain, M., Lubbers, R., & Struthers, W. (2004). The power of love: Mediation of rejection in roommate relationships of dependents and self-critics. *Personality and Social Psychology Bulletin, 30*, 94-105.

Mongrain, M., Vettese, L. C., Shuster, B., & Kendal, N. (1998). Perceptual biases, affect, and behavior in the relationships of dependents and self-critics. *Journal of Personality and Social Psychology, 75*, 230-241.

Mongrain, M., & Zuroff, D. C. (1989). Cognitive vulnerability to depressed affect in dependent and self-critical college women. *Journal of Personality Disorders, 3*, 240-251.

Mongrain, M., & Zuroff, D. C. (1994). Ambivalence over emotional expression and negative life events: Mediators of depressive symptoms in dependent and self-critical individuals. *Personality and Individual Differences, 16*, 447-458.

Mongrain, M., & Zuroff, D. C. (1995). Motivational and affective correlates of dependency and self-criticism. *Personality and Individual Differences, 18*, 347-354.

Monroe, S. M., & Hadjiyannakis, K. (2002). The social environment and depression: Focusing on severe life stress. In I. H. Gotlib & C. L. Hammen (Eds.), *Handbook of depression* (pp. 314-340). New York/London: The Guilford Press.

Moore, R. G., & Blackburn, I-M. (1996). The stability of sociotropy and autonomy in depressed patients undergoing treatment. *Cognitive Therapy and Research, 20*, 69-80.

Morrison, T. L., Urquiza, A. J., & Goodlin-Jones, B. L. (1998). Depressive experiences and romantic relationships in young adulthood. *Psychological Reports, 82*, 339-349.

Morse, J. Q., Robins, C. J., & Gittes-Fox, M. (2002). Sociotropy, autonomy, and personality disorder criteria in psychiatric patients. *Journal of Personality Disorders, 16*, 549-560.

Mulder, R. T. (2002). Personality pathology and treatment outcome in major depression: A review. *American Journal of Psychiatry, 159*, 359-371.

Murphy, B., & Bates, G. W. (1997). Adult attachment style and vulnerability to depression. *Personality and Individual Differences, 22*, 835-844.

Nelson, D. R., Hammen, C., Daley, S. E., Burge, D., & Davila, J. (2001). Sociotropic and autonomous personality styles: Contributions to chronic life stress. *Cognitive Therapy and Research, 25*, 61-76.

Nietzel, M. T., & Harris, M. J. (1990). Relationship of dependency and achievement/autonomy to depression. *Clinical Psychology Review, 10*, 279-297.

Nordahl, H. M., & Stiles, T. C. (2000). The specificity of cognitive personality dimensions in cluster C personality disorders. *Behavioural and Cognitive Psychotherapy, 28*, 235-246.

O'Connor, R. C., & O'Connor, D. B. (2003). Predicting hopelessness and psychological distress: The role of perfectionism and coping. *Journal of Counseling Psychology, 50*, 362-372.

Ouimette, P. C., & Klein, D. N. (1993). Convergence of psychoanalytic and cognitive-behavioral theories of depression: An empirical review and new data on Blatt's and Beck's models. In J. M. Masling & R. F. Bornstein (Eds.), *Psychoanalytic perspectives on psychopathology (Empirical studies of psychoanalytic theories Vol. 4)* (pp. 191-223). Washington, DC: American Psychological Association.

Ouimette, P. C., Klein, D. N., Clark, D. C., & Margolis, E. T. (1992). Personality traits in offspring of parents with unipolar affective disorder: An exploratory study. *Journal of Personality Disorders, 6*, 91-98.

Ouimette, P. C., Klein, D. N., & Pepper, C. M. (1996). Personality traits in the first degree relatives of outpatients with depressive disorders. *Journal of Affective Disorders, 39*, 43-53.

Overholser, J. C., & Freiheit, S. R. (1994). Assessment of interpersonal dependency using the Millon Clinical Multiaxial Inventory-II (MCMI-II) and the Depressive Experiences Questionnaire. *Personality and Individual Differences, 17*, 71-78.

Peselow, E. D., Robins, C. J., Sanfilipo, M. P., Block, P., & Fieve, R. R. (1992). Sociotropy and autonomy: Relationship to antidepressant drug treatment response and endogenous-nonendogenous dichotomy. *Journal of Abnormal Psychology, 101*, 479-486.

Pincus, A. L., & Gurtman, M. B. (1995). The three faces of interpersonal dependency: Structural analyses of self-report dependency measures. *Journal of Personality and Social Psychology, 69*, 744-758.

Piper, W. E., Joyce, A. S., McCallum, M., Azim, H. F., & Ogrodniczuk, J. S. (2001). *Interpretive and supportive psychotherapies: Matching therapy and patient personality*. Washington, DC: American Psychological Association.

Priel, B., & Besser, A. (1999). Vulnerability to postpartum depressive symptomatology: Dependency, self-criticism and the moderating role of antenatal attachment. *Journal of Social and Clinical Psychology, 18*, 240-253.

Priel, B., & Besser, A. (2000). Dependency and self-criticism among first-time mothers: The role of global and specific support. *Journal of Social and Clinical Psychology, 19*, 437-450.

Priel, B., & Shahar, G. (2000). Dependency, self-criticism, social context and distress: Comparing moderating and mediating models. *Personality and Individual Differences, 28*, 515-525.

Raghavan, C., Le, H. N., & Berenbaum, H. (2002). Predicting dysphoria and hostility using the diathesis-stress model of sociotropy and autonomy in a contextualized stress setting. *Cognitive Therapy and Research, 26*, 231-244.

Rector, N. A., Bagby, R. M., Segal, Z. V., Joffe, R. T., & Levitt, A. (2000). Self-criticism and dependency in depressed patients treated with cognitive therapy or pharmacotherapy. *Cognitive Therapy and Research, 24*, 571-584.

Rector, N. A., Zuroff, D. C., & Segal, Z. V. (1999). Cognitive change and the therapeutic alliance: The role of technical and nontechnical factors in cognitive therapy. *Psychotherapy, 36*, 320-328.

Reda, M. A., Carpiniello, B., Secchiaroli, L., & Blanco, S. (1985). Thinking, depression, and antidepressants: Modified and unmodified depressive beliefs during treatment with amitriptyline. *Cognitive Therapy and Research, 9*, 135-143.

Reis, S., & Grenyer, B. F. S. (2002). Pathways to anaclitic and introjective depression. *Psychology and Psychotherapy: Theory, Research and Practice, 75*, 445-459.

Reynolds, S., & Gilbert, P. (1991). Psychological impact of unemployment: Interactive effects of vulnerability and protective factors on depression. *Journal of Counseling Psychology, 38*, 76-84.

Robins, C. J. (1990). Congruence of personality and life events in depression. *Journal of Abnormal Psychology, 99*, 393-397.

Robins, C. J. (1993). Implications of research in the psychopathology of depression for psychotherapy integration. *Journal of Psychotherapy Integration, 3*, 313-330.

Robins, C. J. (1995). Personality-event interaction models of depression. *European Journal of Personality, 9*, 367-378.

Robins, C. J., & Block, P. (1988). Personal vulnerability, life events, and depressive symptoms: A test of a specific interactional model. *Journal of Personality and Social Psychology, 54*, 847-852.

Robins, C. J., Hayes, A. M., Block, P., Kramer, R. J., & Villena, M. (1995). Interpersonal and achievement concerns and the depressive vulnerability and symptom specificity hypotheses: A prospective study. *Cognitive Therapy and Research, 19*, 1-20.

Robins, C. J., Ladd, J., Welkowitz, J., Blaney, P. H., Diaz, R., & Kutcher, G. (1994). The Personal Style Inventory: Preliminary validation studies of new measures of sociotropy and autonomy. *Journal of Psychopathology and Behavioral Assessment, 16*, 277-300.

Rogers, C. R. (1957). The necessary and sufficient conditions of therapeutic personality change. *Journal of Consulting Psychology, 22*, 95-103.

Rosenfarb, I. S., Becker, J., Khan, A., & Mintz, J. (1994). Dependency, self-criticism, and perceptions of socialization experiences. *Journal of Abnormal Psychology, 103*, 669-675.

Rosenfarb, I. S., Becker, J., Khan, A., & Mintz, J. (1998). Dependency and self-criticism in bipolar and unipolar depressed women. *British Journal of Clinical Psychology, 37*, 409-414.

Rude, S. S., & Burnham, B. L. (1993). Do interpersonal and achievement vulnerabilities interact with congruent events to predict depression? Comparison of DEQ, SAS, DAS, and combined scales. *Cognitive Therapy and Research, 17*, 531-548.

Rude, S. S., & Burnham, B. L. (1995). Connectedness and neediness: Factors of the DEQ and SAS dependency scales. *Cognitive Therapy and Research, 19*, 323-340.

Rutter, M., Dunn, J., Plomin, R., Simonoff, E., Pickles, A., Maughan, B., Ormel, J., Meyer, J., & Eaves, L. (1997). Integrating nature and nurture: Implications of person-environment correlations and interactions for developmental psychopathology. *Development and Psychopathology, 9*, 335-364.

Saboonchi, G., & Lundh, L.-G. (2003). Perfectionism, anger, somatic health, and positive affect. *Personality and Individual Differences, 35*, 1585-1599.

Safran, J. D. (1990). Towards a refinement of cognitive therapy in light of interpersonal theory: I. Theory.

Clinical Psychology Review, 10, 87-105.

Sahin, N., Ulusoy, M., & Sahin, N. (1993). Exploring the sociotropy-autonomy dimensions in a sample of Turkish psychiatric inpatients. *Journal of Clinical Psychology, 49*, 751-763.

Sakado, K, Sato, T., Uehara, T., Sakado, M., Kuwabara, H., & Someya, T. (1999). The association between the high interpersonal sensitivity type of personality and a life time history of depression in a sample of employed Japanese adults. *Psychological Medicine, 29*, 1243-1248.

Sanathara, V. A., Gardner, C. O., Prescott, C. A., & Kendler, K. S. (2003). Interpersonal dependence and major depression: Aetiological inter-relationships and gender differences. *Psychological Medicine, 33*, 927-931.

Santor, D. A., & Patterson, R. L. (2003). *Frequency and duration of mood fluctuations: Effects of dependency, self-criticism, and negative events.* Manuscript submitted for publication.

Santor, D. A., Pringle, J. D., & Israeli, A. L. (2000). Enhancing and disrupting cooperative behavior in couples: Effects of dependency and self-criticism following favorable and unfavorable performance feedback. *Cognitive Therapy and Research, 24*, 379-397.

Santor, D. A., & Yazbeck, A. A. (2003). *Soliciting unfavorable social comparisons: Effects of self-criticism.* Manuscript submitted for publication.

Santor, D. A., & Zuroff, D. C. (1997). Interpersonal responses to threats to status and interpersonal relatedness: Effects of dependency and self-criticism. *British Journal of Clinical Psychology, 36*, 521-541.

Santor, D. A., & Zuroff, D. C. (1998). Controlling shared resources: Effects of dependency, self-criticism, and threats to self-worth. *Personality and Individual Differences, 24*, 237-252.

Sato, T., & McCann, D. (1997). Vulnerability factors in depression: The facets of sociotropy and autonomy. *Journal of Psychopathology and Behavioral Assessment, 19*, 41-62.

Sauro, M. D., Jorgensen, R. S., Larson, C. A., Frankowski, J. J., Ewart, C. K., & White, J. (2001). Sociotropic cognition moderates stress-induced cardiovascular responsiveness in college women. *Journal of Behavioral Medicine, 24*, 423-439.

Schachter, E. P., & Zlotogorski, Z. (1995). Self-critical and dependent aspects of loneliness. *Israel Journal of Psychiatry and Related Sciences, 32*, 205-211.

Segal, Z. V., & Ingram, R. E. (1994). Mood priming and construct activation in tests of cognitive vulnerability to unipolar depression. *Clinical Psychology Review, 14*, 663-695.

Segal, Z. V., Shaw, B. F., & Vella, D. D. (1989). Life stress and depression: A test of the congruency hypothesis for life event and depressive subtype. *Canadian Journal of Behavioural Science, 21*, 389-400.

Segal, Z. V., Shaw, B. F., Vella, D. D., & Katz, R. (1992). Cognitive and life stress predictors of relapse in remitted unipolar depressed patients: Test of the congruency hypothesis. *Journal of Abnormal Psychology, 101*, 26-36.

Shafran, R., & Mansell, W. (2001). Perfectionism and psychopathology: A review of research and treatment. *Clinical Psychology Review, 21*, 879-906.

Shahar, G., Blatt, S. J., Zuroff, D. C., & Pilkonis, P. A. (2003). Role of perfectionism and personality disorder features in response to brief treatment for depression. *Journal of Consulting and Clinical Psychology, 71*, 629-633.

Shahar, G., Blatt, S. J., Zuroff, D. C., Krupnick, J. L., & Sotsky, S. M. (2004). Perfectionism impedes social relations and response to brief treatment for depression. *Journal of Social and Clinical Psychology, 23*, 140-154.

Shahar, G., Blatt, S. J., Zuroff, D. C., Kuperminc, G. P., & Leadbeater, B. J. (2004). Reciprocal relations between depressive symptoms and self-criticism (but not dependency) among early adolescent girls (but not boys). *Cognitive Therapy and Research, 28*, 85-103.

Shahar, G., Henrich, C., Blatt, S. J., Ryan, R., & Little, T. D. (2003). Interpersonal relatedness, self-definition, and their motivational orientation during adolescence: A theoretical and empirical integration. *Developmental Psychology, 39*, 470-483.

Shahar, G., Joiner, T. E., Zuroff, D. C., & Blatt, S. J. (2004). Personality, interpersonal behavior, and depression: Co-existence of stress-specific moderating and mediating effects. *Personality and Individual Differences, 36*, 1583-1596.

Shahar, G., & Priel, B. (2003). Active vulnerability, adolescent distress, and the mediating/suppressing role of life events. *Personality and Individual Differences, 35*, 199-218.

Shapiro, J. P. (1988a). Relationships between dimensions of depressive experience and perceptions of the lives of people in general. *Journal of Personality Assessment, 52*, 297-308.

Shapiro, J. P. (1988b). Relationships between dimensions of depressive experience and evaluative beliefs about people in general. *Personality and Social Psychology Bulletin, 14*, 388-400.

Shea, M. T., Pilkonis, P. A., Beckham, E., Collins, J. F., Elkin, I., Sotsky, S. M., & Docherty, J. P. (1990). Personality disorders and treatment outcome in the NIMH Treatment of Depression Collaborative Research Program. *American Journal of Psychiatry, 147*, 711-718.

Sherry, S. B., Hewitt, P. L., Flett, G. L., & Harvey, M. (2003). Perfectionism dimensions, perfectionistic attitudes, dependent attitudes, and depression in psychiatric patients and university students. *Journal of Counseling Psychology, 50*, 373-386.

Simons, A. D., Angell, K. L., Monroe, S. M., & Thase, M. E. (1993). Cognition and life stress in depression: Cognitive factors and the definition, rating, and generation of negative life events. *Journal of Abnormal Psychology, 102*, 584-591.

Smith, T. W., O'Keeffe, J. L., & Jenkins, M. (1988). Dependency and self-criticism: Correlates of depression or moderators of the effects of stressful events? *Journal of Personality Disorders, 2*, 160-169.

Solomon, A., Arnow, B. A., Gotlib, I. H., & Wind, B. (2003). Individualized measurement of irrational beliefs in remitted depressives. *Journal of Clinical Psychology, 59*, 439-455.

Solomon, A., Haaga, D. A. F., Brody, C., Kirk, L., & Friedman, D. G. (1998). Priming irrational beliefs in recovered-depressed people. *Journal of Abnormal Psychology, 107*, 440-449.

Spasojevic, J., & Alloy, L. B. (2001). Rumination as a common mechanism relating depressive risk factors to depression. *Emotion, 1*, 25-37.

Spitzer, R., Endicott, J., & Robins, C. J. (1978). Research Diagnostic Criteria: Rationality and reliability. *Archives of General Psychiatry, 35*, 773-782.

Tennant, C. (2002). Life events, stress and depression: A review of recent findings. *Australian and New Zealand Journal of Psychiatry, 36*, 173-182.

Vettese, L. C., & Mongrain, M. (2000). Communication about the self and partner in relationships of dependents and self-critics. *Cognitive Therapy and Research, 24*, 609-626.

Vogel, P. A., Stiles, T. C., & Nordahl, H. M. (2000). Cognitive personality styles in OCD outpatients compared to depressed outpatients and healthy controls. *Behavioural and Cognitive Psychotherapy, 28*, 247-258.

Voyer, M., & Cappeliez, P. (2002). Congruency between depressogenic schemas and life events for the prediction of depressive relapse in remitted older patients. *Behavioural and Cognitive Psychotherapy, 30*, 165-177.

Wachtel, P. L. (1994). Cyclical processes in personality and psychopathology. *Journal of Abnormal Psychology, 103*, 51-66.

Wampold, B. E. (1997). Methodological problems in identifying efficacious psychotherapies. *Psychotherapy Research, 7*, 21-43.

Westen, D., & Morrison, K. (2001). A multidimensional meta-analysis of treatments for depression, panic, and generalized anxiety disorder: An empirical examination of the status of empirically supported therapies. *Journal of Consulting and Clinical Psychology, 69*, 875-899.

Whiffen, V. E., & Aube, J. A. (1999). Personality, interpersonal context and depression in couples. *Journal of Social and Personal Relationships, 16*, 369-383.

Whiffen, V. E., Aubé, J. A., Thompson, J. M., & Campbell, T. L. (2000). Attachment beliefs and interpersonal contexts associated with Dependency and Self-Criticism. *Journal of Social and Clinical Psychology, 19*, 184-205.

Whisman, M. A., & Friedman, M. A. (1998). Interpersonal problem behaviors associated with dysfunctional attitudes. *Cognitive Therapy and Research, 22*, 149-160.

Wilhelm, K., Boyce, P., & Brownhill, S. (2004). The relationship between interpersonal sensitivity, anxiety disorders and major depression. *Journal of Affective Disorders, 79*, 33-41.

Wiseman, H. (1997). Interpersonal relatedness and self-definition of loneliness during the transition to university. *Personal Relationships, 4*, 285-299.

Woodside, D. B., Bullik, C. M., Halmi, K. A., Fichter, M. M., Kaplan, A., Berrettini, W. H., Strober, M., Treasure, J., Lilenfeld, L., Klump, K., & Kaye, W. H. (2002). Personality, perfectionism, and attitudes toward eating in parents of individuals with eating disorders. *International Journal of Eating Disorders, 31*, 290-299.

Zettle, R. D., Haflich, J. L., & Reynolds, R. A. (1992). Responsivity to cognitive therapy as a function of treatment format and client personality dimensions. *Journal of Clinical Psychology, 48*, 787-797.

Zettle, R. D., & Herring, E. L. (1995). Treatment utility of the sociotropy/autonomy distinction:

Implications for cognitive therapy. *Journal of Clinical Psychology, 51*, 280-289.

Zuroff, D. C. (1992). New directions for cognitive models of depression. *Psychological Inquiry, 3*, 274-277.

Zuroff, D. C., & Blatt, S. J. (2002). Vicissitudes of life after the short-term treatment of depression: Roles of stress, social support, and personality. *Journal of Social and Clinical Psychology, 21*, 473-496.

Zuroff, D. C., Blatt, S. J., Sanislow III, C. A., Bondi, C. M., & Pilkonis, P. A. (1999). Vulnerability to depression: Reexamining state dependence and relative stability. *Journal of Abnormal Psychology, 108*, 76-89.

Zuroff, D. C., Blatt, S. J., Sotsky, S. M., Krupnick, J. L., Martin, D. J., Sanislow III, C. A., & Simmens, S. (2000). Relation of therapeutic alliance and perfectionism to outcome in brief outpatient treatment of depression. *Journal of Consulting and Clinical Psychology, 68*, 114-124.

Zuroff, D. C., & de Lorimier, S. (1989). Ideal and actual romantic partners of women varying in dependency and self-criticism. *Journal of Personality, 57*, 825-846.

Zuroff, D. C., & Duncan, N. (1999). Self-criticism and conflict resolution in romantic couples. *Canadian Journal of Behavioural Science, 31*, 137-149.

Zuroff, D. C., & Fitzpatrick, D. K. (1995). Depressive personality styles: Implications for adult attachment. *Personality and Individual Differences, 18*, 253-265.

Zuroff, D. C., Igreja, I., & Mongrain, M. (1990). Dysfunctional attitudes, dependency, and self-criticism as predictors of depressive mood states: A 12-month longitudinal study. *Cognitive Therapy and Research, 14*, 315-326.

Zuroff, D. C., Koestner, R., & Powers, T. A. (1994). Self-criticism at age 12: A longitudinal study of adjustment. *Cognitive Therapy and Research, 18*, 367-385.

Zuroff, D. C., & Mongrain, M. (1987). Dependency and self-criticism: Vulnerability factors for depressive affective states. *Journal of Abnormal Psychology, 96*, 14-22.

Zuroff, D. C., Moskowitz, D. S., & Côté, S. (1999). Dependency, self-criticism, interpersonal behaviour and affect: Evolutionary perspectives. *British Journal of Clinical Psychology, 38*, 231-250.

Zuroff, D. C., Moskowitz, D. S., Wielgus, M. S., Powers, T. A., & Franko, D. L. (1983). Construct validation of the Dependency and Self-Criticism scales of the Depressive Experiences Questionnaire. *Journal of Research in Personality, 17*, 226-241.

Zuroff, D. C., Stotland, S., Sweetman, E., Craig, J.-A., & Koestner, R. (1995). Dependency, self-criticism and social interactions. *British Journal of Clinical Psychology, 34*, 543-553.

Chapter 5

A Dialectic Model of Personality Development

and Psychopathology: Recent Contributions

to Understanding and Treating Depression

Sidney J. Blatt and Golan Shahar

Personality Development and Psychopathology

Psychological development is often portrayed as a linear, monotonic function, with each developmental phase following and deriving from a prior phase. We believe that psychological development, however, is complex and more aptly described as a dialectic process in which development occurs reciprocally across various developmental lines, such that development in one domain facilitates development in parallel but contrasting domains that then, in turn, facilitate further development in the original domain. The development of concepts of self and of significant others is an example of this reciprocal development, such that a more differentiated relationship with an other contributes to further differentiation within the self and, conversely, further differentiation within the self leads to further differentiation in relationships with others. Self and other are reciprocal constructs that develop in a mutually facilitating dialectic transaction.

Blatt and colleagues (Blatt & Shichman, 1983; Blatt & Blass, 1990, 1996) have articulated this fundamental dialectic between the development of the self and relatedness to others. Based on an elaboration and extension of Erikson's (1950) epigenetic psychosocial developmental model, Blatt and colleagues (e.g., Blatt & Shichman, 1983) identified three levels in the development of interpersonal relatedness: basic trust (vs. mistrust), cooperation (vs. alienation), and intimacy (vs. isolation) which they coordinate with aspects of Erikson's model that they identified as pertinent to the development of the self: autonomy (vs. shame), initiative (vs. guilt), industry (vs. inferiority), identity (vs. role diffusion), genera-tivity (vs. stagnation), and integrity (vs. despair). Blatt and Blass (1990, 1996), in an elaboration of this dialectic developmental model, noted that phases in the development of relatedness (trust, cooperation, and intimacy) are juxtaposed in Erikson's model with their polar attributes (mistrust, alienation, and isolation, respectively). The negative counterparts of each phase in the development of self-definition (e.g., shame, guilt, inferiority), however, are not polar attributes; rather they reflect a more complex developmental process involving both behavioral and experiential components. Erikson identified the negative experiential or affective component of each phase in the development of self-definition (or identity) such that, for example, the counterpart of a failure to develop autonomy is not a lack of autonomy, but shame. Likewise, the experiential or affective component of difficulty in the development of initiative is not a lack of initiative, but guilt. Thus, difficulty in the development of aspects of self-definition can be expressed in affective (experiential) dimensions (e.g., shame, guilt, as specified by Erikson) as well as in behavioral dimensions such as a lack of autonomy, a lack of initiative, or a lack of industry (Blatt & Blass, 1990, 1996).

For development to proceed in the relatedness dimension from a sense of trust to a capacity for cooperation, first in the family and later with peers, the child has to develop a behavioral capacity for autonomy (or separateness) with a sense of pride (or a lack of shame), as well as a behavioral capacity for initiation without feelings of guilt, and a capacity for industry free of feelings of inferiority. Behavioral and affective achievements in these early phases in the development of self enable the child to establish relationships with others in new ways. The process of moving from a sense of basic trust with a caregiving other to an emergent capacity for reciprocal relatedness – to a sense of cooperation (Blatt & Blass, 1992, 1996) – depends on the child's ability to establish a sense of self as autonomous and capable of initiation and industry that facilitates the child's beginning to be able to participate in cooperative relationships (e.g., first in parallel, then interactive, and, eventually, in reciprocal play). And the development of a capacity to participate in cooperative and collaborative relationships, in turn, leads to further refinement of the self. Eventually, with the development of a sense of identity, one has the capacity to form an intimate reciprocal relationship based on the recognition of what one wants to share in a relationship with an appreciation of what one brings to and what one wants from an enduring intimate relationship. Thus, the sense of self and the quality of interpersonal relatedness develop in a reciprocal, mutually facilitating, dialectic transaction. These two dimensions normally develop in a reciprocal dialectic process, such that development in one dimension facilitates development in the other. Throughout life, from infancy to senescence, development in the sense of self leads to refinements in the capacity for interpersonal relatedness, and development in the quality of interpersonal relationships enriches the sense of self (Blatt & Blass, 1990, 1996; Blatt & Shichman, 1983).

As noted in Chapter 3, these processes define two fundamental dimensions in personality development:

(a) development of a differentiated, integrated, realistic, essentially positive sense of self or an identity, and

(b) development of the capacity to form mutually satisfying, reciprocal, interpersonal relationships.

These two dimensions are central in theoretical formulations in psychoanalytic theory (e.g., Freud, 1914/1958, 1926/1959, 1930/1961; Loewald, 1962), and in general conceptual (e.g., Angyal, 1941, 1951; Bakan, 1966), and empirical approaches (e.g., Benjamin, 1974; Wiggins, 1991) to personality theory.

Relatedness and self-definition are central dimensions not only in normal personality development, but they are also central issues in many forms of psychopathology. Most forms of psychopathology emerge from disruptions, at different developmental levels, of this normal developmental dialectic process in the development of self and of a capacity for interpersonal relatedness. Disruptions at different points in this normal dialectic developmental process are expressed in different ways in various forms of psychopathology (e.g., Blatt, 1990; Blatt & Shichman, 1983), including depression. Thus, most forms of psychopathology involve either a one-sided, distorted, intense preoccupation, at different developmental levels, with preserving a sense of self or a one-sided, distorted preoccupation, at different developmental levels, with maintaining interpersonal relatedness. Some individuals, more often women, deal with developmental disruptions by becoming preoccupied with interpersonal relationships at the expense of the development of a sense of self. Other individuals, more often men, deal with developmental disruptions by becoming preoccupied with the issues of self-definition at the expense of relatedness. Thus, two basic configurations of psychopathology can be identified: 1) an anaclitic or relatedness configuration of psychopathology that includes the dependent or infantile personality disorder, anaclitic depression, and the hysterical personality disorder – disorders preoccupied with issues of interpersonal relatedness (e.g., trust, dependability, affection, and love) at various developmental levels; and 2) an introjective or self-definitional configuration of psychopathology that includes the paranoid, obsessive-compulsive, depressive, and phallic narcissistic personality disorders – disorders preoccupied with issues of self-definition (e.g., autonomy, self-control, and self-worth) at different developmental levels (Blatt & Shichman, 1983).

In these formulations, various forms of psychopathology, including depression, are not viewed as separate diseases that derive from presumed, but unspecified and undocumented, biological disturbances, but rather maladaptive modes that individuals develop to deal with severe and persistent disruptions in psychological development. This approach assumes that most biological dimensions create nonspecific vulnerabilities that can gain expression in multiple ways in the vicissitudes of the interpersonal care-giving relationships between parents and child. Extensive research of normal psychological development provides a well-delineated developmental framework for identifying deviations or distortions of normal developmental processes that derive from the interaction of biological vulnerabilities with disrupted parent-child interaction and lead to a variety of psychological disturbances (e.g., Blatt, 1995a; Blatt & Homann, 1992; Goodman & Gotlib, 2002). Freud's insights into melancholia (Freud, 1917/1957), for example, were derived from his contrast of aspects of clinical depression with normal loss and grieving (mourning). Freud's contrast of pathology with normality enabled him to identify central elements in clinical depression. This approach of defining psychopathology as deriving from disruptions of normal psychological development has important potential advantages including avoiding categorical distinctions of psychopathology based on manifest symptoms, maintaining continuity between normal psychological development and various forms of psychopathology, establishing relationships among various forms of psychopathology to deal with complex issues of comorbidity, and of identifying dimensions relevant to various disorders beyond their manifest symptomatic expressions.

The Understanding and Treatment of Depression

Dissatisfaction with symptom-based diagnostic classifications of depression has led several investigators to differentiate types of depression based on a differentiation among the fundamental developmental concerns that contribute to individuals becoming depressed. Our research team (e.g., Blatt, 1974; Blatt, D'Afflitti, & Quinlan, 1976) identified two major foci in depression: (1) disruptions of gratifying interpersonal relationships (e.g., object loss or neglect) and (2) disruptions of an effective and essentially positive sense of self (e.g., feelings of failure or guilt). Extensive clinical and empirical evidence indicates that depression is organized around these two issues – around interpersonal issues such as feelings of abandonment and loneliness, or around an impaired sense of self expressed in preoccupations with personal failure, inadequacy, or transgression (Blatt, 2004; Blatt & Zuroff, 1992). These two themes (abandonment and failure) differentiate two major foci around which depression can be organized: (1) depressive experiences often precipitated by object loss that we have called anaclitic (Blatt, 1974) or dependent (Blatt et al., 1976, Blatt, Quinlan, Chevron, McDonald, & Zuroff, 1982) and (2) introjective (Blatt, 1974) or self-critical (Blatt et al., 1976, 1982) depressive experiences precipitated by feelings of failure, guilt, and other impairments of self-worth.

Based on the assumption that psychopathology is most effectively considered, not as separate diseases deriving from unspecified and undocumented biological disturbances (e.g., such as a clinically undocumented chemical imbalance in depression), but as disruptions of normal psychological development, we (Blatt et al., 1976) reviewed the classic psychoanalytic literature on depression (e.g., Freud's *Mourning and Melancholia* [1917/1957], Edward Bibring's *Mechanisms of Depression* [1953], Mabel Blake Cohen and colleagues' *An Intensive Study of Twelve Cases of Manic Depression Psychosis* [1954]), and gleaned from these reports, not symptoms of depression, but examples of the everyday life experiences of depressed individuals and their families. We eventually identified 66 items from this literature – items that tapped issues like a distorted or depreciated sense of self and others, dependency, helplessness, egocentricity, fear of loss, ambivalence, difficulty dealing with anger, self-blame, guilt, loss of autonomy, and distortions of family relations. These items were not selected from any particular theoretical position on depression, but because they represented a wide range of experiences that were characteristic of the lives of depressed individuals. These 66 items were initially administered to a large sample of college students with the instructions to rate, on a 7-point scale, the degree to which each item characterized their experiences. Based on Principal Components Analysis with a varimax rotation, we found that this questionnaire, which we called the Depressive Experiences Questionnaire (DEQ), was composed of three primary factors (Blatt et al., 1976): a factor containing items primarily focused on issues of loneliness and abandonment (e.g., "I often think about the danger of losing someone who is close to me"), labeled Dependency, 2) a factor comprised of items focused on issues of self-definition and self-worth (e.g., "There is considerable difference between how I am now and how I would like to be"), labeled Self-Criticism, and an Efficacy factor comprised of items reflecting feelings of resilience, competence and personal strength (e. g., "I have many inner resources"). Thus, we serendipitously developed an empirical method (the DEQ; Blatt et al., 1976) that reliably and systematically assesses the two primary sources or foci of depression that Freud (1917/1957) had tried to integrate into a unified conceptualization of depression in *Mourning and Melancholia*: a traditional source of depression derived from superego issues of self-worth, self-blame and guilt, and a source of depression derived from interpersonal concerns of loneliness and fears of abandonment (Blatt, 1974).

A wide range of empirical studies over the past three decades have demonstrated that the three factors of the DEQ are highly stable; they have been replicated in clinical and non-clinical samples of both adolescents and adults in a number of different cultures (e.g., Beutel et al., 2004; Compas, 2002; Frank et al., 1997; Jae Im, 1998; Luyten, 2002; Priel, Besser, & Shahar, 1998; Zuroff, Quinlan, & Blatt, 1990). These studies consistently indicated that the 66 items of the DEQ cluster into three primary factors. The first factor, *Dependency*, reflects wishes to be cared for, loved and protected, and fear of being abandoned. The second factor, *Self-Criticism or Self-Critical Perfectionism*, taps preoccupation with achievement and feelings of inferiority and guilt in the face of perceived failure to meet standards. The third factor, *Efficacy*, represents personal resilience and inner strength. A wide range of research (see summary in Blatt, 2004) has demonstrated that the two primary factors of the DEQ (the Interpersonal or Dependency and the Self-Criticism factors) are relatively independent dimensions of depression that provide understanding of some of the distal as well as proximal factors that contribute to the onset of depression as well as of various expressions of depression in a wide range of clinical and non-clinical samples in a number of cultures.

The empirical confirmation of these two primary dimensions of depressive experiences is consistent with clinical-theoretical formulations about the nature of depression from psychoanalytic (e.g., Arieti & Bemporad, 1978, 1980; Blatt, 1974; Bowlby, 1980) and cognitive-behavioral (Beck, 1983) perspectives. Arieti and Bemporad (1978, 1980) differentiated a depression associated with a preoccupation with the loss of a "dominant other" from a depression provoked by a failure to achieve a "dominant goal." Bowlby (1980) discussed depression as associated with either an anxious attachment or a compulsively self-reliant attachment style. From a cognitive-behavioral perspective, Aaron Beck (1983) articulated a similar distinction in his differentiation of a sociotropic depression, a depression focused around disruptions of interpersonal relationships, from an autonomous depression focused around disruptions of autonomy and self-definition. Thus several groups of psychoanalytic theorists and a preeminent cognitive-behavioral theorist agree about the importance of differentiating between a depression focused on interpersonal issues and a depression focused on issues of self-worth and self-definition (Blatt & Maroudas, 1992).

Several other procedures, in addition to the DEQ, have been developed that assess these two dimensions of depression. Aaron Beck (1983) developed an assessment method similar to the DEQ, the Sociotropy-Autonomy Scale (SAS; Beck, 1983), and several other investigators (e.g., Cane, Olinger, Gotlib, & Kuiper, 1986) found that the Dysfunctional Attitudes Scale (DAS; Weissman & Beck, 1978) also assesses these two dimensions of depression. Robins and Luten (1991) combined elements from the DEQ and the SAS to create the Personal Style Inventory (PSI) to assess these two dimensions of depression in an attempt to develop a scale that might have improved psychometric properties (Robins et al., 1994). Research with all of these scales (e.g., DEQ, SAS, DAS, PSI) has resulted in an impressive extensive research literature that has led to a fuller understanding of some of the early and contemporary life experiences that contribute to the occurrence of depression and of important differences in the clinical expression and treatment of anaclitic (dependent) and introjective (self-critical) types of depression (e.g., Blatt, 2004; Blatt & Homann, 1992; Blatt & Zuroff, 1992; Clark & Beck, 1999; see also Chapter 4, this volume).

In addition to contributing to clarifying aspects of the etiology, clinical expressions, and treatment of depression, the development of the DEQ has contributed to differentiating several developmental levels in the evolution of self-definition and of the capacity for interpersonal relatedness. As discussed earlier, interpersonal relatedness evolves from feelings of trust, to a capacity for cooperation and collaboration, to a capacity for intimacy. Likewise, self-definition or identity evolves from reactive feelings of autonomy, to proactive capacities for initiative and industry, to the formation of a consolidated identity and a capacity for generativity, and ultimately to feelings of integrity.

Developmental Levels of Interpersonal Relatedness and Self-Definition

As noted earlier, interpersonal relatedness and self-definition are central to personality development. Personality development evolves out of a dynamic dialectic tension between these two fundamental developmental processes. An increasingly differentiated, integrated, and mature sense of self is contingent on establishing satisfying interpersonal relationships and, conversely, the continued development of increasingly mature and satisfying interpersonal relationships is contingent on the development of a mature self-concept or identity. In normal personality development, these two developmental processes evolve in an interactive, reciprocally balanced, mutually facilitating fashion from birth through senescence (Blatt, 1990, 1995a; Blatt & Blass, 1990, 1992, 1996; Blatt & Shichman, 1983). If development does not proceed well, however, interpersonal relatedness can be characterized by feelings of mistrust about the dependability of others, by an alienation from others, or by feelings of loneliness and isolation. Likewise, disruptions in the development of a sense of self can involve fears of annihilation; concerns about a loss of control; and feelings of shame, guilt and inferiority; and of a lack of integrity.

Recent research with the DEQ (e.g., Blatt, Zohar, Quinlan, Zuroff, & Mongrain, 1995; Blatt, Zohar, Quinlan, Luthar, & Hart, 1996; Blatt & Shahar, 2003) has differentiated empirically two levels of interpersonal relatedness: (1) a maladaptive desperate *neediness*, in which one feels terrified about abandonment and threatened by feelings of helplessness when alone, and (2) a more adaptive *relatedness*, in which one has meaningful involvement with particular individuals and feels a sense of sadness and loss if these relationships are disrupted. Other recent research with the DEQ (Kuperminc, Blatt, & Leadbeater, 1997) has also identified empirically two levels in the development of the self – a maladaptive, reflective, ruminative, self-critical, evaluative sense of self and an adaptive, proactive, efficacious sense of self. Self-evaluative ruminative concerns about self-worth include feelings of a loss of autonomy, initiative, and industry, and feelings of shame, guilt, and inferiority. These concerns and doubts about self-worth are orthogonal to, and independent of, the second level in the development of the self – feelings of efficacy, identity, integrity, and purpose.

As research with the DEQ has progressed, it has become evident that Factor 2, the Self-Criticism factor, was more effective than Factor I, the Dependency factor, in predicting depressive symptoms and a host of adaptive and maladaptive outcomes (Blatt et al., 1982; Nietzel & Harris, 1990; Priel & Shahar, 2000). We (Blatt, Zohar, et al., 1995, 1996) examined Factor I of the DEQ with the hypothesis that the Dependency factor of the DEQ may actually include two facets or subfactors, one that assesses adaptive interpersonal *relatedness* and the other that assesses a more maladaptive *dependence or neediness*. Using Small Space Analysis (SSA), a theory-driven clustering procedure developed by the research methodologist Louis Guttman, we identified these two facets within the Dependency factor (Factor I) in both adults and adolescents (Blatt, Zohar et al., 1995, 1996; Henrich, Blatt, Kuperminc, Zohar, & Leadbeater, 2001; see also Rude & Burnham, 1995).

One facet, labeled *relatedness*, includes items that assess feelings of loss, sadness, and loneliness in reaction to disruption of relationships with a particular person (e.g., "I would feel like I'd be losing an important part of myself if I lost a very close friend"). These feelings are not undifferentiated and non-specific; rather, they reflect concerns about the loss of a special person to whom one feels attached. These items do not reflect feeling helpless without this relationship, but rather feeling that this particular relationship is valued and therefore loss is accompanied by feelings of sadness and loss. The second facet, labeled *dependence or neediness*, includes items expressing feelings of helplessness, fears and apprehension about separation and rejection, and intense and broad-ranging concerns about a general loss of contact with others, unrelated to a particular relationship (e.g., "I become frightened when I am alone"). These items reflect a desperate need for others but with little differentiation or specification of any particular person or relationship. The primary theme of these items is an intense fear of abandonment and feelings of helplessness. Hence, the results of Small Space Analyses with adolescent and adults indicate that the Dependency or Interpersonal Factor of the DEQ is comprised of two sets of items that assess both adaptive and maladaptive manifestations of interpersonal relatedness.

When the two facets of dependency (i.e., relatedness and dependence or neediness) were used to predict depressive symptoms and psychological well-being, two interesting patterns emerged. First, the *dependence or neediness* facet had significantly higher correlations with measures of depression while the *relatedness* facet had significantly higher correlations with measures of psychological well-being (Blatt, et al. 1995, 1996; Henrich et al., 2001). Second, the intercorrelations between the four DEQ variables (i.e., self-criticism, efficacy, dependence or neediness, and relatedness) no longer reflect the orthogonality found among the three original DEQ factors (i.e., Dependency, Self-criticism and Efficacy). Specifically, Self-criticism correlated positively with *dependence or neediness* and negatively with *relatedness* (e.g., $r = .19$ and $-.10$; respectively; Blatt,

144

et al., 1996). That is, self-criticism, a maladaptive sense of self, correlated positively with the maladaptive dimension of interpersonal relatedness (*neediness*), and negatively with the adaptive dimension of interpersonal relations (*relatedness*). In contrast, Efficacy, an adaptive sense of self, correlated positively with relatedness and negatively with *dependence* or neediness (e.g., $r = .16$ and $-.23$; respectively) (Blatt, et al. 1996).

Two Levels of Self-Definition

The differential correlations of the DEQ Self-Criticism and Efficacy factors with the maladaptive and adaptive dimensions of interpersonal relationships (i.e., neediness and relatedness, respectively) suggested that the Self-Criticism and Efficacy factors of the DEQ assess different levels of the self-concept – a maladaptive and an adaptive view of the self respectively. Thus the DEQ has become more than a measure of two sources of depression, it has also become an effective research instrument for measuring adaptive as well as maladaptive aspects of both interpersonal relations and self-definition. The significant correlations between maladaptive aspects of self-definition and interpersonal relations (self-criticism and neediness) and between adaptive aspects of self-definition and interpersonal relations (efficacy and relatedness) also suggest support for the formulations (Blatt & Blass, 1990, 1996; Blatt & Shichman, 1983) of the parallel dialectic development of self-definition and relatedness.

Self-Criticism: Maladaptive aspects of the self. Extensive research documents the maladaptive aspects of self-criticism (e.g., Blatt, 1974, 2004; Blatt et al., 1976, 1982). Individuals with elevated scores on DEQ Self-Criticism are sensitive to ridicule and are uncomfortable in interpersonal relationships; they tend to be interpersonally isolated and insensitive, formal, ambivalent, reserved, and distant, and they often try to manipulate others through deception and flattery (e.g., Dunkley, Blankstein, & Flett, 1997). They are prone to feelings of guilt, sadness, hopelessness, and depression (e.g., Mongrain, 1998), and at times they can be seriously suicidal (Blatt, 1974, 1995b; Blatt et al., 1982; Beck, 1983; Enns, Cox, & Inayatulla, 2003; Fazaa, 2001; Fazaa & Page, 2003; Shahar, 2001). These feelings of self-criticism are relative resistant to brief therapeutic interventions (Blatt, Quinlan, Pilkonis, & Shea, 1995; Blatt, Zuroff, Bondi, Sanislow, & Pilkonis, 1998) and several studies (e.g., Alden & Bieling, 1966; Zuroff & Fitzpatrick, 1995) demonstrate the avoidant qualities of the individuals with elevated scores on the Self-Criticism factor of the DEQ.

Efficacy: Adaptive aspects of the Self. In contrast to the extensive research on self-criticism as a maladaptive dimension of the self, research on the Efficacy factor of the DEQ has been minimal. Investigators who use the DEQ usually report findings with the Dependency and Self-Criticism factors, mentioning only in passing that the Efficacy factor was not used in the study (cf. Priel & Shahar, 2000). Authors who mention the Efficacy factor usually do so in a few lines, rarely elaborating its negative correlation with depression (Blatt et al., 1976; Blatt, et al., 1982; Klein, 1989). Even when Efficacy was found to be associated with higher levels of functioning over time (Klein, 1989), it was still mentioned only briefly.

Our recent increased interest in the Efficacy factor is primarily the result of our study of risk and resilience in early adolescence (Leadbeater, Kuperminc, Blatt, & Herzog, 1999). A large and diverse sample of early adolescents (230 girls and 230 boys) in an urban middle school (6th to 8th grade), were evaluated over a one-year interval. Although most of the reports from this research project focused on Dependency and Self-Criticism, some interesting findings were obtained with the Efficacy factor. While Self-Criticism was related to maladaptive indicators of social and academic functioning, Efficacy was related to indicators of adaptation (Kuperminc, Blatt, & Leadbeater, 1997), a finding that suggests that Self-Criticism taps ruminative, self-reflective preoccupations with past and current deficits and deficiencies, whereas Efficacy assesses proactive feelings and behavior – positive self-attitudes. Self-Criticism, for example, predicted increases in internalizing and externalizing symptoms over a one-year period whereas Efficacy predicted a reduction in these symptoms over the same time period (Kuperminc, Leadbeater, & Blatt, 2001). Further analyses of the data from the study of these adolescent students (Shahar, Gallagher, Blatt, Kuperminc, & Leadbeater, in press) indicate that Efficacy moderates, or buffers, the adverse effects of Dependency and Self-Criticism on depressive symptoms. Adolescents who had greater levels of vulnerability, as reflected in elevated Dependency and Self-criticism, were even more prone to depression and impaired functioning, especially if they also had reduced levels of personal resilience, as reflected in lower Efficacy. These longitudinal analyses indicated that Efficacy moderated the combined effect of Dependency and Self-Criticism in the development of depression. Specifically, adolescents who had elevated levels of both Dependency and Self-Criticism tended to be more depressed if they also have low, rather than high, levels of Efficacy (see also Blatt et al., 1982).

Adaptive and Maladaptive Levels of Interpersonal Relatedness and Self-Definition and the Social Context

Extensive research has examined the interaction between the four DEQ variables (Neediness, Relatedness, Self-criticism, and Efficacy) and aspects of the social context like stressful life events, social support, and close interpersonal relationships. As noted in Chapter 4, earlier studies that examined the effect of the DEQ variables on depressive symptoms usually treated the social context as a moderator (Blatt & Zuroff, 1992). Contextual variables like stressful events were expected to augment the maladaptive tendencies of self and interpersonal relatedness. According to what has come to be called the "congruency hypothesis" (Blatt & Zuroff, 1992; Coyne & Whiffen, 1995; Robins, 1995), individuals with elevated levels of dependency would become depressed in response to stressful interpersonal events like rejection and loss. Similarly, individuals with elevated levels of self-criticism would become depressed in response to events threatening the self, such as failure. Empirical support has usually been found for the congruency hypothesis with respect to dependency, but only on occasion for self-criticism (for reviews, see Blatt, 2004; Blatt & Zuroff, 1992; Coyne & Whiffen, 1995; Robins, 1995; Shahar, 2001; Chapter 4, this volume).

It is important to note that these various attempts to study the congruency hypothesis usually assumed that individuals are passive in relation to the contextual factors that seem to precipitate their distress (Priel & Shahar, 2000). More recent formulations, however, have come to emphasize that individuals may actively generate the contextual conditions implicated in their distress (Buss, 1987; Coyne, 1976, 1998; Hammen, 1991, 1998; Joiner, 1994; Plomin & Caspi, 1999). Conse-quently, investigators have now begun to focus on the interactions of the DEQ variables with contextual variables like stressful events, social support, and the quality of close relationships (Blatt & Shahar, 2003).

Research findings indicate that self-criticism is a primary instigator of depressive symptoms because it generates a risk-related social environment (Dunkley, Zuroff, & Blankstein, 2003; Shahar, 2001). Specifically, elevated self-criticism inter-feres with close relations: it predicts interpersonal ruptures and tensions (Mongrain, Vettese, Shuster, & Kendal, 1998; Vettese & Mongrain, 2000; Priel & Besser, 2000; Priel & Shahar, 2000; Zuroff & Duncan, 1999) and other interpersonal stressful events (Priel & Shahar, 2000; Shahar, Joiner, Zuroff, & Blatt, 2004; Shahar & Priel, 2003). Self-criticism also predicts reduced levels of social support (Mongrain, 1998; Priel & Shahar, 2000), and fewer positive life events (Shahar & Priel, 2003). Thus, individuals with a maladaptive sense of self appear to generate contextual conditions that render them vulnerable to depression and emotional distress.

Dunkley, Zuroff and Blankstein (2003), studying college men and women, recently examined both personal dispositional and situational factors that contribute to high negative and low positive affect in self-critical individuals. Over a 7-day period, they assessed daily reports of hassles, stress, social support, and coping styles. Using structural equation modeling (SEM), they found that Self-Criticism influenced emotional experiences each day through a number of maladaptive tendencies. Self-Criticism contributed to experiences of negative affect through an increase in daily hassles and the use of an avoidant coping style, and to a reduction of positive affect through a failure to maintain social support. Also, self-critical individuals were particularly reactive to stressors that implied personal failure, loss of control, and criticism from others. They also were relatively ineffective in using more adaptive coping strategies like problem-focused coping.

Another compelling example of the tendency of self-critical individuals to generate a negative social context was obtained in analyses we conducted on data from the Treatment of Depression Collaborative Research Project (TDCRP), a randomized clinical trial that compared three outpatient treatments for major depression: Cognitive-behavioral Therapy (CBT), Interpersonal Therapy (IPT), and Imipramine plus clinical management (IMI-CM), sponsored by the National Institute of Mental Health. These three active treatments were also compared to an inactive placebo plus clinical management (PLA-CM). Original analyses of these data indicated few substantial differences in clinical outcome among the three active treatment groups (Elkin et al., 1989; Imber et al., 1990). Additional analyses that our research team conducted on this data set, however, demonstrated that patients' pretreatment self-criticism or perfectionism had a highly significant negative impact on therapeutic outcome in all three treatments conditions (Blatt, Quinlan et al., 1995; Blatt, Zuroff et al., 1998). Pretreatment Self-Critical Perfectionism impeded the improvement of two-thirds of the patients in this sample, and this impeding of therapeutic progress occurred primarily during the second half of the treatment, between the 9th and the 16th session (Blatt et al., 1998). Further analyses (Zuroff, Blatt, Sotsky, Krupnick, Martin, Sanislow, & Simmens, 2000) indicated that at least part of this adverse effect of pretreatment self-criticism (perfectionism) on treatment outcome was mediated through patients' impaired participation in the therapeutic alliance. Pretreatment Self-Critical Perfectionism predicted lower levels of patients' constructive contribution to the therapeutic alliance. This interference in the formation and maintenance of the therapeutic alliance in turn predicted poorer therapeutic outcome. We (Shahar, Blatt, Zuroff, Krupnick, & Sotsky, 2004) also found that the poorer outcome of self-critical, perfectionist patients resulted not only from their failure to participate in the therapeutic alliance but also from their difficulties in maintaining close interpersonal relationships outside therapy. Specifically, pretreatment Self-Critical Perfectionism predicted reduced interpersonal involvement with the therapist in treatment as well as in the patients' general social network outside of treatment. Both of these, in turn, predicted poorer therapeutic outcome. These adverse effects of pretreatment Self-Critical Perfectionism on the therapeutic alliance and on close relations explained much of the variance of the adverse effect of Self-Critical Perfectionism on therapeutic outcome (Shahar, Blatt et al., 2004; see also Shahar, Blatt, Zuroff, & Pilkonis, 2002). Thus, Self-Critical Perfectionism not only contributes to considerable emotional distress but it also disrupts therapeutic attempts to alleviate this distress.

We (Blatt & Shahar, 2003) believe that self-critical individuals generate a risk-related social context because they have negative representations of self and significant others. Several investigators (e.g., Blatt, 1974; Blatt, Wein, Chevron, & Quinlan, 1979; Mongrain, 1998) have demonstrated that self-critical young adults hold particularly negative representations of parental figures. These negative representations seem to organize self-critical individuals' social exchange, making it difficult for them to respond to positive interpersonal cues (Aubé & Whiffen, 1996), forcing them to avoid intimacy and self-disclosure (Zuroff & Fitzpatrick, 1995) and to act in a hostile manner in close relations (Zuroff & Duncan, 1999), thereby creating conflicts, confrontations, and other stressful events (Priel & Shahar, 2000; Shahar & Priel, 2003). It seems that self-critical individuals project their own self-criticism onto others and therefore expect the condemnation from others that they inflict upon themselves. Ironically, to the extent that these negative representations generate a risk-related environment, this negative interpersonal environment is likely to consolidate and even exacerbate their negative representations of themselves and others, thus contributing to a reciprocal, vicious, interpersonal loop or circle that is frequently observed by clinicians treating depressed patients (Andrews, 1989; Blatt & Zuroff, 1992; Wachtel, 1994; Zuroff, 1992).

In contrast to the disruptive effects of self-criticism on social relationships, the impact of the dependency (or the interpersonal) dimension of the DEQ on social relationships is more complex suggesting that this personality construct contains both elements of risk and resilience (Blatt, Zohar et al., 1995, 1996; Bornstein, 1998; Shahar, 2001; Shahar & Priel, 2003). Though dependency predicts interpersonal problems that contribute to depression, it also predicts a capacity for intimacy (Fichman, Koestner, & Zuroff, 1994) and being able to establish and maintain elevated levels of social support (Mongrain, 1998; Priel & Shahar, 2000). Dependency, like self-criticism, predicts elevated levels of negative events that lead to depression and anxiety; but different than self-criticism, dependency also predicts positive events which partly explains why dependent individuals report lower levels of distress than self-critical individuals (Shahar & Priel, 2002). Dependent women are interested in closeness and intimacy and experience greater feelings of affection and love in their romantic relationships (Zuroff & deLorimier, 1989; Zuroff & Fitzpatrick, 1995). They are more positive about their same-sex relationships – they perceive these relationships as more friendly and tend to more frequently use positive expressions in their same-sex interactions (Zuroff & Franko, 1986). Dependent individuals go to remarkable length to preserve interpersonal harmony (Santor, Pringle, & Israeli, 2000), are uncomfortable with feelings of hostility (Zuroff, Moskowitz, Wieglus, Powers, & Franko, 1983), and have difficulty being assertive (Fichman et al., 1994). Thus, they tend to use compromise in dealing with interpersonal conflicts (Zuroff & Fitzpatrick, 1995). In summary, dependency is correlated with investment in interpersonal relationships. In nonclinical samples it is related to valuing emotional closeness and an active interest in maintaining good interpersonal relationships. In clinical samples, dependency is associated with apprehensions and resentments about loss, neglect, deprivation, and abandonment by parents, spouse, and friends (Blatt et al., 1982).

Studies have only recently begun to investigate the impact of Efficacy, the adaptive dimension of self, on the social context. To address this question, we examined the role of the adaptive and maladaptive sense of self in adolescent development. We examined the role of the Self-Criticism and Efficacy factors of the DEQ in predicting a positive social context in young adolescents (Blatt & Shahar, 2003). The results of this study, derived from a Structural Equation Modeling (SEM; Hoyle & Smith, 1994) analysis examination of the longitudinal effects of Self-Criticism and Efficacy on the social context, indicate that Self-criticism and Efficacy present opposite patterns. Self-Criticism significantly predicted an increasingly negative social context while Efficacy significantly predicted an increasingly positive social context. Also, it was noteworthy that social context at Time 1 strongly predicted Time 2 social context, indicating that the social context of adolescents tends to be stable over time. Thus, the variations in the social context produced by Self-Criticism and Efficacy are impressive.

In summary, empirical research with the Depressive Experiences Questionnaire (DEQ) demonstrates that Self-criticism and Efficacy, which respectively assess maladaptive and adaptive dimensions of the self, are intimately tied to social relations, and in fact generate contextual circumstances in predictable ways. Self-criticism generates a negative, risk-related, social context whereas Efficacy generates a positive, resilience-related context. Thus, the DEQ is an instrument not only for assessing two major foci of depression, but also a method for assessing several levels in the development of interpersonal relations and in the sense of self. This further differentiation of developmental levels within the DEQ should facilitate further research on depression as well as provide a method for systematically studying different phases of personality development. Not only has the development of the DEQ facilitated the differentiation of two primary sources of depression and the systematic investigation of some of the etiological, clinical, and therapeutic issues in these two types of depression (e.g., Blatt, 2004; Blatt & Zuroff, 1992) – the distal and proximal antecedents, as well as the clinical implications of these different types of depression – it now has the potential to contribute to the study of personality development.

Anaclitic and Introjective Configurations of Psychopathology

In addition to the research using the DEQ to assess anaclitic and introjective dimensions in depression and different levels of interpersonal relatedness and self-definition, a fair amount of clinical research has used the anaclitic-introjective distinction categorically to study the differential response of anaclitic and introjective patients in both brief and long term intensive treatment in outpatient and inpatient settings. Judges in several studies (Blatt, 1992; Blatt & Ford, 1994; Blatt & Shahar, 2004b) were able to reliably distinguish between anaclitic and introjective patients. The results of these studies indicate that anaclitic and introjective patients are differentially responsive to different types of therapeutic interventions and express their therapeutic gains in different ways. Introjective patients are relatively unresponsive to brief treatment (e.g., Blatt et al., 1995), but they respond effectively to long-term intensive, psychodynamically oriented treatment (Blatt, 1992; Blatt & Ford, 1994; Blatt & Shahar, 2004a; Fonagy et al., 1996). Further analyses (Blatt 1992; Blatt & Shahar, 2004a) of data from the Menninger Psychotherapy Research Project (MPRP) revealed that introjective patients had a significantly more constructive response to psychoanalysis than to Supportive-Expressive Psychotherapy (SEP). In contrast, anaclitic patients were significantly more responsive to SEP than they were to psychoanalysis (Blatt, 1992). Other studies (Blatt & Ford, 1994) indicate that anaclitic and introjective patients tend to express their therapeutic gains in different ways. Therapeutic progress in introjective patients is usually expressed in change in their cognitive functioning and in the intensity of their manifest symptoms, while therapeutic gain in anaclitic patients is usually expressed in changes in their interpersonal relationships and in their representation of the human form on the Rorschach. Thus, anaclitic and introjective patients seem to change in different dimensions – the dimensions most salient to their character type.

While the anaclitic-introjective distinction has lead to the development of dimensional measures that have been quite productive in research, the question remains about the possibility of a mixed type of individual with both predominant anaclitic and introjective features. We have begun to explore a "mixed group" of individuals, both within clinical and non-clinical samples, who cannot be easily classified within the anaclitic and introjective distinction. We have begun to explore, for example, differences among patients who clearly seem to have primarily an intense primary preoccupation with issues of relatedness or with issues of self-definition (clearly differentiated anaclitic and introjective patients) with a mixed group of patients who are not easily classified within the anaclitic-introjective distinction and who seem to have intense concerns with both dimensions – with issues of both relatedness and self-definition.

Research findings in both clinical and non-clinical samples, using a wide-range of criteria, clearly indicate the validity of the anaclitic and introjective distinction both categorically and dimensionally. Theoretically, it is possible, however, that some individuals can have predominant aspects of both dimensions. In fact, one criterion of normality or high level psychological functioning, such as in self-actualizing individuals (e.g., Maslow, 1954), would be the ability to integrate, at high developmental levels, aspects of both an investment in interpersonal relatedness and in expressions of self-definition – in Eriksonian terms, investment in intimacy and in generativity, or in Freud's terms, in love and work. Thus, high levels of psychological functioning can be defined as a capacity to establish and maintain an effective integration of high levels of both anaclitic and introjective dimensions – to maintain a capacity of reciprocal relatedness with a clear and effective identity. As discussed earlier, the capacity for mutuality and interpersonal reciprocity requires a clear and effective sense of self – an identity in which one clearly recognizes what one can contribute to, as well as gain from, a relationship.

Mixed Anaclitic and Introjective Features

Some patients are less amenable to the anaclitic-introjective categorization because they demonstrate intense and extreme preoccupations in both domains – with issues of both self-definition and with interpersonal relatedness. Although the number of mixed-type patients is usually relatively small, they raise important clinical and theoretical issues. Further analyses (Shahar, Blatt, & Ford, 2003) of the data from the study of long-term, intensive psychodynamically oriented inpatient treatment of ninety seriously disturbed, treatment resistant patients (the Riggs-Yale Project [R-YP]; Blatt & Ford, 1994) revealed important differences between the "mixed group" of patients and patients clearly and confidently classified as either anaclitic or introjective. Two judges, in rating these 90 patients as either anaclitic or introjective, also indicated, on a 100-point scale, their certainty or confidence in making these ratings. We assumed that patients received lower certainty scores because they had both anaclitic and introjective features. Using these clarity/confidence ratings, we were able to divide the 90 patients in the Riggs-Yale sample into three groups. The mixed-type group consisted of the 13 anaclitic patients and the 14 introjective patients with the lowest scores of clarity/conviction. The mean certainty of the 13 "previously anaclitics", now mixed-group, patients was $M = 57.53$ ($SD = 3.07$, range = 52-60) and the mean certainty of the 14 "previously introjectives", now mixed-group, patients was $M = 57.53$ ($SD = 2.49$, range = 55-60). These two groups did not differ in terms of the level of their clarity/conviction ratings ($t[25] = .16$, ns). Neither did the remaining 29 anaclitic and 34 introjective patients differ in the average of clarity/conviction assigned to them (M's = 73.13 vs. 76.70, SD's = 7.85 and 10.99, ranges = 63-90 and 63-98; for anaclitics and introjectives, respectively; $t[61] = 1.45$, ns).

The mixed-type patients were significantly more distressed and vulnerable at admission than their anaclitic and introjective counterparts. They had significantly more psychiatric symptoms, greater thought disorder, lower Performance and Full Scale IQ, less accurate object representations (among men), and had greater utilization of maladaptive defense mechanisms (projection [among men], and identification [among women]). The findings that the mixed group of patients with both anaclitic and introjective features had significantly higher indications of psychopathology, is consistent with earlier findings (Blatt et al., 1982) based on a comparison of three groups of depressed inpatients – patients with elevated scores on DEQ Dependency, a group of patients with elevated scores of DEQ self-Criticism, and a third group of patients with elevated scores on both DEQ dimensions – that found that the mixed group had significantly higher levels of depression. Contrary to expectations, however, the mixed-group evidenced significantly greater therapeutic gain over the course of long-term intensive, inpatient treatment. Mixed group men improved significantly in terms of psychiatric symptoms and mixed group men and women had significantly greater increase in performance IQ and less frequent utilization of projection as a defense mechanism (Shahar et al., 2003).

These findings raise several important theoretical and clinical issues. These results suggest that the intense focus of anaclitic and introjective individuals on issues of interpersonal relatedness or self-definition, respectively, indicates their capacity to construct a relatively focal mode of adaptation that enables them to function more effectively at admission than less clearly organized patients. The mixed-type patients appear not to have achieved the same level of personality consolidation as either of the "pure" type of individuals. But this consolidated mode of adaptation of clearly defined anaclitic and introjective inpatients appears to impair significantly their accessibility to treatment and to limit the extent of their therapeutic gain. The lack of consolidation of a well-articulated defensive organization in mixed group inpatients, at least in the seriously disturbed, treatment-resistant inpatients evaluated in this study, appears to make them more accessible to therapeutic intervention (Shahar et al., 2003).

Anaclitic and Introjective Dimensions in Dynamic Interaction

Theoretical formulations and research investigations have generally viewed anaclitic and introjective features as a basic character or personality trait that usually occurs as a predominant quality or, somewhat less frequently, in combination. This assumption of an anaclitic and an introjective personality organization has been supported by the results of a wide-range of empirical research (see summary in Blatt, 2004; see also Chapter 4, this volume). Recent research (Shahar et al., 2003) indicates, as discussed above, that the mixed group also defines another type of personality organization. But recent clinical experience also suggests that on occasion these character or personality qualities can also co-occur in a dynamic constellation in which one set of qualities serves as a defense against recognizing and experiencing the other set of qualities. Thus, an exaggerated emphasis on introjective issues of self-worth, power, and agency can serve as a defense against recognizing and experiencing intense and painful interpersonal longings, or, conversely, intense preoccupation with issues of interpersonal relatedness and always seeking to be with others can serve as a defense against self-reflection and the painful recognition of intense feelings of dissatisfaction with oneself because of profound feelings of failure or guilt.

A clinical example of an impressively powerful, agentic woman demonstrates how her exaggerated emphasis on these introjective qualities served as a defense against recognizing and acknowledging the intensity of her depressive longings for closeness with her mother, a relationship she had long-sought but had never been able to achieve. These desperate longings for a close relationship with her very distant, aloof, and unavailable mother unconsciously dominated her psychological organization and were part of her marked vulnerability to depression and possibly to suicide.

Madeline, a highly successful 35 year-old attorney, volunteered to be the subject in a study of the contributions of different approaches to psychological assessment, conducted by Jerry Wiggins (2003). As part of this project, Madeline visited with several senior psychologists, each of whom had expertise in a particular approach to psychological assessment. Assessment of Madeline from a psychodynamic perspective was conducted by Behrends and Blatt (2003) and material from that assessment demonstrated how her intense and highly effective introjective personality organization also served as a defense against profoundly painful, relatively unconscious, anaclitic needs. The recent analysis of Madeline's psychological test protocols (Behrends & Blatt, 2003) as part of a book on paradigms of psychological assessment (Wiggins, 2003) provides an excellent example of this more dynamic interaction of anaclitic and introjective personality dimensions.

Madeline, a 35-year old, single, Native American woman, grew up in a highly disrupted environment, raised by seriously abusive, alcoholic parents. She left home at the age of 12, lived in a series of foster placements, and in her late adolescence and young adulthood spent several years in prison. During her incarceration, she was placed in solitary confinement after seriously assaulting a fellow female prisoner. After discharge from prison, Madeline changed her life profoundly. She received a high school diploma through equivalency examination and eventually graduated law school. Despite her criminal record, she successfully petitioned the state bar association to sit for the bar examination, and, after much dispute, was eventually admitted to the bar in her state. She established an extensive legal practice, successfully defending over 50 clients in criminal proceedings. In her community, she was considered a most impressive and powerful individual who had overcome considerable adversity to establish a very successful career. She was much admired by friends and colleagues, so much so, that Wiggins (2003) selected her to be the subject of his book on psychological assessment.

Psychodynamic psychological assessment with the Rorschach, Thematic Apperception Test (TAT), Wechsler Intelligence Test, and the Object Relations Inventory (ORI; e.g., Blatt, Stayner, Auerbach, & Behrends, 1996), consistent with findings independently reported from other assessment procedures (e.g., MMPI, NEO-FFI, etc), noted Madeline's remarkable agentic strengths which were vividly portrayed in her opening response to the Rorschach on Card I and in a response to Card V. Equally impressive in Madeline's Rorschach protocol were responses that indicated her intense vulnerability to threat as expressed in her response to Card IV. The intensity of these responses suggested that Madeline's agentic capacities also served as a counter phobic defense to deal with intense fears and apprehensions. But even more basic was the function of these intense agentic qualities to also ward off vulnerability to largely unconscious, profoundly painful, feelings of loneliness and loss as expressed in her continued longing to establish a relationship with her mother. Thus in many ways, Madeline's impressive introjective qualities and powerful agentic strengths were the basis not only for her developing very important adaptive capacities, but they also provide important defensive functions to protect her from introjective fears and apprehensions about attack and assault, and, more importantly, from recognizing and experiencing powerful unfilled, but deeply repressed, anaclitic longings for a close, need-gratifying relationship with a maternal object.

Madeline, according to Behrends and Blatt (2003), presented an extremely complex diagnostic picture of being head-strong and fiercely independent as well as achingly tender and vulnerable. During psychological assessment she was provocatively oppositional and defiant as well as selfless and generous with a capacity for empathy and mutuality. In her psychological test protocols (WAIS, TAT, and Rorschach), Madeline communicated a sense of power and strength that was expressed in her functioning as a highly competent and successful attorney who has made remarkable achievements despite an extraordinarily painful and difficult, even traumatic, childhood and adolescence. Her power, strength, and accomplishment were conveyed in Rorschach responses like the well-perceived response of a woman in the center of Card I who was seen as "holding her hands up, got great big wings. Like she's professing! Very powerful! I like that…her back is to you. She's facing the crowd. She'd have to be giving them information…. Someone important in front of all these people! Like she'd have something important to say," or in Madeline's response to Card V of the Rorschach, "A butterfly in flight, quite majestic, out for an afternoon flight."

These responses of power, strength, independence, beauty, and majesty were juxtaposed with responses indicating intense vulnerability as well as a profound sense of loneliness and emptiness. Madeline's intense vulnerability was expressed in her response to Card IV of the Rorschach of a "Scary monster. Great big monster, getting sick! Huge feet, small head, claws. Oh, it's like fire, burning this little person. Poor bugger. Very imposing figure! Tiny head, not very smart, dangerous!" She elaborated the response further by noting that "top is his head, looking down, spraying from the mouth. First looks like he's getting sick. Then looks like fire, very dark….Fire from guy's mouth. Burning him on purpose! Little bugger didn't stand a chance! …. Like it wasn't accidental. His back is to us. He's inside of the fire. Little arms hanging down there …. Don't you see that? God, I hope so! It's so obvious! I need to put some dancing pandas in that picture!" (Referring back to one of her more positive, playful responses to Card II of the Rorschach).

These Rorschach responses express the polarity of Madeline's experience from a sense of personal strength and power, to feelings that the world is dangerous and destructive in which a poor vulnerable little person can be tortured and destroyed. And Madeline's powerful agentic (introjective) qualities clearly offered her a considerable sense of strength in this highly destructive and dangerous world. But it is important to note that Madeline was not only vulnerable to feelings of danger in a hostile destructive world, but also to a profound sense of loneliness, emptiness, and abandonment – an active yearning for her mother that was expressed in her comments when asked to describe herself that "there was never a baby in our family. The first time I ever kissed my mother was when she was lying in the hospital, having just slit her wrists on the kitchen table. I saw my cousin brushing her hair, and I was green with envy." And in describing her mother, Madeline notes that "She wouldn't let you know her, so your questions remain questions. If you ask her about her childhood, she just gets up and leaves! So I'm left with just blanks."

Madeline's unfulfilled longings and needs for a close relationship and a primary attachment with her mother was vividly expressed in several of her responses to Card X of the Rorschach, "It looks like a party in a psychedelic aquarium. A party! They're having fun. Everybody's smiling. They live in an ecosystem, all in someway attached. Fine, so no one's trying to get away. All are enjoying themselves at the party. All so very, very, very, different. Having a great time." Madeline then notes that there is a blue crab on the side, "This blue crab. Guy's forlorn, defeated. There is the eye and a big ole nose. Not so much sad as hopeless. This (on the other side) is not a mirror image. Otherwise, an underwater circus! A great thing going on!" (The examiner noted feeling sad and tearful herself in reaction to these responses).

The response of pleasure and excitement in the comfort, stability, and security in being "attached" to others within a containing ecosystem seems to express a deep longing for a primary reunion with her mother. Thus, Madeline's exaggerated introjective assertion of autonomy, freedom, independence, and power seem to have both important adaptive and defensive functions. These introjective strivings and expressions of agency are not only expressed in her successful career and her remarkable resilience in coping with severe adversity in a potentially dangerous and destructive world, but they also serve to defend Madeline from the painful recognition of the intensity of her profound depressive anaclitic longings for a primary relationship with her mother. This complex diagnostic picture illustrates how, in some individuals, exaggerated emphasis on one configuration (in this case, on qualities of the introjective configuration) can serve to defend against recognizing and experiencing profound involvement with the warded-off elements of more painful and threatening anaclitic issues.

Future clinical and empirical research needs to identify ways to differentiate when anaclitic and introjective qualities define basic personality or character features and when these two sets of qualities have a more dynamic relationship in which intense emphasis on one set of attributes serves to defend against recognizing and experiencing the intensity of concerns in the other domain. This dynamic defensive interplay between introjective and anaclitic issues can be identified in clinical evaluations. But subsequent research on this phenomenon will depend on our ability to develop methods that might enable us to differentiate between anaclitic and introjective character or personality organization from when these two types of personality organization occur in a more dynamic context.

The findings with Madeline also suggest that the primary differentiation of anaclitic and introjective dimensions on the Rorschach, and possibly on other unstructured assessment procedures like the Thematic Apperception Test (TAT; Morgan & Murray, 1935), may occur primarily in the thematic content rather than the structural organization of the responses (see also, for example, the contributions of McAdams, 1993). This would explain why Blatt (1992) and Blatt and Ford (1994) found so few significant pretreatment differences between anaclitic and introjective patients on the Rorschach variables they used to empirically assess therapeutic change. The structural variables on the Rorschach, like F+% (i.e., the degree of reality testing), degree and type of thought disorder (Allison, Blatt, & Zimet, 1988), and the differentiation, articulation, and integration of human responses (Blatt, Brenneis, Schimek, & Glick, 1976), may not be effective in differentiating anaclitic from introjective personality organization, but they may be very useful in defining the developmental level of the anaclitic and introjective personality organization. The content of responses to the Rorschach and the TAT (whether they focus on issues of relatedness or self-definition), however, may provide a reliable basis for differentiating between anaclitic and introjective personality organization, while the structural variables, like the type and degree of cognitive organization, may define the developmental level at which the different behavioral and symptomatic expressions of an anaclitic or introjective personality organization are expressed. Thus, less differentiated and integrated anaclitic individuals would have more infantile and dependent features – in DEQ terms, have greater neediness; while anaclitic patients with greater differentiation and integration would have more oedipal features – in DEQ terms, greater relatedness with greater adaptive potential. And less differentiated and integrated introjective individuals would have more paranoid, obsessive, and depressive features – in DEQ terms, a more self-critical focus, while more differentiated and integrated introjective individuals would have, in DEQ terms, a greater sense of personal efficacy with greater adaptive potential. These formulations await systematic investigation.

Conclusions

In summary, our recent empirical research and clinical observations indicate that refinements of the anaclitic-introjective distinction have facilitated the study of normal development as well as aspects of the clinical process. The formulations of the importance of issues of interpersonal relatedness and self-definition as two fundamental dimensions of psychological development appears to be applicable to understanding normal development, disruptions in development that are expressed in different forms of psychopathology, and in the processes of therapeutic change, thus supporting the fundamental assumption of this work that much can be gained by considering psychological disturbances, not as separate diseases that may have some as yet unspecified and undocumented biological causes, but as expressions of severe disruptions of normal psychological development.

References

Alden, L. E., & Bieling, P. J. (1996). Interpersonal convergence of personality constructs in dynamic and cognitive models of depression. *Journal of Research in Personality, 30*, 60-75.

Allison, J., Blatt, S. J., & Zimet, C. N. (1968). *The Interpretation of Psychological Tests*. New York: Harper and Row. Second edition: reprinted in 1988, Hemisphere Publishing Company.

Andrews, J. D. W. (1989). Psychotherapy of depression: A self-confirmation model. *Psychological Review, 96*, 576-607.

Angyal, A. (1941). *Foundations for a science of personality*. New York: Viking Press.

Angyal, A. (1951). *Neurosis and treatment: A holistic theory*. New York: Wiley.

Arieti, S., & Bemporad, J. R. (1978). *Severe and mild depression: The therapeutic approach*. New York: Basic Books.

Arieti, S., & Bemporad, J. R. (1980). The psychological organization of depression. *American Journal of Psychiatry, 137*, 1360-1365.

Aubé, J., & Whiffen, V. E. (1996). Depressive styles and social acuity: Further evidence for distinct interpersonal correlates of dependency and self-criticism. *Communication Research, 23*, 407-424.

Bakan, D. (1966). *The duality of human existence: An essay on psychology and religion*. Chicago, IL: Rand McNally.

Beck, A. T. (1983). Cognitive therapy of depression: New perspectives. In P. J. Clayton & J. E. Barrett (Eds.), *Treatment of depression: Old controversies and new approaches* (pp. 265-290). New York: Raven.

Behrends, R. S., & Blatt, S. J. (2003). Psychodynamic assessment. In J. Wiggins & K. Trobst (Eds.), *Paradigms of Personality Assessment* (pp. 226-342). New York: Guilford Press.

Benjamin, L. S. (1974). Structural analysis of social behavior. *Psychological Review, 81,* 392-425.

Beutel, M. E., Wiltink, J., Hafner, C., Reiner, I., Bleichner, F., & Blatt, S. J. (2004). Abhangigkeit und Selbstkritik als psychologische dimensionen der depression – validierung der deutschsprachigen version des Depressive Experiences Questionnaire (DEQ) [Dependency and Self-Criticism as psychological dimensions in depression: Validation of the German version of the Depressive Experiences Questionnaire (DEQ)]. *Zeitschrift für Klinische Psychologie, Psychiatrie und Psychotherapie, 1,* 1-14.

Bibring, E. (1953). The mechanism of depression. In P. Greenacre (Ed.), *Affective disorders* (pp. 13-48). New York: International Universities Press.

Blatt, S. J. (1974). Levels of object representation in anaclitic and introjective depression. *Psychoanalytic Study of the Child, 29,* 107-157.

Blatt, S. J. (1990). Interpersonal relatedness and self-definition: Two personality configurations and their implications for psychopathology and psychotherapy. In J. L. Singer (Ed.), *Repression and dissociation: Implications for personality theory, psychopathology & health* (pp. 299-335). Chicago: University of Chicago Press.

Blatt, S. J. (1992). The differential effect of psychotherapy and psychoanalysis on anaclitic and introjective patients: The Menninger Psychotherapy Research Project revisited. *Journal of the American Psychoanalytic Association, 40,* 691-724.

Blatt, S. J. (1995a). Representational structures in psychopathology. In D. Cicchetti & S. Toth (Eds.), *Rochester Symposium on Developmental Psychopathology: Vol. 6. Emotion, Cognition, and Representation* (pp. 1-33). Rochester, NY: University of Rochester Press.

Blatt, S. J. (1995b). The destructiveness of perfectionism: Implications for the treatment of depression. *American Psychologist, 50,* 1003-1020.

Blatt, S. J. (2004). *Experiences of depression: Theoretical, clinical and research perspectives*. Washington, DC: American Psychological Association.

Blatt, S. J., & Blass, R. (1996). Relatedness and self-definition: A dialectic model of personality development. In G. G. Noam & K. W. Fischer (Eds.), *Development and vulnerabilities in close relationships* (pp. 309-338). Hillsdale, NJ: Lawrence Erlbaum Associates.

Blatt, S. J., & Blass, R. B. (1990). Attachment and separateness: A dialectic model of the products and processes of psychological development. *Psychoanalytic Study of the Child, 45,* 107-127.

Blatt, S. J., & Blass, R. B. (1992). Relatedness and self-definition: Two primary dimensions in personality development, psychopathology, and psychotherapy. In J. Barron, M. Eagle, & D. Wolitsky (Eds.), *The interface of psychoanalysis and psychology* (pp. 399-428). Washington, DC: American Psychological Association.

Blatt, S. J., Brenneis, C. B., Schimek, J. G., & Glick, M. (1976). The normal development and psychopathological impairment of the concept of the object on Rorschach. *Journal of Abnormal Psychology, 85,* 364-373.

Blatt, S. J., D'Afflitti, J. P., & Quinlan, D. M. (1976). Experiences of depression in normal young adults. *Journal of Abnormal Psychology, 85,* 383-389.

Blatt, S. J., & Ford, R. (1994). *Therapeutic Change: An object relations perspective*. New York: Plenum.

Blatt, S. J., & Homann, E. (1992). Parent-child interaction in the etiology of dependent and self-critical depression. *Clinical Psychology Review, 12,* 47-91.

Blatt, S. J., & Maroudas, C. (1992). Convergence among psychoanalytic and cognitive-behavioral theories of depression. *Psychoanalytic Psychology, 9,* 157-190.

Blatt, S. J., Quinlan, D. M., Chevron, E. S., McDonald, C., & Zuroff, D. (1982). Dependency and self-criticism: Psychological dimensions of depression. *Journal of Consulting and Clinical Psychology, 50,* 113-124.

Blatt, S. J., Quinlan, D. M., Pilkonis, P. A., & Shea, T. (1995). Impact of perfectionism and need for approval on the brief treatment of depression: The National Institute of Mental Health Treatment of Depression Collaborative Research Program Revisited. *Journal of Consulting and Clinical Psychology,*

63, 125-132.

Blatt, S. J., & Shahar, G. (2003). Das dialogische Selbst: Adaptive und maladaptive Dimensionen. In P. Giampieri-Deutsch (Ed.), *Psychoanalyse im Dialog der Wissenschaften. Band 2, Anglo-Amerikanische Perspektiven* (pp. 285-309). Stuttgart: Kohlhammer.

Blatt, S. J., & Shahar, G. (2004a). Psychoanalysis: With whom, for what, and how? Comparisons with psychotherapy. *Journal of the American Psychoanalytic Association, 52*, 393-447.

Blatt, S. J., & Shahar, G. (2004b). Stability of the patient by treatment interactions in the Menninger Psychotherapy Research Project. *Bulletin of Menninger Clinic, 68*, 23-36.

Blatt, S. J., & Shichman, S. (1983). Two primary configurations of psychopathology. *Psychoanalysis and Contemporary Thought, 6*, 187-254.

Blatt, S. J., Stayner, D., Auerbach, J., & Behrends, R. S. (1996). Change in object and self representations in long-term, intensive, inpatient treatment of seriously disturbed adolescents and young adults. *Psychiatry: Interpersonal and Biological Processes, 59*, 82-107

Blatt, S. J., Wein, S. J., Chevron, E. S., & Quinlan, D. M. (1979). Parental representations and depression in normal young adults. *Journal of Abnormal Psychology, 88*, 388-397.

Blatt, S. J., Zohar, A. H., Quinlan, D. M., Zuroff, D. C., & Mongrain, M. (1995). Subscales within the dependency factor of the Depressive Experiences Questionnaire. *Journal of Personality Assessment, 64*, 319-339.

Blatt, S. J., Zohar, A., Quinlan, D. M., Luthar, S. S., & Hart, B. (1996). Levels of relatedness within the dependency factor of the Depressive Experiences Questionnaire for adolescents. *Journal of Personality Assessment, 67*, 52-71.

Blatt, S. J., & Zuroff, D. C. (1992). Interpersonal relatedness and self-definition: Two prototypes for depression. *Clinical Psychology Review, 12*, 527-562.

Blatt, S. J., Zuroff, D. C., Bondi, C. M., Sanislow, C., & Pilkonis, P. (1998). When and how perfectionism impedes the brief treatment of depression: Further analyses of the NIMH TDCRP. *Journal of Consulting and Clinical Psychology, 66*, 423-428.

Bornstein, R. F. (1998). Depathologizing dependency. *Journal of Nervous and Mental Diseases, 186*, 67-73.

Bowlby, J. (1980). *Attachment and loss: Volume 3. Loss: Sadness and depression.* New York: Basic Books.

Buss, D. M. (1987). Selection, evocation, and manipulation. *Journal of Personality and Social Psychology, 53*, 1214-1221.

Cane, D. B., Olinger, L. J., Gotlib, I. H., & Kuiper, N. A. (1986). Factor structure of the Dysfunctional Attitude Scale in a student population. *Journal of Clinical Psychology, 42*, 307-309.

Clark, D. A., & Beck, A. T. (1999). *Scientific foundations of cognitive theory and therapy of depression.* New York: John Wiley & Sons.

Cohen, M. B., Baker, G., Cohen, R. A., Fromm-Reichman, F., & Weigert, E. V. (1954). An intensive study of twelve cases of manic depressive psychosis. *Psychiatry, 17*, 103-137.

Compas, R. C. (2002). Manifestations of dependent and self-critical personality styles in Rorschach: An exploratory study. *Journal of Projective Psychology and Mental Health, 9*, 93-104.

Coyne, J. C. (1976). Toward an interactional description of depression. *Psychiatry, 39*, 28-40.

Coyne, J. C. (1998). Thinking interactionally about depresssion: A radical restatement. In T. Joiner & J. C. Coyne (Eds.), *The interactional nature of depression.* Washington, DC: American Psychological Association.

Coyne, J. C., & Whiffen, V. E. (1995). Issues in personality as diathesis for depression: The case of sociotropy-dependency and autonomy self-criticism. *Psychological Bulletin, 118*, 358-378.

Dunkley, D. M., Blankstein, K. R., & Flett, G. L. (1997). Specific cognitive-personality vulnerability styles in depression and the five-factor model of personality. *Personality and Individual Differences, 23*, 1041-1053.

Dunkley, D. M., Zuroff, D. C., & Blankstein, K. R. (2003). Self-Critical perfectionism and daily affect: Dispositional and situational influences on stress and coping. *Journal of Personality and Social Psychology, 84*, 234-252.

Elkin, I., Shea, M. T., Watkins, J. T., Imber, S. D., Sotsky, S. M., Collins, J. F., Glass, D. R., Pilkonis, P. A., Leber, W. R., Docherty, J. P., Fiester, S. J., & Parloff, M. B. (1989). NIMH Treatment of Depression Collaborative Research Program: General effectiveness of treatments. *Archives of General Psychiatry, 46*, 971-983.

Enns, M. W., Cox, B., & Inayatulla, M. (2003). Personality predictors of outcome for adolescents hospitalized for suicidal ideation. *Journal of the American Academy of Child & Adolescent Psychiatry,*

42, 720-727.

Erikson, E. H. (1950). *Childhood and society* (2nd ed.). New York: Norton.

Fazaa, N. (2001). *Dependency, Self-criticism and suicidal behavior.* Unpublished thesis, University of Windsor, Windsor, Ontario.

Fazaa, N., & Page, S. (2003). Dependency and self-criticism as predictors of suicidal behavior. *Suicide & Life-Threatening Behavior, 33*, 172-185.

Fichman, L., Koestner, R., & Zuroff, D. C. (1994). Depressive styles in adolescence: Assessment, relation to social functioning, and developmental trends. *Journal of Youth and Adolescence, 23*, 315-330.

Fonagy, P., Leigh, T., Steele, M., Steele, H., Kennedy, R., Mattoon, G., Target, M., & Gerber, A. (1996). The relation of attachment status, psychiatric classification, and response to psychotherapy. *Journal of Consulting and Clinical Psychology, 64*, 22-31.

Frank, S. J., Van Egeren, L. A., Paul, J. S., Poorman, M. O., Sanford, K., Williams, O. B., & Field, D. T. (1997). Measuring self-critical and interpersonal preoccupations in an adolescent inpatient sample. *Psychological Assessment, 9*, 185-195.

Freud, S. (1957). Mourning and melancholia. In J. Strachey (Ed. and Trans.), *The standard edition of the complete psychological works of Sigmund Freud* (Vol. 14, 243-258). London: Hogarth Press. (Original work published 1917)

Freud, S. (1958). On narcissism: An introduction. In J. Strachey (Ed. and Trans.), *The standard edition of the complete psychological works of Sigmund Freud* (Vol. 14, 73-102). London: Hogarth Press. (Original work published 1914)

Freud, S. (1959). Inhibitions, symptoms and anxiety. In J. Strachey (Ed. and Trans.), *The standard edition of the complete psychological works of Sigmund Freud* (Vol. 20, 87-174). London: Hogarth Press. (Original work published 1926)

Freud, S. (1961). Civilization and its discontents. In J. Strachey (Ed. and Trans.), *The standard edition of the complete psychological works of Sigmund Freud* (Vol. 21, 64-145). London: Hogarth Press. (Original work published 1930)

Goodman, S., & Gotlib, I. (2002). *Children of depressed parents. Mechanisms of risk and implications for treatment.* Washington, DC: American Psychological Association.

Hammen, C. (1991). Generation of stress in the course of unipolar depression. *Journal of Abnormal Psychology, 100*, 555-561.

Hammen, C. (1998). The emergence of an interpersonal approach to depression. In T. E. Joiner & J. C. Coyne (Eds.), *The interpersonal nature of depression* (pp. 21-35). Washington, DC: American Psychological Association.

Henrich, C., Blatt, S. J., Kuperminc, G. P., Zohar, A., & Leadbeater, B. J. (2001). Levels of interpersonal concerns and social functioning in early adolescent boys and girls. *Journal of Personality Assessment, 76*, 48-67.

Hoyle, R.H., & Smith, G.T. (1994). Formulating clinical research hypotheses as structural equation models: A conceptual overview. *Journal of Consulting and Clinical Psychology, 3*, 429-440.

Imber, S. D., Pilkonis, P. A., Sotsky, S. M., Elkin, I., Watkins, J. T., Collins, J. F., Shea, M. T., Leber, W. R., & Glass, D. R. (1990). Mode-specific effects among three treatments for depression. *Journal of Consulting and Clinical Psychology, 58*, 352-359.

Jae Im, C. (1996). *The characteristics of two depressive dimensions.* Unpublished master's thesis. University of Korea.

Joiner, Jr., T. E. (1994). Contagious depression: Existence, specificity to depressive symptoms, and the role of reassurance-seeking. *Journal of Personality and Social Psychology, 67*, 287-296.

Klein, D. F. (1989). The revised DEQ: A further evaluation. *Journal of Personality Assessment, 53*, 703-715.

Kuperminc, G. P., Blatt, S. J., & Leadbeater, B. J. (1997). Relatedness, self-definition and early adolescent adjustment. *Cognitive Therapy and Research, 21*, 301-320.

Kuperminc, G. P., Leadbeater, B. J, & Blatt, S. J. (2001). School social climate and individual differences in vulnerability to psychopathology among middle school students. *Journal of School Psychology, 39*, 141-159.

Leadbeater, B. J., Kuperminc, G. P., Blatt, S. J., & Hertzog, C. (1999). A multivariate mode of gender differences in adolescent's internalizing and externalizing problems. *Developmental Psychology, 35*, 1268-1282.

Loewald, H. W. (1962). Internalization, separation, mourning, and the superego. *Psychoanalytic Quarterly, 31*, 483-504.

Luyten, P. (2002). *Normbesef en depressie: Aanzet tot een integratief theoretisch kader en een empirisch onderzoek aan de hand van de depressietheorie van S. J. Blatt* [Personal standards and depression: An integrative psychodynamic framework, and an empirical investigation of S. J. Blatt's theory of depression]. Unpublished doctoral dissertation, University of Leuven, Leuven, Belgium.

Maslow, H. (1954). *Motivation and personality*. New York: Harper & Row.

McAdams, D. P. (1993). *The stories we live by: Personal myths and the making of the self*. New York: Morrow

Mongrain, M. (1998). Parental representations and support-seeking behavior related to dependency and self-criticism. *Journal of Personality, 66*, 151-173.

Mongrain, M., Vettese, L. C., Shuster, B., & Kendal, N. (1998). Perceptual biases, affect, and behavior in the relationships of dependents and self-critics. *Journal of Personality, 75*, 230-241.

Morgan, C. D., & Murray, H. A. (1935). A method for investigating fantasies: The Thematic Apperception Test. *Archives of Neurology and Psychiatry, 34*, 289-306.

Nietzel, M. T., & Harris, M. J. (1990). Relationship of dependency and achievement/autonomy to depression. *Clinical Psychology Review, 10*, 279-297

Plomin, R., & Caspi, A. (1999). Behavioral genetics and personality. In L. A. Pervin & O. P. John (Eds.), *Handbook of personality theory and research* (2nd ed., pp. 251-276). New York: Guilford.

Priel, B., & Besser, A. (2000). Dependency and self-criticism among first-time mothers: The role of global and specific support. *Journal of Social and Clinical Psychology, 19*, 437-450.

Priel, B., & Shahar, G. (2000). Dependency, self-criticism, social context and distress: Comparing moderating and mediating models. *Personality and Individual Differences, 28*, 515-525.

Priel, B., Besser, A., & Shahar, G. (1998). *Israeli Adaptation of the DEQ: Psychometric properties*. Unpublished Manuscript. Behavioral Sciences Department, Ben-Gurion University of the Negev, Beer-Sheva, Israel.

Robins, C. J. (1995). Personality-event interaction models of depression. *European Journal of Personality, 9*, 367-378.

Robins, C. J., & Luten, A. G. (1991). Sociotropy and autonomy: Differential patterns of clinical presentation in unipolar depression. *Journal of Abnormal Psychology, 100*, 74-77.

Robins, C. J., Ladd, J., Welkowitz, J., Blaney, P. H., Diaz, R., & Kutcher, G. (1994). The Personal Style Inventory: Preliminary validation studies of new measures of sociotropy and autonomy. *Journal of Psychopathology and Behavioral Assessment, 16*, 277-300.

Rude, S. S., & Burnham, B. L. (1995). Connectedness and neediness: Factors of the DEQ and SAS dependency scales. *Cognitive Therapy and Research, 19*, 323-340.

Santor, D. A., Pringle, J. D., & Israeli, A. L. (2000). Enhancing and disrupting cooperative behavior in couples: Effects of dependency and self-criticism following favorable and unfavorable performance feedback. *Cognitive Therapy and Research, 24*, 379-397.

Shahar, G. (2001). Commentary on "Shame and community: Social components of depression." Personality, shame, and the breakdown of social ties: The voice of quantitative depression research. *Psychiatry, 64*, 228-239.

Shahar, G., Blatt, S. J., & Ford, R. Q. (2003). Mixed anaclitic-introjective psychopathology in treatment resistant inpatients undergoing psychoanalytic psychotherapy. *Psychoanalytic Psychology, 20*, 84-102.

Shahar, G., Blatt, S. J., Zuroff, D. C., Krupnick, J. L., & Sotsky, S. M. (2004). Perfectionism impedes social relations and response to brief treatment for depression. *Journal of Social and Clinical Psychology, 23*, 140-154.

Shahar, G., Blatt, S. J., Zuroff, D. C., & Pilkonis, P. A. (2002). Role of perfectionism and personality disorder features in response to brief treatment for depression. *Journal of Consulting and Clinical Psychology, 71*, 229-233.

Shahar, G., Gallagher, L. F., Blatt, S. J., Kuperminc, G. P., & Leadbeater, B. J. (in press). An interactive-synergetic approach to the assessment of personality vulnerability to depression: Illustration with the adolescent version of the Depressive Experiences Questionnaire. *Journal of Clinical Psychology*.

Shahar, G., Joiner, T. E. Jr., Zuroff, D. C., & Blatt, S. J. (2004). Personality, interpersonal behavior, and depression. Co-existence of stress-specific moderating and mediating effects. *Personality and Individual Differences, 36*, 1583-1596.

Shahar, G., & Priel, B. (2003). Active vulnerability, adolescent distress, and the mediating/suppressing role of life events. *Personality and Individual Differences, 35*, 199-218.

Vettese, L. C., & Mongrain, M. (2000). Communication about the self and partner in the relationships of dependents and self-critics. *Cognitive Therapy and Research, 24*, 609-626.

161

Wachtel, P. L. (1994). Cyclical processes in personality and psychopathology. *Journal of Abnormal Psychology, 103*, 51-66.

Weissman, A. N., & Beck, A. T. (1978, August-September). *Development and validation of the Dysfunctional Attitudes Scale: A preliminary investigation.* Paper presented at the 86th Annual Convention of the American Psychological Association, Toronto.

Wiggins, J. S. (1991). Agency and communion as conceptual coordinates for the understanding and measurement of interpersonal behavior. In W. W. Grove & D. Cicchetti (Eds.), *Thinking clearly about psychology, Vol. 2: Personality and psychotherapy* (pp. 89-113). Minneapolis: University of Minnesota Press.

Wiggins, J. S. (Ed.). (2003). *Paradigms of personality assessment.* New York: Guilford Press.

Zuroff, D. C. (1992). New directions for cognitive models of depression. *Psychological Inquiry, 3*, 274-277.

Zuroff, D. C., Blatt, S. J., Sotsky, S. M., Krupnick, J. L., Martin, D. J., Sanislow, C. A., & Simmens, S. (2000). Relation of therapeutic alliance and perfectionism to outcome in brief outpatient treatment of depression. *Journal of Consulting and Clinical Psychology, 68*, 114-124.

Zuroff, D. C., & deLorimier, S. (1989). Ideal and actual romantic partners of women varying in dependency and self-criticism. *Journal of Personality, 57*, 825-846.

Zuroff, D. C., & Duncan, N. (1999). Self-criticism and conflict resolution in romantic couples. *Canadian Journal of Behavioral Science, 31*, 137-149.

Zuroff, D. C., & Fitzpatrick, D. (1995). Depressive personality styles: Implications for adult attachment. *Personality and Individual Differences, 18*, 253-265.

Zuroff, D. C., & Franko, D. L. (1986, April). *Depressed and test anxious subjects' interactions with friends: Effects of dependency and self-criticism.* Paper presented at the meeting of the Eastern Psychological Association, New York.

Zuroff, D. C., Moskowitz, D. S., Wielgus, M. S., Powers, T. A., & Franko, D. L. (1983). Construct validation of the Dependency and Self-Criticism scales of the Depressive Experiences Questionnaire. *Journal of Research in Personality, 17*, 226-241.

Zuroff, D. C., Quinlan, D. M., & Blatt, S. J. (1990). Psychometric properties of the Depressive Experiences Questionnaire. *Journal of Personality Assessment, 55*, 65-72.

Chapter 6

'Closed Doors and Landscapes in the Mist' 1.

Childhood and Adolescent Depression

in Developmental Psychopathology

Nicole Vliegen, Patrick Meurs, & Gaston Cluckers

In the following two chapters, we will focus on depression in childhood and adolescence. Chapter 6 presents theoretical perspectives and empirical research from the domain of developmental psychopathology in general, summarizing the knowledge that has been acquired since childhood depression became recognized as an important clinical problem, some 25 years ago. We will describe the major developments in this area and we discuss recent integrative theories of childhood depression. Chapter 7 focuses more specifically on psychodynamic developmental psychopathology. It treats, from a historical point of view, the contribution psychoanalysis can make to the domain of developmental psychopathology today, and it reflects on how psychoanalytic developmental psychopathology can benefit from the broader current of developmental psychopathology.

Both chapters refer in their title to "closed doors and landscapes in the mist", an image from a play therapy of a depressive child. We will introduce this image in chapter 6 and work it out at the end of chapter 7.

From the first sessions on, eight-year-old Jan[1] establishes a positive and differentiated contact with his therapist. He says that he likes to come to the playroom and is able to symbolize his thoughts and affects in different ways: by talking, playing, drawing, etc. Once the therapeutic alliance is well formed, he starts to bring in more depressive contents, signalling an important element he will have to work through in the course of the therapy. In session 8, Jan makes a very significant drawing about "silhouettes in the mist". These silhouettes have no arms and cannot reach each other. Their faces lack any reference to senses. Because of this, the facial expressions of these figures are rather flat.

In the same session, Jan also plays a boy, longing to go to a house, but the house is really far away. When the boy reaches the house at last, the door is closed. The boy waits on the doorstep. He stays there, waiting and waiting for the door to open. But the boy is unsure whether or when others will come to let him in, and, whether they will like his initiative at all.

This is the kind of material we can meet in play therapy with depressed children. Elements of the developmental psychopathological perspective constructed in the next two chapters, will be used to think about certain vulnerabilities and signs of resilience in this schoolboy named Jan. In addition to this, we will extensively return to the introjective and anaclitic elements in Jan's play material and try to understand them from a "developmental pathways perspective". Some elements of intervention, sensitive to the specificities of introjective and anaclitic themes, will be shown.

But firstly, in this chapter, we will summarize some of the main results from mainstream developmental psychopathological research on depression. We discuss the specificities of the symptomatology of depression in children and its age-related manifestations; we treat classification issues, prevalence, course and comorbidity. We discuss epidemiological findings and consider some major theoretical formulations about childhood depression and development. By the end, we will come to an integration of perspectives with authors such as Cicchetti and Toth (1998) and Goodman and Gotlib (1999); we also point out the importance of Blatt's contribution (Blatt, 2004; Blatt & Homann, 1992) on the developmental origins of depression. By doing so, we will have worked out a broad framework against which the addition of a psychodynamic developmental psychopathology will become clear in the next chapter. In the following chapter, we sketch a developmental line of normal and maladaptive depressive phenomena in childhood, bringing together some anchor points of the most important psychoanalytic theories of depression. At the end of the next chapter, we will then return to the playroom, in the presence of eight-year-old Jan. Some illustrations from later parts of his therapy will highlight how one can work with depressed

---

[1] The therapist in this case is Patrick Meurs. Jan's process has been described extensively by Meurs and Cluckers (1999). Some aspects that are illustrative of our clinical work with childhood depression will be described in the next chapter of this book.

children in different phases of treatment and with different kinds of depressive phenomena.

Depression in Developmental Psychopathology: Research Findings

From Denial to Recognition

For the past twenty-five years, childhood depression has been recognized as an important problem. Cees de Wit (1997) describes the important change that has taken place in the overall attitude on this topic. A firm denial gave way into a general and strong conviction about the importance of depressive syndromes in childhood and of the implications throughout the life course. This recognition made it possible for therapeutic interventions and prevention programs to be developed and set up for depressive children, and to have these programs financed and evaluated on a scientific basis. However, only recently, a multidisciplinary workgroup preparing the Strategic Plan for Mood Disorders Research of the National Institute of Mental Health (NIMH), still noted important gaps in our understanding of the onset, course, and recurrence of mood disorders in children and adolescents (Costello, et al., 2002).

Several factors have facilitated this evolution concerning the recognition of childhood depression. Firstly, society is confronted with the enormous cost of untreated childhood depression later on in life. The few follow-up studies that exist show that prepubertal-onset depressive children have more substance abuse/dependence and conduct disorder/antisocial personality disorder in adulthood as well as impaired functioning in important roles (Weissman, et al., 1999a, b; Hammen & Garber, 2001). Major depressive disorder (MDD) in particular shows remarkable continuity from childhood to adulthood and is associated with high morbidity and potential mortality through suicide (Pine, Cohen, Gurley, Brook, & Ma, 1998; Weissman, et al., 1999a, b).

Secondly, there is increased recognition of the fact that depression cannot only occur in puberty and adolescence, but also in grade-school children, and even in toddlers and infants (de Wit, 1997; Garber & Flynn, 2001; Kolvin & Sadovski, 2001; Lazarus, 2002; Luby, 2000; Shaffer & Waslick 2002). One can only be struck by the tragic suicides of depressed children, reported in our newspapers from time to time:

A twelve-year-old boy ended his life Thursday night at his school in the neighborhood of Liège. He hanged himself in the playground and left a note about being disappointed in love. Suicide at this age is rather exceptional, but depression in young children is increasing.

Belga, De Standaard, March 2003

165

Is childhood depression the same as or comparable to depression in adulthood? Are the symptoms and the course identical? To answer these questions, we will first of all differentiate between core symptoms and age-specific symptoms of childhood depression.

Core Symptoms. The DSM-IV criteria (American Psychiatric Association, 1994) for depressive disorders are essentially identical for all developmental levels or phases. There are only two minor variations for children and adolescents, with regard to the duration of the symptoms and the understanding of irritability in children with depressive symptoms (see also below).

Core symptoms that are typical of depression across one's life span are mentioned in the DSM-IV, as well as by several important researchers; they include loss of the capacity to enjoy, decreased interest and motivation, and enduring dysthymia (Harrington, 1993; Poznanski & Mokros, 1994; De Wit, 1997).

Age-specific manifestations. Developmental psychopathologists (Cicchetti & Toth, 1998; de Wit, 1997) suggest that manifestations of depression might depend considerably on the level of cognitive, social, emotional, moral and physiological development. This means that some of the symptoms of depression are different during childhood and throughout one's lifespan.

Weiss and Garber (2003) suggested two explanations for developmental differences in depressive symptoms. First, children and adults differ in how they express particular symptoms of depression, although the very nature of these symptoms would be similar at all ages. For example, dysphoric mood might be expressed by excessive crying in very young children, by nonverbal sadness in grade-school children, by irritability in adolescents and by depressed mood in adults, but the core mood symptom is essentially the same across these age-specific expressions (Garber & Flynn, 2001).

Another possibility is that the symptoms of the depressive illness really differ in nature, due to the developmental level. Some depressive symptoms require a certain level of cognitive, emotional, moral or social development. Under the age of eight, for example, suicidal ideation is not really possible; one will only observe these thoughts later in childhood. Another example is that of guilt, which becomes observable only in older toddlers (de Wit, 1997).

Based upon clinical observation and developmentally based research in 3 to 6 year olds, de Wit (1997) has proposed a model that includes both core symptoms of depression that are invariable across the life span and age or 'developmental phase specific' depressive symptoms. This model, which subsequently underwent a series of revisions based on later research findings (Lous, de Wit, De Bruynn & Riksen-Walraven, 2002; Lous, de Wit, De Bruyn, Riksen-Walraven, & Rost, 2000) is presented in Table 1.

TABLE 1
Differential age-specific symptoms of depression (Based on de Wit, 1997, pp. 169-170; Lous, de Wit, De Bruyn & Riksen-Walraven, 2002; Lous, de Wit, De Bruyn, Riksen-Walraven, & Rost, 2000).

Infant	Toddler/preschooler	Grade-school children	Adolescent
Anaclitic depression - Crying - Searching - Protest - Despair - Withdrawal - Apathy	*Sad facial expression and posture concerning play and playfulness:* - Inability to experience pleasure - Lack of playfulness - Absence of symbolic play - More nonplay behaviors	*Sad mood* *Concerning activity* - Inability to experience pleasure - Apathy - Decreased activity *Concerning emotionality* - Feelings of guilt	*Sad mood* *Concerning activity* - Inability to experience pleasure - Apathy - Decreased activity - Withdrawal - Boredom - Decreased achieve- ment motivation
Infant depression - Inconsolable and frequent crying - Failure to thrive - Sleep and eating disorders - Retarded growth	*Concerning growth* - Failure to thrive - Retarded growth *Concerning emotionality* - Separation anxiety - 'magic' feelings of guilt (from 4 years on) - Absence of other cognitive symptoms of depression	- Feelings of being bad - Negative self-esteem - Negative thoughts about the future - Preoccupation with illness and death - Preliminary suicidal thoughts *Secondary* - Social problems - Problems with aggression - Problems with regard to school adjustment - Somatic problems	- Lack of appetite - Weariness - Sleep disorders *Concerning emotionality* - Feelings of guilt - Feelings of being bad - Negative self-esteem - Feeling uneasy and uncomfortable about one's own body, sexuality, relationships with peers - Suicidal plans and/or attempts *Sometimes* - Drug/alcohol abuse - Conduct disorders - Truancy/ absenteeism

Based on research on children of depressed mothers, Goodman and Gotlib (1999) offer a view that is even more developmentally guided. These authors not only take into account symptoms of depression, but they also look at what happens in the further development of children of depressed mothers. Although these findings may perhaps not be generalizable to all depressed children, they are nevertheless very interesting.[2] Compared with children of non-depressed controls:
• Infants of depressed mothers have been found to be more fussy, to obtain lower scores on measures of mental and motor development, and to have more difficult temperaments and less secure attachments to their mothers.

---

[2] Research on children of depressed mothers is discussed in more detail below.

- Toddlers of depressed mothers have been found to react more negatively to stress and to be delayed in their acquisition of effective self-regulation strategies.
- School-aged children and adolescents of depressed mothers experience more school problems, are less socially competent and have lower levels of self-esteem and more behavior problems (Goodman & Gotlib, 1999).

Blatt (2004, p. 174) states that behavioral disorders in adolescence are often symptomatic expressions of an enduring subclinical depression that has not reached a level of severity intense enough to warrant being diagnosed as depression. Goodman and Gotlib (2002) hypothesize that these developmental disturbances are part of the vulnerability for depression. We will return to this issue later on in this chapter.

Classification

In the DSM-IV, depression in childhood and adolescence is not mentioned in the section on specific childhood disorders, but is discussed in the section on mood disorders in adults. According to DSM-IV, criteria for depression in childhood and adolescence are essentially the same as for diagnosing major depression or dysthymic disorder in adulthood, with two minor differences:
- First, irritability is mentioned as an important manifestation of dysphoric mood.
- Second, in order to diagnose dysthymic disorder in children and adolescents, the minimal duration of a depressive mood is one year instead of two years for adults.

Further indications of age-specific manifestations are not mentioned in the DSM-IV. This is considered highly problematic by many authors in the field of developmental psychopathology. There remains an important gap between descriptions of childhood and adolescent depression in DSM-IV and clinical and research knowledge concerning age-specific expressions of depression. One important attempt to fill this gap is the DC: 0-3, a diagnostic classification manual of the zero to three ages (Zero to three's Diagnostic Classification Task Force, 1999). This classification is intended to complement the DSM-IV categorization, particularly in clinical settings where interventions are set up for (very) young children and their families because the DSM-IV lacks any criteria for diagnosing depression in these early developmental phases. The DC describes three types of mood disorders in infants and toddlers: (1) prolonged bereavement/grief reaction; (2) depression of infancy and early childhood, and (3) mixed disorder of emotional expressiveness:
- ***Prolonged bereavement/grief reaction*** is typically seen after the loss of a primary caregiver. Symptoms include:
  - Crying, calling, searching, refusing the attempts of others to offer comfort
  - Emotional withdrawal, lethargy, sad facial expression, lack of interest in age-appropriate activities

- Eating and sleep disorders
- Regression/loss of previously achieved developmental milestones
- Constricted range of affect
- Detachment/seeming indifference toward reminders of the lost caregiver versus extreme sensitivity to any reminder of the caregiver
- ***Depression of infancy and early childhood*** is a type of depression in infants and young children who exhibit a pattern of sadness or irritable mood with diminished interest and/or pleasure in developmentally appropriate activities, diminished capacity to protest, excessive whining, and a diminished repertory of social interactions and initiative. These symptoms may be accompanied by disturbances in sleep or eating behavior, including weight loss. The symptoms must be present for a period of at least two weeks.
- ***Mixed disorder of emotional expressiveness*** should be used for infants and young children who have an ongoing difficulty expressing developmentally appropriate emotions. The difficulties reflect problems in their affective development and experiences.

Prevalence

Traditionally, prevalence studies provide different prevalence estimates. According to de Wit (1997) and Garber and Flynn (2001) depression is quite rare in young children, less common during childhood, but its frequency increases clearly in adolescence. Among children under five, about 0.9% are depressed (Poznanski & Mokros, 1994). Among grade-school children, approximately 2% are depressed (Anderson, Williams, McGee, & Silva, 1987; Kashani & Simonds, 1979). In adolescence, the prevalence of depression ranges from 3% to 18%. Heuves (1990) found in a study in the Netherlands that 3% to 8% were depressed. Birmaher et al. (1996) reviewed ten years of American research and found comparable rates ranging between 0.4% and 8.3%. Lewinsohn, Hops, Roberts, Seeley and Andrews (1993) found a range from 8.3% to 18.5%. Cicchetti and Toth (1998) argue that some developmental constraints on cognition, language, memory and self-understanding may compromise the accuracy of an assessment of depression in children. Hankin and colleagues (1998) state that it is likely that most mood disorders in adults began during middle to late adolescence, which might be a vulnerable period for the first depressive episode.

From adolescence on, results of research also show a significant gender difference (Hankin & Abramson, 1999). From the age of 13 on, girls are about twice as vulnerable to depression as boys, specifically when one considers "pure" childhood depression, with no co-morbidity with other diagnoses. When co-morbidity with other internalizing or externalizing disorders is taken into account, sex differences are less clear. In pre-puberty, the rate of depression is about equal in boys and girls (Garber & Flynn, 2001), but in some studies – especially those on early childhood depression – the prevalence of depression is higher among boys (de Wit, 1997). This raises the question whether depression in pubertal and adolescent boys is often unrecognized and may express itself in other symptoms such as irritability, difficult behavior, hyperactivity, learning problems and even conduct disorders (Blatt, 2004).

Course

When we look in detail at clinical psychological research on depression in children, we find that major depressive disorders in childhood last on average about nine months before recovery, while dysthymic disorders (DD) endure for a period of approximately four years (Kovacs et al., 1984b). This is very similar to the duration of depressive episodes in adults (Coryell et al., 1994). Because of the important developmental tasks that children face during childhood and adolescence, these are considerable periods of time. Taking into account the amount of new developmental capacities a child has to master in several domains at the same time, we should bear in mind that nine months is almost the length of time a school year lasts and that four years is a big part of a child's school life.

With regard to prognosis, most children with major depression recover but the probability of relapse is considerable. The cumulative probability of a new depressive episode within two years is 40%, within five years about 70% (Birmaher et al., 1996; Kovacs, 1996; Kovacs, Feinberg, Crouse-Novak, Paulauskas, & Finkelstein, 1984a; Kovacs et al., 1984b). The course of dysthymic disorder in children is different and less spectacular than in childhood major depression, but still exhibits plenty of pitfalls. Seventy percent of the children that recovered from dysthymic disorder develop a major depressive disorder within a time span of two to three years (Kovacs et al. 1984a; Kovacs et al. 1984b). This subgroup – depressed children with the longer but less intense course of depression – is also at increased risk of relapse within two years after recovery: 50% to 70% show relapse if not treated, and have a less positive clinical picture and outcome when treated.

Comorbidity

Comorbidity is a very common phenomenon and a particular problem for depressed children and adolescents (de Wit, 1997; Garber & Flynn, 2001). Co-morbidity rates between depression and other disorders in childhood are estimated

170

at 40% to 90%, which is very high. The most frequent comorbid disorders include dysthymic disorder, anxiety disorders, oppositional defiant disorder, antisocial conduct disorders, ADHD, eating disorders, obsessive-compulsive disorders and, in adolescence, substance abuse.

Of special interest from a clinical point of view is the comorbidity of depression and antisocial behavior (Harrington, Fudge, Rutter, Pickles, & Hill, 1991). The problems facing depressed children with antisocial behavior clearly differ from those of children with depression only. Running away from home, setting fires, and destroying other people's property are symptoms that occur more frequently in antisocial children with depression than in antisocial children without depression. Blatt (2004) argues that many of these behavioral disturbances may be expressions of depression or *depressive equivalents*. Depressed children with comorbid anti-social behavior typically also show more severe depression. From a clinical and therapeutic point of view, it is very important to keep this potential comorbidity in mind in the assessment and treatment of children, especially in those children with antisocial features. Antisocial behavior is often the most obvious and visible problem, and thus underlying depressive problems are not recognized and therefore left untreated. In addition, antisocial behavioral problems such as impulse control problems and the regulation of aggression clearly can have a different meaning in the case of an underlying depression.

In general, child psychiatric literature considers comorbidity as an important phenomenon, one that is associated with more severe psychopathology and a worse prognosis (de Wit, 1997; Harrington, Rutter, & Fombonne, 1996)

Etiology

It is quite difficult to describe the complexity of etiological factors and processes involved in childhood and adolescent depression. Most research is restricted to one of these etiological factors, such as:
• genetic factors
• neurobiological factors
• environmental and interpersonal factors
• stressful life events
• temperament
• cognitive distortions

Garber and Flynn (2001) offer an exhaustive overview of research into these etiological factors that contribute to the vulnerability of depression in childhood and adolescence. In what follows, we briefly highlight some of these research findings.

Children of depressed parents are three times more likely to experience an episode of depression than children of a reference group without parental depression. Among children of depressed parents, 40% experience a depressive episode of at least six months' duration before they are 18, compared to only 12% of the children in the control group (Beardslee et al., 1998). Furthermore, the onset of depression is earlier in these children than in a control group (Weissman et al., 1987).

Research findings provide evidence for both genetic and environmental effects (Plomin, 1990). Children of depressed parents are genetically more vulnerable but are also exposed to higher levels of stressful life events, including marital and family conflict and financial problems (Blatt & Homann, 1992; Hammen et al., 1987). Furthermore, children of depressed parents seem to be less competent in dealing with stressors (Garber, Braafladt, & Zeman, 1991).

Phares, Duhig and Watkins (2002) identified 19 studies that explored paternal depression in relation to their children's functioning. The differences between the effects of paternal and maternal depression are relatively few. Children of depressed fathers and those of depressed mothers have about the same risk of developing emotional and behavioral problems. Research has also shown that the father can have either a protective or a risk-enhancing role when the mother is depressed, depending upon his abilities to offer the child interaction and communication that is more healthy, playful and vital.

Children who, from very early on, grow up in an atmosphere of parental mood changes that not have been diagnosed have a greater probability of suffering from dysthymic disorder (DD) and major depressive disorder (MDD) throughout childhood. These unrecognized recurring mood changes in one or both parents usually pass, but they can have a serious influence on several domains of child development, especially when the other parent also suffers from psychological problems or is little involved in raising the child. The younger the child is when faced with parental mood disorders, the more it is at risk of developing depressive symptoms later in childhood or in adult life. This means that treating depression in adults also can prevent later depression in their offspring by decreasing the probability of the intergenerational transmission of mood disorders. Furthermore, this implies that clinicians engaged in the treatment of depressed adults have to take into account the children of these patients. This can be done in various ways, ranging from inviting the children to talk about what is happening to their mother or father, to bringing the family in contact with child guidance workers who can support the family.

Interactions of depressed mothers with their children are more negative, more controlling and less responsive or affectively involved. From their exhaustive review of the literature, Garber and Flynn (2001) conclude that non-supportive and negative family interactions increase the child's vulnerability for depression in two ways. Firstly, through modelling and direct feedback from the depressed parent, the child learns inadequate patterns of social interaction, problem solving and affect regulation. For instance, a mother's flat and apathic response to her toddler's proudly showing that he can handle his spoon may lead to feelings of unworthiness and guilt, and/or a comparable flat expressiveness in the child, through processes of imitation and identification, especially when this is the mother's habitual way of responding to the child's moments of pride. Radke-Yarrow and Zahn-Wachsler (1990) noted that depressed mothers are more hostile, less affectionate or less consistent in their affection. They are less communicative, less skilful in managing their children, and try to avoid discipline and punishment, but are at the same time more negative and critical towards their children.

Second, these negative interactions between child and parent have negative consequences for the development of the self. To begin with, they tend to undermine the development of a sense of basic trust in the child. The experience that others are there or will be available for sensitive parenting or as "a secure home base" is missing. This also makes the child more vulnerable in interaction with others in general. The child develops a poor capacity to count upon reliable others, becomes less communicative about what is difficult for him or her, and does not develop the skills that can help him find other supportive adults in school or other contexts.

Stressful life events contribute to the onset of childhood depression and to an increase in depressive symptoms. There is a significant association between stressful life events and depression in children (Compas, Grant, & Ey, 1994). Although there is not one single specific type of stressful life event that causes depression, research findings indicate that depressed children have experienced more loss, separation and interpersonal conflict (e.g., Monroe, Rohde, Seeley, & Lewinsohn, 1999; Rueter, Scaramella, Wallace, & Conger, 1999).

For example, in life histories of depressed adolescents, the death of a parent or the divorce of parents are more often mentioned than in the life histories of nondepressed adolescents. But this is also true for early academic failure in grade school and for first love relationships that were broken off early in puberty. It seems that several different life events, in interaction with one another, increase the probability of depression in children. The life histories of children with recurrent depressive episodes also show an accumulation of parental conflicts, maltreatment, rejection, separation, several removals, unemployment of both parents, etc. (Garber & Flynn, 2003)

Blatt, Quinlan, Chevron, McDonald and Zuroff (1982) and Beck (1983) developed the *personality-event congruency hypothesis.* When a stressor falls into an individual's particular area of vulnerability, this would increase the likelihood of depression. For example, individuals whose sense of psychological well-being is primarily derived from interpersonal relationships (dependent/sociotropic individuals) have an increased risk of depression when they experience stressors within the social domain. Those who derive their self-esteem from achievement-related goals (self-critical/autonomous individuals) are at greater risk of depression when they encounter failure or an inability to live up to the standards and ideals they had set up for themselves. However, as in adults (see Blatt, 2004; see also Chapter 4, this volume), support for the congruency hypothesis in children is mainly limited to Dependency/Sociotropy (e.g., Fichman, Koestner, & Zuroff, 1997; Hammen & Goodman-Brown, 1990; Little & Garber, 2000).

Depression in childhood and adolescence is the result of an interaction between genetic and contextual factors that confront the child with an adversity that cannot be worked through. There appears to be a "scarring" effect (Garber & Flynn, 2001) of depression on the explanatory style of the child. Children with a history of depression tend to develop a so-called "depressive" style of giving meaning to experiences and of interpreting events. Predominant in this style are feelings of rejection, of being unloved, not accepted, and inferior to others. These feelings of insufficiency are associated with a greater sensitivity to signs of rejection and they influence the way information is processed (i.e., the depressive child only recalls or reacts to real or fantasized events that confirm his "lack of self-worth"). Furthermore, this negative style can provoke more rejection and social isolation. On the other hand, even the very minimal amount of negativity that is present in an otherwise good and positive experience will immediately be picked up and experienced as a confirmation of all the bad aspects of the self. In that sense, one negative aspect will have much more of an impact on a depressive child than several positive experiences, because it is easily linked with and fits in with the negative expectations of the child. As noted, this explanatory style persists after recovery from depression. Or, as Nolen-Hoeksema et al. (1992, p. 418) put it: "a period of depression during childhood can lead to the development of a fixed and more pessimistic explanatory style, which remains with a child after his or her depression has begun to subside".

One of the strongest predictors of subsequent depression is previous depression. Compas, Ey and Grant (1993) suggest that depressed mood might be a marker for subsequent depressive symptoms. Subsyndromal levels of depressive symptoms in childhood significantly increase the risk of a full major depression in adolescence (Lewinsohn, Allen, Seeley, & Gotlib, 1999; Pine, Cohen, Cohen, & Brook, 1999; Rueter et al., 1999) and in adulthood (Howarth, Johnson, Klerman, & Weissman, 1992; Judd, Akiskal, & Paulus, 1997). This means that depression in childhood should be treated until full remission is achieved.

Depressotypic organization (Cicchetti & Toth, 1998). Although much research has been done into the factors that contribute to childhood depression, still little is known about how these factors contribute to the onset of depression, and about how these episodes of depression influence further development.

Cicchetti and Toth (1998) developed the concept of *depressotypic organization* to describe how distortions in the cognitive, socio-emotional, representational and biological functions (see Figure 1) are present to varying degrees among individuals with mood disorders and how different etiological factors interact with one another. In individuals functioning in an adaptive way, there is a coherent organization among these domains. This means that these individuals usually are able to consider their thoughts, emotions and representations in the perspective of the context of experiences and are also able to adapt them to socio-emotional experiences and relational events. There is a balanced interaction among the different domains of the internal world and external experience, and when mismatches or disturbances occur, there is a possibility to change and to adjust. In depressed individuals one can find either an incoherent organization among these systems or an organization with one clearly distorted function. The different structures and domains are not interacting in a balanced and attuned way, i.e., some intense persistent negative feelings or deeply anchored thoughts about themselves or the world are leading and influencing all other domains and structures, and there is little possibility to learn from new experiences. All new experiences fall into the same track, confirming what already was thought and felt.

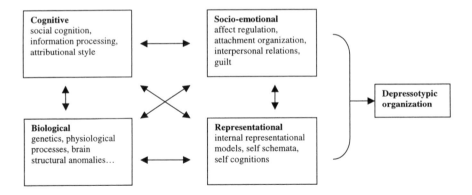

FIGURE 1.
Integration of biological and psychological systems in the emergence of depressotypic organization
(Based on Cicchetti & Toth, 1998).

As noted in the introduction to this chapter, whereas childhood depression was not recognized as such in the literature until recently, there is now a growing body of knowledge concerning the prevalence, course, comorbidity and general etiological factors contributing to depression in childhood and adolescence. One striking characteristic of this literature is that it often followed and sometimes still follows research lines and theoretical points of view relevant to adult depression. We still have little understanding of *why* children become depressive, *how* the depression influences further development and *how* these children grow up into adulthood. What is needed is a more developmental psychopathological model that is dimensional. Therefore, in the remainder of this chapter we review some recent attempts to integrate research findings and developmental theory into developmentally based and developmentally sensitive models of childhood depression (e.g., de Wit, 1997; Cicchetti & Toth, 1998; Goodman & Gotlib, 1999).

Depression Interfering With Normal Development

De Wit (1997) emphasizes that depressed children not only are at risk because of the probability of relapse. Depressive disorders can also interfere seriously with various developmental tasks during different phases of childhood and adolescence. In this way, depression can undermine the developmental capacities that are required for further emotional, cognitive and social growth and health. For instance, ongoing socialization can stagnate when the child withdraws and feels uncomfortable in relationships with peers; apathy and increased inactivity can contribute to being an "underachiever" and to delay in educational achievement or to strong feelings of incompetence. Moreover, as we will show further on in this chapter, depression can be "transmitted" from parent to child (Goodman & Gotlib, 1999).

According to De Wit (1997), a complex model for understanding the interaction among biological vulnerabilities, temperament, emotional immaturity, specific educational styles of the parents and cognitive biases is needed. In the context of this interaction, affect-regulation or mood-regulation problems that are typical of childhood depression can take place. A typical element of these regulatory problems is that negative experiences tend to have long-lasting consequences and their influence is not easily moderated by later experiences. Moreover, even then, early negative experiences tend to be associated with increased vulnerability when faced with stress later on in life.

Cicchetti and Toth (1998) propose an even more complex model to understand the development of depression in children. In this model, the multiple transactions among environment, caregiver and child are not only represented, but they are perceived of as dynamic, reciprocal factors contributing to the likelihood of a depressotypic organization and the emergence of depressive disorder (see Figure 2). Moreover, whether depression occurs is determined not only by the presence or absence of specific vulnerabilities or protective factors. The interplay between these factors and current and previous levels of adaptation as well as the developmental period during which risk factors and stressors are experienced are considered to be important determinants in the pathogenesis of childhood and adolescent depression.

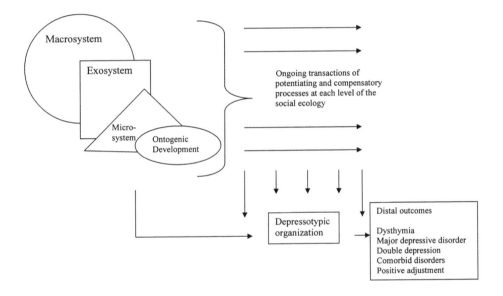

FIGURE 2.
The interplay of multiple transactions among environmental forces, caregiver and child characteristics as contributing to a depressotypic organization and to the likelihood of depression (Based on Cicchetti & Toth, 1998).

---

[3] The model proposed by Cicchetti and Toth (1998) is even more complex than our brief summary suggests. However, even this brief sketch highlights the need for integrative theoretical models that are able to account for a wide variety of theoretical and empirical findings concerning depression in childhood and adolescence.

In this *transactional approach*, ongoing transactions of risk and protective processes are seen as contributing to the emergence and development of a depressotypic organization and thus to the onset and recurrence of depressive disorder. *Potentiating factors* increase the likelihood that a depressotypic organization and a depressive illness occur, while *compensatory factors* decrease the probability of their occurrence. Potentiating and compensatory factors are associated with four different levels:

- the *macrosystem* which contains the beliefs and values of the culture
- the *exosystem* which includes aspects of the community in which children and families live
- the *microsystem* which concerns the immediate environment, mostly the family
- *ontogenic development*: those factors within the person that affect his or her adaptation. In ontogenic development, one can differentiate still further between the developmental biological system on the one hand and the resolution of developmental tasks on the other hand. Maladaptive resolutions of early developmental tasks can contribute to the development of pathways to depression through depressotypic organizations of developmental structures. According to Cicchetti and Toth (1998), four developmental issues are of specific importance for the emergence of a depressotypic organization and a depressive disorder:
  - The development of homeostatic and physiological regulation
  - Affect differentiation and the modulation of attention and arousal
  - The development of a secure attachment relationship
  - The development of the self-system

Child Development in the Context of Parental Depressive Psychopathology

Goodman and Gotlib's (1999) Integrative Model

As we pointed out before, much research has focused on the adverse effects on offspring of parents with depression. Recently, Goodman and Gotlib (1999) proposed an integrative model with the purpose of identifying mediating and moderating factors in the relationship between parental depression and maladaptive developmental pathways.

According to Goodman and Gotlib, such an integrative model should incorporate reciprocal and transactional relationships and should take into account a developmental point of view. Researchers have increasingly recognized the importance of such *reciprocal and transactional relationships* within families. The child's characteristics, such as gender and temperament, can strongly influence the developmental course as a function of the complex interplay between parent and child (Gotlib & Wheaton, 1997). A *developmental perspective*, in turn, is to a certain extent still lacking in most studies of children of depressed mothers. Yet, Cicchetti and Schneider-Rosen (1986) already argued that knowledge of developmental processes is essential when studying risk factors for the development of psychopathology in children and to subsequently develop prevention programs. Most researchers studied children of depressed mothers in one developmental phase or across a broad range of developmental phases, which limited the extent to which their findings could be generalized. For instance, conclusions drawn from studies of children in one developmental stage cannot be automatically generalized to children of other developmental stages. Moreover, studies that select children with a different age can mask important developmental issues. Hence, many studies failed to address developmental issues. In addition, from a developmental perspective, it appears essential to take into account the timing of the mother's depression, especially of the first depressive episode during the child's lifetime. Hence, a developmental theory must be sensitive to the maturational tasks the child has to master at the time of the exposure to the depression and its consequences.

Finally, from a developmental perspective, one can see that adult depression usually is not a single, time-limited event (see also Chapter 1, this volume). As many depressions are chronic or recurrent, few children are exposed to only one episode of maternal depression. Research often fails to take into account the specific moment in his development at which the child is confronted with parental depression.

General Principles of Goodman and Gotlib's Integrative Risk Model

Goodman and Gotlib (1999) describe four possible transmission mechanisms involved in the transgenerational transmission of depression from mother to child.[4] Two of these mechanisms are mainly of a biological nature, such as heritability of depression and innate dysfunctional neuroregulatory mechanisms. The other mechanisms have to do with disturbances in the interaction between the child of a depressed mother and his/her environment, including the exposure to maternal negative and/or maladaptive cognitions, behaviors and affects and the exposure to a stressful environment in general (see Figure 3). When the mother is depressed, one or, in most cases, a combination of these transmission mechanisms is present. The occurrence of one or more of these transmission mechanisms is also hypothesized to be associated with the emergence of vulnerabilities in several domains of the child's functioning: psychobiological, cognitive, affective and behavioral/interpersonal. These vulnerabilities should not be considered as discrete

---

[4] Although Goodman and Gotlib (1999) discuss the effects of depression in the mother on the child, as noted earlier, there are few differences between paternal and maternal depression with regard to their effects on child development (Phares et al., 2002)

domains, but as interacting with each other. Finally, Goodman and Gotlib propose that these vulnerabilities interact with three potential moderators: the role of the father, the timing and the course of maternal depression and different child characteristics.

This theoretical model allows Goodman and Gotlib to summarize a wide variety of research on children of depressed mothers. In the next section, we briefly discuss the main transmission mechanisms as well as moderators of this transmission described by Goodman and Gotlib.

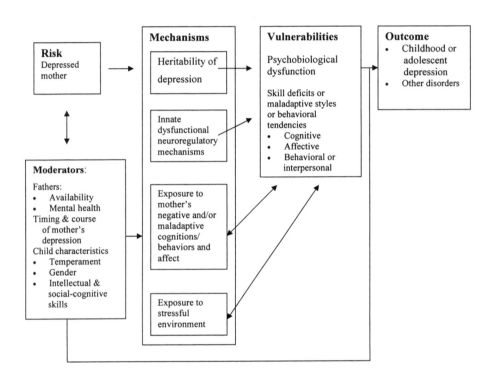

FIGURE 3.
An integrative model for the transmission of risk to children of depressed mothers
(Based on Goodman & Gotlib, 1999).

Mechanisms of Transmission

Mechanism 1: Having a depressed mother confers on the child a genetic predisposition to depression. Genetic vulnerability for depression may be either indirect, direct, or both. First, children of depressed mothers may inherit depression directly. They may inherit DNA that regulates the biological mechanisms of the child in a way that is different from that of children of nondepressed mothers. Secondly, genetic liability might be indirect, by inheriting vulnerability factors for depression, such as particular personality traits or cognitive or interpersonal styles that increase the risk of depression.

Summarizing the large amount of empirical support for this mechanism, we can say that there is less clear support for childhood-onset and adolescence-onset depression than there is for adult-onset depression. Furthermore, the genetic contribution seems to be greater for early than for late-onset depression. Heritability has further been found to be stronger for less severe childhood depression and for girls, in contrast to more severe levels of depression and in boys, where environmental factors seem to have a stronger influence.

Mechanism 2: Infants of depressed mothers are born with dysfunctional neuroregulatory mechanisms that interfere with emotional regulation processes and consequently increase vulnerability to depression. This mechanism assumes that inheritance of dysfunctional neuroregulatory mechanisms is due to genetic factors or to negative prenatal experiences. This can be the case when the mother was depressed during or before pregnancy. The foetus is then exposed to neuroendocrine alterations associated with the mother's depression, to constricted blood flow, etc. However, much of this research is new and has yet to be replicated. Goodman and Gotlib also remark that none of these studies tested the role of early behavior and interaction as mediating the association between maternal depression and depression in children.

Mechanism 3: Depressed mothers expose their children to negative or maladaptive cognitions, behaviors, and affect, which places the children at elevated risk of developing depression. This mechanism consists of several components. First, parental depression is associated with negative thoughts, behaviors and affect. This can have a serious impact on the quality of mothering. Depressed mothers typically show inadequate, non-supportive parenting behaviors, and are unable to attune to the child's developmentally dependent social and emotional needs. This in turn will influence the child's social, cognitive and emotional development. Through identification, modelling, and social learning, the child often acquires ways of thinking, behaving and feeling that resemble those of the depressed mother, putting the child at increased risk of depression.

Goodman and Gotlib (1999) state that there is little question that depressed mothers are characterized by negative affect, cognition and behavior, leaving them unable to meet the social and emotional needs of their children. These unmet needs limit the children's social, emotional and cognitive development. Although there is little research examining whether this negative way of feeling, thinking and behaving in children of depressed mothers leads to the development of depression, there is evidence from human and animal studies that this negative functioning places the children at an elevated risk of depression.

Mechanism 4: Contextual features in families with depressed mothers, particularly some specific stressors, contribute significantly to the development of psychopathology in children. As noted in Chapters 4 and 8 in this volume, the relationship between stress and depression is well documented in adults. Children of depressed mothers are not only exposed to their mother's depression, but also to a variety of stressors associated with their mother's depression in the domains of marital and social relationships, job, finances, etc. These elevated levels of exposure to stress, in comparison with children of normal parents, further elevate the risk of depression. Despite the general finding that children of depressed mothers are living in a more stressful environment, little research has examined the potential mediating role of stress.

Moderators

Moderator 1: Fathers may increase the risk of psychopathology in children of depressed mothers if they are absent or if they also show psychopathology. Similarly, fathers may represent a protective factor if they are healthy, involved and supportive. According to Goodman and Gotlib (1999), there is growing evidence that fathers have an important role in families with a maternal depression. They can either increase or decrease the risk of psychopathology in their offspring. When fathers are absent and/or suffer from mental disorders themselves, they are not able to offer supportive, corrective, healthier relational experiences, nor are they able to support the child's healthy social relationships with others such as peers. From a clinical point of view, for the child, the absence of a healthy adult often implies the absence of recognition of the child's need for sensitive, responsive and caring parenting by adults. In contrast, although research has not always yielded consistent results, taken together, existing studies suggest that normal, involved fathers may protect the child from future psychopathology.

Moderator 2: The timing and evolution of maternal depression. In general, the younger the child is at the time of maternal depression, the bigger the impact. Because the first year of life represents an important critical period characterized by rapid development in the physiological, affective and cognitive domains, maternal depression at this age (e.g., postpartum depression) has particularly serious consequences for subsequent development. Parental regulation of the

182

infant's emotions, for example, is a very important part of relational exchange, and postpartum depression can make the mother incapable of noticing the child's needs and responding to them in a helpful and regulating way.

Another important moderator is the *course of maternal depression.* As with most depressed patients, depressed mothers recover from their depression sooner or later. However, little is known about the response of children to this recovery. Yet, the patterns the child has acquired while the mother was depressed, and which can be seen as adaptive reactions in dealing with a depressive key figure, may already become generalized. Hence, these "ways of being with a depressed mother" (Stern, 1995) may have become generalized to other relationships. For instance, while a withdrawal reaction can be adaptive in the context of inconsistent, unresponsive or harsh parenting, it can prevent the child from finding supportive interactions with others: with healthy adults or with friends in one's peer groups. This can further contribute to feelings of loneliness and social incompetence. Moreover, when depression in the mother is more chronic or recurrent, which is often the case given the fact that relapse in depression is the rule rather than the exception (Belsher & Costello, 1988), the adverse impact on the child's functioning can be expected to be even bigger. Clearly, more research is needed to find out more about the impact of the timing and the course of depression in mothers on the subsequent development of their offspring.

Moderator 3: Characteristics of the child, such as temperament, gender, intellectual and social-cognitive skills, can moderate the association of maternal depression and developmental child outcomes. From a transactional and clinical point of view, one could argue that *temperament* could play an important moderating role in the relationship between maternal depression and child dysfunction. Empirical research, however, has found no support for this assumption (Goodman & Gotlib, 1999).

Research on the impact of *gender* has yielded conflicting results. Most research on children of depressed mothers does not report gender differences. However, some studies have found that maternal depression has more of a negative impact on the development of girls as compared with boys, while other studies have found the reverse. Goodman and Gotlib (1999) wonder whether these conflicting findings could be explained by gender-specific models of the impact of maternal depression. Based on Murray's (1992) findings that there is a significant increase in insecure attachment in boys due to a non-sensitive environment, Hay (1997), for instance, suggested that boys may be more vulnerable to mothers' noncontingent responsiveness and negative affect than girls. Other research (e.g., Klimes-Dougan & Bolger, 1998) found different coping strategies in boys and girls. Leadbeater, Kuperminc, Blatt and Hertzog (1999) found in a group of early adolescent boys and girls (age 11-13) that self-critical vulnerability predicted internalizing and externalizing problems for both boys and girls. Interpersonal vulnerability predicted increases in internalizing problems. These authors found also that the quality of adolescent relationships with parents and peers influenced the adjustment of girls. Girls with positive relationships with their parents showed a lower level of internalizing and externalizing problems, had fewer stressful life events, and less self-critical vulnerability. For boys, positive relationships were associated with less self-critical vulnerability and fewer stressful life events but paradoxically with a higher level of interpersonal vulnerability. However, further research is needed to investigate the impact of gender.

Intelligence as well as level of social-cognitive functioning seems to protect the child against adverse outcome. Radke-Yarrow and Sherman (1990), for instance, found in two different age groups that children characterized by three protective factors (above-average intelligence, socially engaged and "having a special positive place in the family") did not meet criteria for any psychiatric diagnosis, even when the mother clearly suffered from major depression.

To summarize, the theoretical model proposed by Goodman and Gotlib (1999) not only integrates a wide variety of research on maternal depression, but it also sets a research agenda for the coming years. In our view, one particular point that deserves future research attention concerns the mechanisms by which specific child characteristics exert a moderating effect on the relationship between maternal depression and child development. These mechanisms might also include interactions between child and life stress (see also Chapter 4, this volume).

Summary and Conclusions

Depression in childhood and adolescence has long been a neglected topic in theory and research. Research in this domain originated only about 25 years ago, and coincided more or less with the birth of developmental psychopathology. In these 25 years and mainly under the influence of developmental psychopathology, the notion of "depression" in childhood and adolescence evolved from a static condition that was described with clear and delineated symptoms, towards a developmentally based disorder that can affect people throughout their lives, from early infancy to later life. Childhood and adolescent depression are not only associated with a risk of relapse in later life, but also with a more broad, possibly enduring vulnerability for psychopathology in general. However, at the same time, the presence of protective factors both in the child and his/her environment might moderate this vulnerability.

In this chapter, we reviewed some of the main research findings and theoretical models that integrate these findings from a developmental psychopathological perspective. As noted, although our insights into childhood and adolescent depression and the factors contributing to it are already considerable, much more theoretical and empirical research is needed. Ultimately, this knowledge should be able to inform both preventive and therapeutic programs that are specifically tailored to the developmental needs of depressed children and adults.

In the next chapter, we will focus on one specific orientation within developmental psychopathology, namely a psychoanalytic developmental psychopathological perspective. As psychoanalytic thinking concerning depression has always focused on childhood factors as contributing to depression, and even considers depression as an inherent part of human development, a comparison of psychoanalytic developmental psychopathology with the theory and research reviewed in this chapter could prove to be a fruitful endeavor to further our understanding of depression in childhood and adolescence.

References

American Psychiatric Association (1994). *Diagnostic and statistical manual of mental disorders* (4th ed.). Washington, DC: Author.

Anderson, J., Williams, S., McGee, R., & Silva, P. (1987). DSM-III disorders in pre-adolescent children: Prevalence in a large sample from the general population. *Archives of General Psychiatry, 44,* 69-76.

Beardslee, W., Versage, E., & Gladstone, T. (1998). Children of affectively ill parents: A review of the past ten years. *Journal of the American Academy of Adolescent Psychiatry, 37,* 1134-1141.

Beck, A. (1983). Cognitive therapy of depression: New perspectives. In P. Clayton & J. Barrett (Eds.), *Treatment of depression: old controversies and new approaches* (pp. 265-290). New York: Raven Press.

Belga (2003). Twaalfjarige verhangt zich op school. [Twelve year old hangs himself]. *De Standaard, 01/03/2003.*

Belsher, G., & Costello, C. (1988). Relapse after recovery from unipolar depression: A critical review. *Psychological Bulletin, 104,* 84-96.

Birmaher, B., Ryan, N., Williamson, D., Brent, D., Kaufman, J., Dahl, R., et al. (1996). Childhood and adolescent depression: A review of the past ten years. Part I. *Journal of the American Academy of Child and Adolescent Psychiatry, 35,* 1427-1439.

Blatt, S. J. (2004). *Experiences of depression. Theoretical, clinical, and research perspectives.* Washington, DC: American Psychological Association.

Blatt, S. J., & Homann, E. (1992). Parent-child interaction in the etiology of dependent and self-critical depression. *Clinical Psychology Review, 12,* 47-91.

Blatt, S., Quinlan, D., Chevron, E., McDonald, C., & Zuroff, D. (1982). Dependency and self-criticism: Psychological dimensions of depression. *Journal of Consulting and Clinical Psychology, 50,* 113-124.

Cicchetti, D., & Schneider-Rosen, K. (1986). An organizational approach to childhood depression. In M. Rutter, C. Izard & P. Read (Eds.), *Depression in young people: Developmental and clinical perspectives* (pp. 71-134). New York: Guilford Press.

Cicchetti, D., & Toth, S. (1998). The development of depression in children and adolescents. *American Psychologist, 53,* 221-241.

Compas, B., Ey, S., & Grant, K. (1993). Taxonomy, assessment and diagnosis of depression during adolescence. *Psychological Bulletin, 114,* 323-344.

Compas, B., Grant, K., & Ey, S. (1994). Psychological stress and child/adolescent depression: Can we be more specific? In W. Reynolds & H. Johnston (Eds.), *Handbook of depression in children and adolescents* (pp. 509-523). New York: Plenum.

Coryell, W., Akiskal, H., Leon, A., Winokur, G., Maser, J., Mueller, T., et al. (1994). The time course of non-chronic major depressive disorder: Uniformity across episodes and samples. *Archives of General Psychiatry, 51,* 405-410.

Costello, E., Pine, D., Hammen, C., March, J., Plotsky, P., Weissman, M., et al. (2002). Development and natural history of mood disorders. *Biological Psychiatry, 52,* 529-542.

de Wit, C. (1997). Depressies bij kinderen en adolescenten. De stand van zaken na vijfentwintig jaar onderzoek. [Depression in children and adolescents. State of the art after twenty-five years of research]. *Kind en Adolescent, 4,* 166-184.

Fichman, L., Koestner, R., & Zuroff, D. C. (1997). Dependency and distress at summer camp. *Journal of Youth and Adolescence, 26,* 217-232.

Garber, J., Braafladt, N., & Zeman, J. (1991). The regulation of sad affect: An information processing perspective. In J. Garber & K. Dodge (Eds.), *The development of affect regulation and dysregulation* (pp. 208-240). New York: Cambridge University Press.

Garber, J., & Flynn, C. (2001). Vulnerability to depression in childhood and adolescence. In R. Ingram & J. Price (Eds.), *Vulnerability to Psychopathology. Risk across the lifespan* (pp. 175-225). New York/London: The Guilford Press.

Goodman, S., & Gotlib, I. (1999). Risk for psychopathology in the children of depressed mothers: A developmental model for understanding mechanisms of transmission. *Psychological Review, 106,* 458-490.

Goodman, S., & Gotlib, I. (2002). *Children of depressed parents. Mechanisms of risk and implications for treatment.* Washington, DC: American Psychological Association.

Gotlib, I., & Wheaton, B. (Eds.). (1997). *Stress and adversity over the life course: Trajectories and turning points.* New York: Cambridge University Press.

Hammen, C., & Garber, J. (2001). Vulnerability to depression across the life span. In R. Ingram & J. Price (Eds.), *Vulnerability to Psychopathology. Risk across the lifespan* (pp. 258-267). New York/ London: The Guilford Press.

Hammen, C., & Goodman-Brown, T. (1990). Self-schemas and vulnerability to specific life stress in children at risk for depression. *Cognitive Therapy and Research, 14,* 215-227.

Hammen, C., Gordon, D., Burge, D., Adrian, C., Jaenicke, C., & Hiroto, D. (1987). Maternal affective disorders, illness and stress: Risk for children's psychopathology. *American Journal of Psychiatry, 144,* 736-741.

Hankin, B., & Abramson, L. (1999). Development of gender differences: Description and possible explanations. *Annals of Medicine, 31,* 372-379.

Hankin, B., Abramson, L., Moffit, T., Silva, P., McGee, R., & Angell, K. (1998). Development of depression from preadolescence to young adulthood: Emerging gender differences in a 10-year longitudinal study. *Journal of Abnormal Psychology, 107,* 128-140.

Harrington, R. (1993). *Depressive disorder in childhood and adolescence.* Chichester: John Wiley and Sons.

Harrington, R., Fudge, H., Rutter, M., Pickles, A., & Hill, J. (1991). Adult outcomes of childhood and adolescent depression. II. Links with antisocial disorders. *Journal of the American Academy of Child and Adolescent Psychiatry, 30,* 434-439.

Harrington, R., Rutter, M., & Fombonne, E. (1996). Developmental pathways in depression: Multiple meanings, antecedents, and endpoints. *Development and Psychopathology, 8,* 601-616.

Hay, D. (1997). Postpartum depression and cognitive development. In P. Murray (Ed.), *Postpartum depression and child development* (pp. 85-110). New York: Guilford Press.

Heuves, W. (1990). *Depression in young male adolescents. Theoretical and clinical aspects.* Unpublished doctoral dissertation. Rijksuniversiteit Leiden, Leiden, The Netherlands.

Howarth, E., Johnson, J., Klerman, G., & Weissman, M. (1992). Depressive symptoms as relative and attributable risk factors for first onset major depression. *Archives of General Psychiatry, 49,* 817-823.

Judd, L., Akiskal, H., & Paulus, M. (1997). The role and clinical significance of subsyndromal depressive symptoms (SSD) in unipolar major depressive disorder. *Journal of Affective Disorders, 45,* 5-18.

Kashani, J., & Simonds, J. (1979). The incidence of depression in children. *American Journal of Psychotherapy, 136,* 1203-1205.

Klimes-Dougan, B., & Bolger, A. (1998). Coping with maternal depressed affect and depression: Adolescent children of depressed and well mothers. *Journal of Youth and Adolescence, 27,* 1-15.

Kolvin, I., & Sadovski, H. (2001). Childhood depression: Clinical phenomenology and classification. In I. Goodyear (Ed.), *The depressed child and adolescent (2nd ed.). Cambridge Child and Adolescent Psychiatry* (pp. 119-142). New York: Cambridge University Press.

Kovacs, M. (1996). Presentation and course of major depressive disorder during childhood and later years of the life span. *Journal of the American Academy of Child and Adolescent Psychiatry, 35,* 705-715.

Kovacs, M., Feinberg, T., Crouse-Novak, M., Paulauskas, S., & Finkelstein, R. (1984a). Depressive disorders in childhood: I. A longitudinal perspective study of characteristics and recovery. *Archives of General Psychiatry, 41,* 229-237.

Kovacs, M., Feinberg, T., Crouse-Novak, M., Paulauskas, S., Pollock, M., & Finkelstein, R. (1984b). Depressive disorders in childhood: II. A longitudinal study of the risk for subsequent major depression. *Archives of General Psychiatry, 41,* 643-649.

Lazarus, A. (2002). Depression in primary care: Where psyche meets soma. *Psychiatric Annals, 32,* 505-506.

Leadbeater, B. J., Kuperminc, G. P., Blatt, S. J., & Hertzog, C. (1999). A multivariate model of gender differences in adolescents' internalizing and externalizing problems. *Developmental Psychology, 35,* 1268-1282.

Lewinsohn, P., Allen, N., Seeley, J., & Gotlib, I. (1999). First onset versus recurrence of depression: Differential processes of psychological risk. *Journal of Abnormal Psychology, 108,* 483-489.

Lewinsohn, P., Hops, H., Roberts, R., Seeley, J., & Andrews, J. (1993). Adolescent psychopathology: I. Prevalence and incidence of depression and other DSM-III-R disorders in high school students. *Journal of Abnormal Psychology, 102,* 133-144.

Little, S. A., & Garber, J. (2000). Interpersonal and achievement orientations and specific stressors predicting depressive and aggressive symptoms in children. *Cognitive Therapy and Research, 24,* 651-670.

Lous, A., de Wit, C., de Bruyn, E., & Riksen-Walraven, M. (2002). Depression markers in young children's play: A comparison between depressed and non-depressed 3- to 6-year-olds in various play situations. *Journal of Child Psychology and Psychiatry and Allied Disciplines, 43,* 1029-1038.

Lous, A., de Wit, C., de Bruyn, E., Riksen-Walraven, M., & Rost, H. (2000). Depression and play in early childhood: Play behavior of depressed and non-depressed 3- to 6-year-olds in various play situations. *Journal of Emotional and Behavioral Disorders, 8,* 249-260.

Meurs, P., & Cluckers, G. (1999). Psychosomatic symptoms, embodiment and affect. Weaving threads to the affectively experienced body in therapy with a neurotic and a borderline child. *Journal of Child Psychotherapy, 25,* 71-91.

Monroe, S., Rohde, P., Seeley, J., & Lewinsohn, P. (1999). Life events and depression in adolescence: Relationship loss as a prospective risk factor for first-onset of major depressive disorder. *Journal of Abnormal Psychology, 108,* 606-614.

Murray, L. (1992). The impact of postnatal depression on infant development. *Journal of Child Psychology and Psychiatry and Allied Disciplines, 33,* 543-561.

Nolen-Hoeksema, S., Girgus J., & Seligman, M. (1992). Predictors and consequences of childhood depressive symptoms: A 5-year longitudinal study. *Journal of Abnormal Psychology, 101,* 405-422.

Phares, V., Duhig, A., & Watkins, M. (2002). Family context: Fathers and other supports. In S. Goodman & I. Gotlib (Eds.), *Children of depressed parents, mechanisms of risk and implications of treatment* (pp. 203-225). Washington, DC: American Psychological Association.

Pine, D., Cohen, E., Cohen, P., & Brook, J. (1999). Adolescent depressive symptoms as predictors of adult depression: Moodiness or mood disorder? *American Journal of Psychiatry, 156,* 133-135.

Pine, D., Cohen, P., Gurley, D., Brook, J., & Ma, Y. (1998). The risk for early-adulthood anxiety and depressive disorders in adolescents with anxiety and depressive disorders. *Archives of General Psychiatry, 55,* 56-64.

Plomin, R. (1990). *Nature and nurture: An introduction to human behavioral genetics.* Pacific Grove, CA: Brooks/Cole.

Poznanski, E., & Mokros, H. (1994). Phenomenology and epidemiology of mood disorders in children and adolescents. In W. Reynolds & H. Johnston (Eds.), *Handbook of depression in children and adolescents* (pp. 19-39). New York: Plenum Press.

Radke-Yarrow, M., & Sherman, T. (1990). Hard growing: Children who survive. In J. Rolf, A. Masten, D. Cicchetti, K. Nuechterlein & S. Weintraub (Eds.), *Risk and protective factors in the development of psychopathology* (pp. 97-119). Cambridge: Cambridge University Press.

Radke-Yarrow, M., & Zahn-Waxler, C. (1990). Research on affectively ill parents: Some considerations for theory and research on normal development. *Development and Psychopathology, 2,* 349-366.

Rueter, M., Scaramella, L., Wallace, L., & Conger, R. (1999). First onset of depressive or anxiety disorders predicted by the longitudinal course of internalizing symptoms and parent-adolescent disagreements. *Archives of General Psychiatry, 34,* 1618-1628.

Shaffer, D., & Waslick, B. (2002). The many faces of depression in children and adolescents. *Review of Psychiatry, 21,* 1-36.

Stern, D. (1995). *The motherhood constellation: A unified view of parent-infant psychotherapy*. New York: Basic Books.

Weiss, B., & Garber, J. (2003). Developmental differences in the phenomenology of depression. *Development and Psychopathology, 15,* 403-430.

Weissman, M. M., Gammen, G. D., John, K., Merikangas, K. R., Warner, V., Prusoff, B. A., & Sholomskas, D. (1987). Children of depressed mothers: Increased psychopathology and early onset of depression. *Archives of General Psychiatry, 44,* 847-853.

Weissman, M., Wolk, S., Goldstein, R., Moreau, D., Adams, P., Greenwald, S., et al. (1999a). Depressed adolescents grown up. *Journal of the American Medical Association, 281,* 1707-1713.

Weissman, M., Wolk, S., Wickramaratne, P., Goldstein, R., Adams, P., Greenwald, et al. (1999b). Children with prepubertal-onset major depressive disorder and anxiety grown up. *Archives of General Psychiatry, 56,* 794-801.

Zero to three Diagnostic Classification Task Force (1999). *Diagnostic Classification of Mental Health and Developmental Disorders of Infancy and Early Childhood*. Washington, DC: National Centre for infants, toddlers and families.

Chapter 7

'Closed Doors and Landscapes in the Mist' 2.

Depression in Psychoanalytic Developmental

Psychopathology: From Single Track Models

to Complex Developmental Pathways

Patrick Meurs, Nicole Vliegen, & Gaston Cluckers

Developmental psychopathology focuses on charting processes of, or pathways into, psychopathology. It examines the biological, contextual and psychosocial processes involved in the development of psychopathology, as well as the spontaneous or therapy-induced processes of recovery and its biological, contextual and psychological correlates.

Cicchetti and Cohen (1995) indicate that the joint study of normal and pathological development forms a crucial aspect of developmental psychopathology:

"Because all psychopathology can be conceived as a distortion, disturbance, or degeneration of normal functioning, it follows that, if one wishes to understand pathology more fully, then one must understand normal functioning against which psychopathology is compared. Not only is knowledge of normal processes very helpful for understanding, preventing, and treating psychopathology, (…) but also the deviations from and distortions of normal development that are seen in pathological processes indicate in exciting ways how normal ontogenesis may be better investigated and understood. (…) Indeed, for many thinkers, the very essence and uniqueness of a developmental psychopathology approach lies in its focus on both normal and abnormal, adaptive and maladaptive, ontogenetic processes." (Cicchetti & Cohen, 1995, p. 3-4).

In this sense, this discipline represents the study of unfolding illness processes (paths of deviant, maladaptive development) in contrast to normally unfolding development (paths of normal, adaptive development).

First, we will trace the development of this simultaneous approach to normality and pathology in psychoanalytic thinking. Next, we will discuss the strengths and weaknesses of the blueprint of this early developmental psychopathology project in psychoanalysis. In the third section we will briefly outline the renewed interest in developmental psychopathology within psychoanalysis. This is followed by an illustration of the principles of a psychodynamic developmental psychopathology of depression by means of a clinical vignette. Finally, future challenges for psychodynamic developmental psychopathology are discussed.

Rise and Stagnation of the Developmental Psychopathology Project in Psychoanalysis

The simultaneous approach to normal and pathological development is deeply rooted in psychoanalytic thinking. We can see this in a quotation from *A psycho-analytic perspective on developmental psychopathology* (A. Freud, 1974, p. 63-64):

"We have broken with the tradition according to which every mental difficulty is seen and explained by comparison with severe pathological patterns, and, in-stead, try to see it against the background of the *norm*, expectable for the particular child's age, and to measure its distance from it. (…) I have attempted to do this in 1966, in my book *Normality and Pathology in Childhood: Assessment of Development*, by introducing the concept of Lines of Development."

The psychoanalytic contribution to developmental psychopathology, however, is less well known than one might expect from this quotation. In order to understand this, we will first make a historical digression.

The term "developmental psychopathology" was coined in 1974, both by Anna Freud in psychoanalytic literature and by Achenbach (1974) – author of the "Child Behavior Checklist" (Achenbach, 1991) – in experimental clinical child psychology. As a result, it is not immediately clear who can assume the copyright to the term. However, a central concept of developmental psychopathology – *developmental lines* – is without a doubt attributable to Anna Freud. It had already appeared in an article of hers dating from 1963. The above quotation from 1974 also makes it clear that the idea of developmental psychopathology – with the simultaneous study of normal and pathological lines of development – was already firmly entrenched in the research supported by Anna Freud.

The roots of the developmental psychopathology notion in psychoanalysis do indeed go back a long way. While Anna Freud (1966) used the concept of *developmental lines* as a key concept in one of her principal works – *Normality and pathology in childhood* – she had previously used the term *developmental disturbances* quite frequently. This was still a fairly wide concept, referring mainly to a "disturbance, characterized by deviation from normal development" (A. Freud, 1963, p. 44-45). Anna Freud had already started using this concept during the Second World War. Since 1942, she had been observing large groups of children who had been orphaned by war violence, as well as children who presented problems after having been temporarily separated from their parents and placed in foster homes in the countryside in order to escape from the German bombing of major British cities. She learned to look, in these children, for the first signs of psychological problems, the further evolution of these symptoms, both in their spontaneous course and under the influence of more specific care and help. What particularly interested her – and here our historical digression moves closer to the question of depression – were the mourning responses and the responses to separation and loss, more specifically early childhood expressions of grief and depression due to separation from and loss of the beloved care figure. She also searched for a better understanding of the influence of certain characteristics in the child or the environment, leading to an elimination or neutralizing of previous depressive symptoms or, on the contrary, to their emphasis and fixation (Burlingham & Freud, 1944). Within the context of numerous case descriptions, all kinds of familial and individual antecedents are described, which could promote or impede the processing of the complex feelings regarding separation from or loss of the parents. In that sense, Anna Freud had a good feel for the protective and risk factors in the socio-emotional development of these "children without families". Early vulnerabilities and sources of resilience, as well as their influence on the subsequent evolution of the mourning process or on the child's further development, are also extensively covered. Research into the normal and deviant developmental pathways of sad or mourning children, as well as into the factors influencing this and into the widely varying expressions of depression throughout childhood, was central to Anna Freud's work in that period.

Her observational research, which began during the 1940s, was to a certain extent a crystallization of an academic project for psychoanalysis written by Heinz Hartmann (1939) in *Ego psychology and the problem of adaptation*. To Hartmann, the simultaneous study of normal and deviant development was an absolute priority.[1] At the same time as Anna Freud's interpretation of this project, within psychoanalytically inspired developmental psychology we find this emphasis on the simultaneous study of normal and deviant phenomena in *The first year of life: Normal and deviant development of object relations,* the basic work of Spitz and Cobliner (1965).

In one of Anna Freud's latest papers, dated 1981, she indicates how much importance she attaches to the study of early development and to the recognition of early signs of deviance. The possibilities of prevention or early intervention were already widely known at that time, but for refinement and adaptation of early developmentally oriented preventive guidance and child psychotherapy, an ongoing and far-reaching research project covering normal and deviant development was needed. Anna Freud was to construct an extensive dataset for this project, among others, in the form of the Hampstead Clinical Index, which is certainly under-exploited even today. By using observation methods and setting up datasets in several developmental domains, Anna Freud became keenly aware of the sticking points in this academic project; for example, she organized the data of the Clinical Index in such a way that they could be used for group research or for multiple measurements within single cases, being aware of the need to undertake statistical research procedures within psychoanalysis. She also points out how difficult it is to make a distinction between normality and deviance during earliest child development and, certainly, during the first phases of a process that could be the onset of a maladaptive developmental line. She therefore advocates in no uncertain terms an intensification of research into this aspect:

"What concerns us today are the many characteristics expected from the average adult which (…) are described as to their end products, but for which no developmental prestages are itemized. This omission not only leaves a gap in developmental theory; it creates also the false impression that such achievements are come by easily, in fact that they are simply the result of smooth, undisputed, i.e. nonconflictual maturation." (A. Freud, 1981, p. 14)

Another important concern of Anna Freud is to demonstrate that development does not progress in a linear fashion, but with saltatorial developmental changes or shifts. After such a change, the child needs some time to adapt to a new, more complex way of functioning. Throughout these changes, development is progressive or it is being transformed and organized in a complex, hierarchical way, but it also has normal moments of stagnation, contributing to a sense of homeostasis. Nor is development synchronous in all domains or along all of its lines, as is clear from the developmental profiles of children. Moreover, development is embedded in

---

[1] "His interest in the conflict-free aspects of the ego, relates, he emphasizes time and again, to this desire that psychoanalysis becomes a general psychology, and not merely a special theory of psychopathology." (Yankelovich & Barrett, 1970, p. 108).

affective-relational dynamics and complexes from childhood, making temporary stagnation or even regression more understandable. Despite the great effort Anna Freud had made on the level of developmental psychopathology, her approach had insufficient following in psychoanalysis. She complained about this at the end of her life:

"(...) I have attempted to do this by introducing the concept of Lines of Development. (...) But the list given was by no means considered to be complete; rather, it was in fact meant as an invitation to the readers of the book to make their own additions to it. This challenge has so far not been taken up by any other author." (A. Freud, 1974, p. 64)

Contrary to what Anna Freud suggests, there have been important publications on developmental psychopathology within psychoanalysis in that period (e.g., see Nagera, 1970, 1981). But she felt that the domain of psychoanalytic developmental psychopathology had not evolved into a unified research project. Within certain influential circles in psychoanalysis, observation studies of children remained highly controversial until very recently. This empirical methodology on which John Bowlby (1981), in addition to Anna Freud and René Spitz (1945), also based his work on separation and loss of the attachment figure, and which Robert Emde (1981) and Daniel Stern (1985) also used as a basis for their work on socio-emotional development and on the development of the self in contact with the other, is unfortunately still not accepted in some schools in psychoanalysis today. This methodological problem in psychoanalysis has been addressed more systematically in recent years, while empirical research is also strongly advocated by a growing number of "scientist-practitioners" in psychoanalysis (Barron, Eagle, & Wolitzsky, 1990; Shapiro & Emde, 1995; Emde, 1999; Fonagy & Target, 2003).

Moreover, in the 1960s and 1970s, psychoanalysis lost its dominant position within mental health care, as a result of which the knowledge acquired within earlier psychodynamic developmental psychopathology was not adequately disseminated nor fully exploited or valued. This "political" element, together with the large methodological differences between psychoanalysis and other theoretical approaches in psychology meant that psychoanalytic developmental psychopatho-logy was either left out of the picture or was only quoted as an aside – an historically interesting footnote – within the broad and well known research domain which developmental psychopathology – at the intersection between child psychiatry, developmental psychology and clinical psychology – had now become, outside psychoanalysis.

Only recently, Peter Fonagy and Mary Target have placed psychoanalytic developmental psychopathology more accurately and systematically on the map, initially through specific psychoanalytic contributions to handbooks of developmental psychopathology (see Fonagy, 1995a, b; Fonagy & Target, 1997), and subsequently with their book, *Psychoanalytic theories: Perspectives from developmental psychopathology* (Fonagy & Target, 2003).

Inspired by these trailblazers, we are setting out in search of the foundations for a psychoanalytic developmental psychopathology of depression with the aim of taking up the dialogue with mainstream developmental psychopathology. Our starting point is formed by the two dimensions of depression – anaclitic and introjective – as described by Blatt (1974), who recently re-emphasized the need to work out a developmental psychopathological perspective on these dimensions (Blatt, 2004).

We are looking more specifically for the developmental line of normal anaclitic attachment and of maladaptive anaclitic depression as well as for the developmental line of normal introjection of moral imperatives and ideals (normal normative functioning) and of maladaptive introjective depression (pathological normative function).

Emergence of the Blueprint for Psychoanalytic Developmental Psychopathology

Historical Background: Some Founding Moments

Freud's introductory lectures to a developmental perspective on psychopathology. The developmental perspective – referred to in the early years of psychoanalysis as the "genetic perspective" – did not form one of the three key principles quoted by Freud (1900) in his first model of the human psyche, in which he distinguished a dynamic, economic and topographical perspective. The structural and genetic perspectives were added later. This "late" addition means that the developmental perspective is not regarded as obvious in psychoanalytic theory. This is undoubtedly one of the reasons why in some psychoanalytic theories pathways of depression are not automatically developmental pathways (cfr. infra) and why developmental psychopathology was not given an enthusiastic welcome in all psychoanalytic circles.

Freud's innovation was to place the emphasis on early childhood, with the Oedipus complex as the core complex. His first case studies were aimed at demonstrating that psychopathology in adulthood is the result – by deferred action (*Nachträglichkeit*) – of a long and complex pathogenesis. Some systematically repressed wishes remained active in the deeper layers of the psyche and could determine, in a complex way, neurotic difficulties later on in life: the Oedipal dramas from childhood are repeated and worked through in the context of mature adult psychosexuality.

While female neurotic patients originally played an important and inspiring role in developing psychoanalytic models, in case discussions from 1909 onwards Freud describes chiefly male patients. Once Freud concentrates on the psychosexual development of men, he becomes aware not only of the great importance of the aggressive sub-component of psychosexual development, but also of the previous history of it in the earliest Oedipal phase.

In the case description of Little Hans (Freud, 1909a), for example, the libidinal origin of Hans' fears and phobias is set in the broader context of the Oedipus complex. This core complex appears to imply a genuine development, a path throughout the Oedipal phase, from the earliest Oedipal strivings to the later Oedipal phase: Freud makes several remarks on the previous period in which the symptoms of five-year-old Hans already existed in a milder version. Sexual curiosity, problems with aggressive feelings and a somewhat anxious or shy attitude were already present in three-year-old Hans, from the beginnings of the Oedipus complex on.

This pathway perspective throughout the Oedipus complex cannot yet be detected in the case study of Dora published in 1905 (Freud, 1905). In the case study of the Rat Man, published also in 1909, the developmental perspective had become already very clear: the extreme repression of the aggression toward the father, activated in the context of the Rat Man's sexual desire for his mother, can only be understood when in the more archaic early phases of development other defensive operations against the sexual and aggressive impulses must have been activated. In this text, Freud (1909b) is rather vague on the exact timing of these "archaic" mechanisms preceding the extreme repression of the early Oedipus complex.

When Freud again writes about female psychosexuality in 1931, toward the end of his life, this developmental perspective has become even more evident, and more broad: the same word "archaic" now explicitly refers to the pre-Oedipal development (see Assoun, 1981). Consequently, the developmental line is considerably expanded again: from pre-Oedipal roots through early and late Oedipal influences, to ultimate symptom formation (by "deferred action"). At the same time, Freud has noticeable difficulty imagining the continuity in this developmental line. He presents it as if two discontinuous worlds are involved: the pre-Oedipal and the Oedipal development as "two civilizations from different times in history" (Freud, 1932, p. 225-226). A cut-off point or fracture exists between these two "worlds". Freud leaves us with this image of discontinuity in psychosexual development, at least in his later writings, which deal explicitly with female sexuality and, again, hysteria.

In papers dealing with other clinical syndromes, we implicitly find a different view of continuity and discontinuity throughout development. In his work on paranoid psychosis for instance (Freud, 1911, 1922), but definitely in his work on depression and melancholia (Freud, 1917a), the question is raised of the influence of pre-Oedipal and Oedipal development on the emergence of psychopathology. Moreover, in this period important theoretical adjustments occur – the reformulation of the drive theory (Freud, 1920) and the description of the structural model in his second topographical model of the human psyche (Freud, 1923) – which cause him to give more weight to the pre-Oedipal preliminary phase. For example, the formation of moral consciousness, which Freud originally (e.g., Freud, 1905) situated at the end of the Oedipus complex, is situated much earlier. In his writings between 1925 and 1930, continuity between the pre-Oedipal and Oedipal contributions to superego development is suggested.

We can say that Freud worked hard to construct a developmental perspective, rethought it several times, developed it, frequently hesitated and was even sometimes contradictory about it, depending on the context within which he was discussing it. We will now look in more detail at his developmental perspective of depression itself.

We start with his *Mourning and Melancholia* (Freud, 1917a). Here, he distinguishes two types of depression: neurotic and narcissistic depression. The role of aggression in the onset of depression receives much of Freud's attention. More specifically, the fundamental characteristic of affective ambivalence – the fact that human love is never perfect, never fully positive – is referred to by Freud as the key aspect in the psychodynamics of depression. People suffer from depression because of their ambivalence, because of the aggressive component of their love.

Usually, people can tolerate this imperfection in their love lives (ambivalence tolerance). They can keep the aggressive component of their love in the background (and yet remain sufficiently in touch with it to mobilize aggression against the love object, where necessary) or use the aggression constructively, for example to make their loving feelings powerful and assertive. Furthermore, in 1917 Freud (Freud, 1917a) describes another way of making constructive use of ambivalence: people use their aggression to go through the process of mourning. Just like separation, mourning demands some aggression: in protesting against the loss, in assigning the blame for having been left alone, in daring to feel the gift of still being alive, in accepting that the link with the lost object does not have to be idealized. However, depressive people cannot tolerate the imperfection of their love. When they are confronted with loss or even the threat of it, they massively suppress aggressive feelings toward the beloved object. Moreover, these feelings are turned against the self and only in this way, in the form of self-reproach, can they resurface. Aggression, therefore, can only be experienced at a conscious level if it is aimed at the self.

Self-reproach and self-criticism for not having taken good enough care of the loved one, the feeling that I am responsible for the loss of the other, that I did not do enough to prevent the loss – these are clinical manifestations of turning aggression toward the self although it was originally aimed at the other.

Freud's text from 1917 may well be criticized because of its rather limited view of the etiology of depression, but from a phenomenological point of view the text is still highly relevant. Particularly the comparison between normal, neurotic and melancholic (narcissistic) mourning processes is of the utmost importance to the developmental psychopathology perspective we have in mind. In melancholia — labelled a narcissistic neurosis by Freud — aggression against the loved one and the self is primitive (oral) in nature. As a result, the aggression is even more destructive than in psychoneuroses, as an example of which Freud uses obsessional neurosis in this text. In obsessional neurosis, the aggression is of an Oedipal nature, with possible regression to the anal-sadistic realm. The primitive nature of oral aggression can lead to more destructive self-punishment and self-criticism in melancholic patients, which increases the likelihood of suicide compared to obsessional neurotics without melancholic psychopathology, according to Freud (1917a).

In another text from 1917, Freud (1917b) clearly indicates that unfortunately he is not yet in a position to give us more information about the difference between these two levels of pathological ambivalence, the neurotic and the narcissistic. They produce different mourning processes, while the aggression involved has another developmental origin (oral versus Oedipal). In a certain sense, in this text Freud set out a program for further theoretical and empirical research on depression due to primitive (oral) sadistic love or to ambivalent (Oedipal) neurotic love. Other authors have attempted to fill in the theoretical gaps which Freud (1917b) left at the time, citing the influence of "earlier" oral themes and "later" Oedipal aspects in depression, the difference between neurotic and pre-neurotic depression, and the assumption that another developmental layer is associated with every form of depression. Freud was the first to suggest that two levels of depressive psychopathology are linked to two different developmental stages: depression in narcissistic disorders is about oral sadism while depression in neurotic disorders is about Oedipal ambivalence. We will now see how Abraham and Klein continued this line of thinking.

Abraham and Klein: Expansion of Freud's developmental perspective into the earliest developmental phases. For Freud, moral conflicts about aggression towards the beloved object should be placed within the context of the Oedipal phase of psychosexual development. At the end of this phase, the child is usually able to understand in a certain way the emotional contradiction in the fact that the beloved object is also treated aggressively. The child evaluates his love and hate self-critically and sees that it has not met the ego ideal or the normative standards of the superego. The Oedipal phase is the period during which the child can gradually grasp the contradiction between love and hate, as well as the conflict between sexual desire and prohibition. Normally, at the end of the Oedipal phase, the child makes a judgement of condemnation. Freud (1909a) described this mild mechanism of defense only once. It is a mechanism that is almost conscious in nature: henceforth, the normally developing child is better able to make a judgement and to rein in aggression towards the parents. Pathological development is characterized by repression, occurring early in Oedipal development, as is the case with the phobic problems of little Hans (repression as a more extreme mechanism of defense, unconscious in nature), possibly even preceded by a primitive isolation or separation of both tendencies of love and aggression, as is the case with the obsessional neurosis of the Rat Man. In this latter case, the anal-sadistic component of the love was of a particular kind already in the pre-Oedipal development phases. But Freud hasn't given us a further answer about these early pre-Oedipal precursors of problems with aggression and their influence on self-reproach and self-evaluation. He only knew that this raised important questions, since he gave a lot of thought to the pre-Oedipal love-hate balance in texts on paranoia (Freud, 1911, 1922).

Since 1917, other authors have looked at these precursors in particular, more specifically at aggression and its role in early moral functioning. For instance, Karl Abraham (1921/1953a, 1924/1953b) and Melanie Klein (1928) described, respectively, the *sphincter morality of the anal phase* and *the depressive crises in the context of archaic Oedipal anxieties* in the second and third years of life.

Once the child realizes for the first time that its sadism is targeted at the same vitally necessary and beloved object (e.g., the mother) and that the child itself consequently has not only loving, positive tendencies within him, but also aggressive, negative tendencies, the child reaches the depressive position. At a certain moment in development – Abraham and Klein originally place this in the second part of the second year of life – it is possible to see in most children that aggression towards the beloved objects no longer remains without moral conflicts or critical self-evaluation. As a consequence of this early moral reaction, the child can protect the mother from its aggression.

These first moral reactions are an expression of an awareness of the gap between the (extreme) ideal self-image and the "harsh" reality of the "ambivalent" self: the child not only loves the mother but also causes her harm. Moreover, the child gradually realizes that it previously did this in an unconcerned and sometimes ruthless way (to use one of Winnicott's concepts; Winnicott, 1945/1958). The capacity for empathy or concern begins to develop, while aggression is better neutralized, channelled and merged with love.

Klein (1935, 1940) describes these first moral reactions in child development within the context of her theory of the depressive position. The first time a child realizes that the object towards which love and hate are targeted is one and the same, it leads to a painful affective crisis which prompts the child towards reparational tendencies. From then on, the mother becomes more acknowledged and accepted as a differentiated person with her own rights (a whole object); she is no longer an object in the service of the self (a partial object). The central fear of the child at this age – Klein has placed this moment gradually earlier in development – is depressive in nature: the child fears having injured the mother object, banished it from himself or even destroyed it, and now more keenly realizes that he is not a perfectly loving child. The child first realizes his affective ambivalence when he has a certain sense of the consequences of his aggression. He now sees that the mother is not perfect and does not entirely coincide or merge with the child; therefore she cannot be controlled in an omnipotent way. Moreover, the child realizes that a gap exists between the real self and the ideal self. This leads to feelings of guilt, moral reflexes and a genuine desire to repair, initially in the form of perfectionism or of a misunderstanding of the gravity of the consequences of the ambivalence (obsessive versus manic defenses against depressive pain), later in more realistic attempts at reparation.

The desire for perfection – the obsessive defense – is an understandable first attempt to deal with the ambivalences and to close the gap between ideal and real self. In normal development, this quickly assumes the form of "wanting to be as perfect as possible but also accepting that this can never succeed: a certain tolerance of imperfection and ambivalence, a negative capability" (Bion, 1962, p. 118). Or, as Ricoeur (1971, p. 34) has put it: "accepting the best possible human world" instead of "reaching after a perfect world, beyond our human capabilities". In the acceptance process, the ideals of the child, step by step, become more realistic and have a motivating effect, while the reality of imperfection becomes less dramatic and less de-motivating.

The Emerging Model: Single Developmental Lines into Pathology and One-To-One Associations Between Development and Pathology

In *New Introductory Lectures on Psychoanalysis,* Freud (1932) praised Abraham for the distinctions he made within the pre-Oedipal developmental phases. He particularly emphasized the developmental changes in the aggressive aspect of psychosexual ontogenesis and the implications these changes have on the development of guilt, morality and prosocial tendencies. Important steps in moral development are clearly observable in the middle of the anal phase and toward the latter part of the Oedipal phase.

In the middle of the anal phase, the child can no longer approach the loved object in an unconcerned ruthless (and sometimes aggressive[2]) way. Abraham's theory of the first development of guilt as a depressive anxiety, and as a motivating element for reparational tendencies in the latter anal phase, has been taken up by Klein in her theory of the onset of the depressive position, situated in the earliest moments of the Oedipus complex (in her theory coinciding with what traditionally had been described as later oral phase and anal phase).

These first moral reactions are joined in a subsequent developmental phase by guilt and concerns over the Oedipal ambivalence. In this sub-phase, when libidinal tendencies have become dominant in a genital sexual organization, moral consciousness is strengthened to such an extent that the object is better safeguarded from aggressive impulses. Ambivalence is diminished.

In Abraham's theory, the concepts of pre-ambivalent, ambivalent and post-ambivalent phases became associated with this threefold division: the pre-ambivalent development from birth to the middle of the oral phase; the ambivalent development from the middle of the oral phase to the later Oedipal phase; the post-ambivalent development from the later Oedipal phase onward. This blueprint was initially adopted as such by Klein in 1935 (the paranoid phase that precedes the

---

[2] Aggression in this sense means a non-intentional epiphenomenon of the narcissistic phases of development. In the middle of the anal phase, an enormous shift is made towards object relatedness. This brings it about that aggression can be kept at bay and that it can be used more intentionally. This developmental change in the line of aggression is associated with a stronger awareness of one's own responsibility for aggressive acts of the self against the object: a first clear sign of moral development.

depressive position that is passed through toward a post-depressive position). The fact that Klein and other psychoanalysts subsequently changed the timetable of this and adjusted their conceptual framework does not eliminate the threefold structure (functioning according to a paranoid-schizoid mode, a depressive mode and a post-depressive mode). We will now explain this threefold division in early childhood development which is still widespread in psychoanalysis and which has been linked to levels of psychopathology.

General idea: Three developmental phases connected to three levels of psychopathology. The idea persists in both Abraham and Klein that, at a certain point in development, the perception of the aggressive sub-component of the libido brings about a morally inspired self-evaluation and a depressive reaction. They place this in the ambivalent phase of libidinal development. A series of well-known psychoanalysts such as Jacobson (1953), Zetzel (1965), Mahler (1972), Parens (1979) and Kernberg (1984) each described this threefold division in the developmental perspective in their own way. As a result, this three-phase model – of which Abraham is the "godfather" – recurs in variants in many authors who link a developmental perspective to their psychopathological theory. For example, Winnicott (1960/1984) links various forms of psychopathology to either the phase of absolute dependence, to the phase of relative dependence or to the Oedipal phase. Fairbairn (1941/1952a) distinguishes between the phase of infantile dependence, the transitory phase and the phase of complexity in relationships, three moments on the developmental line from infantile to mature dependence. Mahler (1972) and Mahler, Pine and Bergman (1975) refer to the pre-rapprochement phase, the rapprochement phase and the Oedipal phase, while Blatt (1974) distinguishes between psychopathology associated with problems with object permanency, object constancy and affect constancy. Parens (1991) talks of the first precursors of ambivalence, the first (pre-Oedipal) and the second (Oedipal) generation of ambivalence conflicts.

These three compartments in development are not always comparable at the level of content and time, but they are in terms of structure. Psychoanalytic psychopathology theory depends on this structure: for the psychoses, borderline conditions and neuroses, crucial factors are sought in, respectively, the earliest, central and later phases of early childhood development. The underlying assumption is: the more serious the psychopathological syndrome, the earlier in development the deviation from a normal path must have occurred. This three-level framework certainly is a strong element of psychoanalytic theory; the way they are associated to levels of psychopathology raises important questions, as we will argue further on. The strengths and limitations of this framework will be discussed later in this chapter. However, we first discuss the work of two authors (Glazer, 1979; Antonovsky, 1991) who have tried to link depression to the different developmental steps at which deviance from normal development can occur. Their work can be situated in the low-profile period of psychoanalytic developmental psychopathology, between the mid-seventies and the early nineties. Both authors situate the etiology of depression within the perspective of the development of personal standards, more specifically the ego ideal and the superego.

Glazer's Theory of the Developmental Trajectory Towards Object-Related or Narcissistic Depression

Glazer (1979) distinguishes two levels of depression, "object-related depression" and "narcissistic depression". His attempt to understand the pathogenesis which leads to two levels of depression in a developmental context immediately brings us a step closer to the developmental psychopathology project we are seeking.

Glazer's starting point is that ideal and reality are not the same. One possible reaction to this is depressive in nature, heralded by the helplessness of the self which is confronted with the gap between ideal and reality, as well as by the possible aggression which is provoked as a result, or which is involved in some other way. Moreover, this aggression can be turned against the self because in the ideal self image, for example, there is no place for anger towards the object.

Glazer also raises the question of how we can understand, from the helplessness of the self, that depression can be narcissistic or object-related in nature. He argues that the two deviations in the direction of depression start from the same developmental line (the normative function line), but from different locations or developmental moments. Particularly as a result of the latter, the pathway into different levels of depression takes on the nature of a true developmental line. According to Glazer, the central aspect of object-related depression is that the ambivalence with respect to the object is too conflicting. In order to avoid helplessness with respect to this ambivalence, the self will coincide with the object in an extremely positive symbiotic relation within which aggression is no longer present. However, the helplessness does not disappear because the self feels restrained (inhibited) and the possibility is lost of making creative use of aggression within an individualized relation of an autonomous self with the differentiated other. The object relationship itself is now no longer at risk, but its differentiated nature is. In other words, the object relationship is distorted because certain aspects of it are unbearable.

By contrast, in narcissistic depression, helplessness in the self arises as a result of the threat of loss or destruction of a relationship with a self-object. That self-object is vitally necessary to the homeostasis of the self; moreover, it is an object with which the person was previously merged. In this form of depression, the object relationship itself is at issue: it is not a question of a distortion of the object relationship between a differentiated self and object, but rather of the loss of an undifferentiated link with an object, as a result of which the self is also damaged or emptied.

Glazer emphasizes that, in the developmentally more advanced object-related depression, helplessness and inhibition are a consequence of affective ambivalence, which is a source of conflict for the self. More realistic individuation should be worked on during therapy, within which positive and negative components can be present simultaneously or can be integrated. In the developmentally more primitive narcissistic depression, the helplessness is much more of a reaction to the threat that the link with an as yet unseparated but vitally necessary self-object will be lost. Treatment in this case will primarily focus on safe separation, with the presence of the object in the background, rather than on more complex individuation with a differentiated relationship to whole objects and with an integration of negative and positive elements.

As can be seen from the terms used, Mahler's developmental framework is introduced by Glazer in order to put the cause of the helplessness into its proper context: unbearable aspects of individuation (aggression and ambivalence) lead to object-related depression characterized by the fear of loss of approval by the superego or the moral authority; unbearable aspects of separation lead to narcissistic depression characterized by the fear of loss of the relation with the self-object. In other words, while a normative conflict comparable to the conflicts from the *rapprochement subphase* forms the basis for object-related depression, narcissistic depression is linked to an unbearable loss of a self-object, set within the context of the development of the *pre-rapprochement subphase*.

The developmental perspective is not taken further by Glazer. He stops with the role of the normative function in the emergence of the two levels of depression. In object-related depression, the ideal is disrupted by ambivalence, which is inevitable in a complex, integrated picture of self and other; in narcissistic depression the ideal is disrupted by aggression, which could destroy the vitally necessary extremely idealized merger, but which is also needed to come to any differentiation between self and other. In object-related depression, the discordant aggression is repressed; in narcissistic depression unbearable aggression is isolated and split off. In Glazer's words, it is a matter of two forms and levels of deviance of the same developmental line: that of moral development. On this developmental line, aggression is averted in a phase-specific way – in one case because the moral conscience rejects the affective contradiction of love and hate (due to unbearable guilt anxiety), in the other case because, within the most primitive form of moral consciousness, aggression evokes fear of revenge and destruction (annihilation anxiety).

Antonovsky's Theory of the Depressive Experiential Process

Anna Antonovsky (1991) discussed the emergence of depression in a summary article about "the holding of ideals and idealization". In this article, she emphasized how important it is to be able to make the transition from idealization to the holding of ideals, from extreme to realistic ideals or moral standards.

The first love of the child for the parental figures and the self is highly idealizing, but this idealization of self and others is gradually tempered in normal development, giving way to the holding of ideals. Holding ideals is, in other words, more realistic than idealization. According to Antonovsky, a primordial etiological factor in depression is found in problems related to making the transition from (extreme) idealization to tempered, more realistic ideals. Personal standards and moral judgement remain strict as a result, rather than presenting a mildness; people suffer from these extreme, unrealistic ideals, while self-reproach and self-punishing trends are prominently present. In depressive illness, people become stuck on the line from extreme idealization to the holding of realistic ideals.

Ego psychology chiefly stressed the adaptive aspects of covering the path from idealization to the holding of ideals. By the holding of ideals, development is facilitated and a better sense of reality is established as well as a more integrated superego in which the complexity of a mature personality structure can be expressed.

From a clinical point of view, Jacobson (1964, 1971) is of the opinion that the development of the normative function is driven by a back-and-forth movement on this line between "idealization" and "the holding of ideals", from idealizing love towards holding realistic ideals concerning the other or the self. On the other hand, there is the reverse trend in which a continued longing for more idealistic circum-stances and representations of self and other is expressed. The first movement (from extreme to realistic ideals) is never completed; the second (from realism to extreme idealism) is doomed to disillusionment. What is crucial is that, in normal development, de-idealization becomes acceptable, thereby tolerating the tension brought by the realization of imperfection. After having longed for more perfect conditions, gradually a re-libidinalization of the imperfect picture of the self and the other occurs, described by Jacobson as a more mature kind of idealization, and regarded by Antonovsky as "holding ideals in an adaptive way". This new libidinal cathexis of "the fallible other" or "the fallible self" is an adequate counterbalance to the yearning for the perfect situation. Against this background of sufficient love for the imperfect, the gap with the perfect ideal is tolerated, people feel happy enough with the reality of imperfections, without misrepresenting them too much, but with the possibility of striving for certain unfulfilled objectives which lie within the bounds of possibility and of evaluating endeavours and possibilities sufficiently realistically.

A crucial change, which launches the subject on the path to depression, is that the tension which brings the necessary disillusionment of idealization is not tolerated. It is replaced by a feeling of helplessness. Moreover, aggression can also be present within this helplessness in the form of reproach against the self and the other. The helplessness of the self, confronted with the inability to reach or maintain a highly ideal situation, opens up the way to depression.

Among other psychoanalysts, who chiefly stress the drive-related background of depression, even more attention will be devoted to the aggressive component in the etiology of depression. According to Melanie Klein (1945), for example, the idealized object arises as a result of splitting, the mechanism which helps to defend against aggressive impulses. These are then attributed to a persecutory ("bad") object, while the beloved object appears perfect or highly ideal. In a normal experience process, integration of both parts of self and other will then follow in the depressive position. In this integration, the extreme idealization of the good object can be renounced. Goodness is no longer attributed to a bad other; bad aspects in the good object are no longer defended against. The representations of the self and the other become less extreme and more subtle or complex; they become more realistic too. The bad sides of the self and the object become regarded as an inevitable part of the whole and are also less unbearable. However, this is only true in the case of normal integration of the aggressive, negative self and object parts into the loving, positive parts. In the depressive crisis, by contrast, people experience helplessness, a complex affective crisis of guilt, shame, pining and self-reproach about their own aggression and imperfections. More than anything, they want to cure the crisis but believe that this can only be done by returning to the perfect situation and by undoing the imperfection in an omnipotent way, rather than by accepting imperfection and negativity in love or by acknowledging that this imperfection is simply an inevitable component of human relationships. Imperfection is still harshly judged. It is impossible to reach the desired perfect situation and this realization leads to the feeling of helplessness; in that case, the depressive position cannot be tolerated, leading to depressive illness.

While ego psychology primarily regards depression as a reaction to a situation of extreme helplessness of the self (Bibring, 1953), drive psychology places more emphasis on the role of aggressive impulses in the induction of this helplessness. However, ego psychology and drive psychology concur on what they refer to as crucial etiological factors. The emergence of depression is situated in the intervening moment of disillusion with extreme idealization, the inevitably associated helplessness and the (lack of) tolerance for ambivalence associated with this process of disillusionment.

The experiential line of depression therefore runs from extreme idealization to the holding of realistic ideals, with several steps in the development of tolerance of disillusionment and of ambivalence along the way. The line leading to depression crosses clear problems of disillusionment with extreme idealization. These are expressed in ambivalence-intolerance. The imperfection and ambivalence are not tolerated and, at the same time, one realizes that the extremely ideal situation is no longer attainable. This conflict becomes a trap; the self feels helpless because it has no way out since the extreme idealistic images are unrealistic and the realistic images are intolerable.

Antonovsky offers us a "developmental line perspective" on depression in the sense that she describes in great detail the course or development of the experiential processes leading to depression. In principle, the experiential pathway she mentions is applicable to several moments in the development from more extreme to more realistic moral or normative structures. However, the object of study is not about the critical points in this developmental line from idealization to the holding of ideals: Antonovsky's brilliant study is about lines of depressive experience.

Comparing Glazer and Antonovsky, we could say that in a certain way a change in emphasis has occurred, from a developmental psychopathology at the end of the seventies to a theory of dynamic and experiential pathogenesis. Both contributions are situated within another context: Glazer was writing at a period when searching for the crucial developmental line of a psychopathological syndrome was still in vogue, Antonovsky at a period where this focus was less of a concern.

Guiding Principles for an Up-To-Date Psychoanalytic Developmental Psychopathology: From Single Trajectory to Complex Interacting Developmental Lines

Several events inside and outside psychoanalysis brought the developmental psychopathological project back into prominence. The broader acceptance of empirical research methods in psychoanalysis is one of these events: complexity in longitudinal processes can be investigated, combining data from several variables (for example, different developmental domains or pathways). This broadens the existing model of developmental psychopathology: pathological outcomes can be understood as the results of changes and deviations on several developmental pathways and on several crucial moments on these pathways. This carries psychoanalytic developmental psychopathology away from the idea of one single track into psychopathology, possibly from one crucial moment of deviance on. This evolution in psychoanalysis is nurtured to a large extent by the vigour of empirical (experimental) developmental psychopathology within clinical psychology, developmental psychology and (child) psychiatry from the second half of the eighties on (Cicchetti, 1984, 1989; Cicchetti & Toth, 1992; Sroufe & Rutter, 1984).

In the field of the psychoanalytic depression literature Blatt (1974) already advocated this new line of thinking in the mid-seventies; it is no accident that this developmental psychopathological element of Blatt's work received an enormous new impetus from the nineties on.

Blatt's Perspective on Depression as a Pathological Outcome of Two Developmental Lines: Introjection and Anaclitic Relatedness

Blatt expands upon the developmental perspective formulated by Glazer in two ways. On the one hand, he specifies that two developmental lines leading to two forms of depression are involved, rather than talking about two levels of deviance from one and the same developmental line (i.e., the development of personal standards). *Introjective* (self-critical) depression is conceived as a deviation from the line of development of self-definition, including the development of personal standards and morality; *anaclitic* (dependent) depression as a curve on the line of object relational development (Blatt & Shichman, 1983). Subsequently, he even talks about two dimensions which are present in every depressive problem, albeit to a variable extent and often with one of them dominating: the introjective (structural) and the anaclitic (object relational) dimensions of depressive illness. The idea exists of a dominant depressive style (structural/introjective or relational/anaclitic), but in no way are these styles exclusive (Blatt, 1998).

With his theory of two kinds of depressive experiences, Blatt gives full weight to an aspect that in Glazer's theory remained in the background. Specifically, Glazer points to the possibility of depressive reactions as a result of loss of the approval by the moral conscience (falling short with respect to norm and ideal in "object-related depression") as well as resulting from loss of the self-object (the ideal link with it would be lost by the aggression of separation, which would give rise to "narcissistic depression"). Blatt will give more weight to the (object) relational components in what Glazer calls narcissistic depression, as we shall see, without neglecting the possible influence of the superego aspects in these relational depressions, and also, by hinting at relational depressive illness in a broader area than that of the narcissistic level.

As an intermediate consideration, we should also mention here that the use of both sets of terminology can confuse the reader: Glazer's object-related depression corresponds mostly to the introjective depression of Blatt[3] while the narcissistic depression of Glazer chiefly relates to what Blatt calls (object) relational depression (although Blatt clearly sees this relational component more broadly than Glazer: not only dyadic, but just as much triadic).[4]

Blatt also does justice to an object-relational origin of a pathological superego structure in depression, while most of the theories of depression in psychoanalysis stress the ego-psychological origin of depression (the helplessness of the ego), whether or not in interaction with aggressive impulses (Bibring, 1953).

As summarized in Chapter 3, in contrast to Glazer, Blatt distinguishes two developmental lines and he indicates that development into normality or pathology is the result of a dialectic interaction between these two lines. The end result of normal development along the anaclitic developmental line becomes clear in the capacity for satisfactory, intimate, interpersonal relationships; the end result along the introjective line takes the form of a stable, positive feeling of autonomy and identity. In this latter line, the genesis of the ego is central and the formation of ego ideal and superego also plays an important role, more specifically through processes of identification and introjection. Essentially, this second line is concerned with self-definition, self-evaluation, a sense of self-competence and identity.

---

[3] In Glazer, object-related depression refers to depression within the context of whole object relations and complex personality structures with a distinct id, ego, superego, while at this level of depression, Blatt chiefly emphasizes the structural characteristics (the introjection leading to the emergence of the ego ideal and superego). Glazer's narcissistic depression is then located at the level of partial relationships or self-object relationships, while Blatt's relational depression additionally concerns the loss of whole object relationships.

[4] Blatt's approach covers the whole range of personality functioning, from psychotic to normal-neurotic. At each level, depression can occur within which both dimensions (introjection and anaclitic relatedness) can be intermingled. Glazer's approach seems to refer to a more restricted level of pathology: object-related depression is Oedipal in nature and associated to neurotic illness, narcissistic depression is pre-Oedipal and related to pre-neurotic character pathology.

Based on this view of development – development as interaction between several developmental lines – Blatt has also described two clusters of psychopathology (Blatt & Shichman, 1983; Blatt & Zuroff, 1992): the anaclitic and the introjective. Influenced by many types of biological, contextual and/or psychological factors, the subject "chooses" one of the two. This "symptom choice" is, as many before us have indicated, still largely uncharted territory. It is perhaps more important to know that Blatt indicates that whichever "developmental line" and "pathology cluster" is "chosen", the other line can also be entwined with it alongside this dominant line and cluster.

In anaclitic psychopathology, the focus is on problems with interpersonal relationships, merger and individuality, dependence and autonomy, whether within relations of a dyadic or triadic nature. In introjective psychopathology, the focus is on difficulties with self-experience, self-appraisal, self-definition, self-criticism and identity. Introjective aspects will also resonate within dominant anaclitic problems, just as relational aspects will play a role within dominant introjective problems.

Just as we can speak of anaclitic and introjective psychopathology, we can also refer to anaclitic and introjective depression. Anaclitic depression is related to conflicts in the interpersonal realm, particularly relating to dependence and (threatened or real) object loss. Feelings of loneliness, helplessness and weakness dominate. There is a highly intense longing for love and approval, but just as great a fear of rejection and loss of contact. Aggression is largely repressed, in order to protect the longed-for relationship or the necessary dependence. Repressed or denied aggression not infrequently finds an outlet in psychosomatic symptoms. Introjective depression is linked rather to problems concerning the sense of self, self-evaluation and self-appreciation. Feelings of guilt and self-deprecation are prominent. The criticism targeted at the self is strong: the drive of mastery and extreme perfectionism do not permit failure in attaining the strict ideals. Aggression towards the self or the other occasionally comes clearly to the surface, certainly when ideals are not attained by the self or ideal expectations are not met by the other.

Blatt and Zuroff (1992) also link gender considerations to both forms of psychopathology and depression: women present more anaclitic problems, men tend towards introjective problems. Also, it is possible that in ego-oriented Western societies, depressions tend to be introjective, while in societies where identity is determined much more socially, depressions are more likely to be anaclitic or relational. The appearance or phenotype of a psychopathological syndrome may also be determined by the culture of the patient. This aspect is referred to in cross-cultural psychology as the *pathoplasticity of a syndrome* (Kleinman & Good, 1985; Kortmann, 1995). Culture is one element in this plasticity. Markus and Kitayama (1991) were among the first cross-cultural psychologists to argue that instruments that are more sensitive to culture-specific idioms of distress and psychopathology are urgently needed. In this respect, Blatt's *Depressive Experiences Questionnaire* (Blatt, D'Afflitti, & Quinlan, 1976) – with an emphasis on self-critical introjective and on socially oriented relational depression – could have enormous benefits for depression research in multicultural societies. For example, not all depression will have a connotation of a downward movement of the self. This self-evaluative emphasis has been identified by Littlewood (2003) as a typically Western or European idiom for distress or a typical Western format for depressive illness from the 18th century on. Kareem (1992) argues that depression in non-Western immigrants is as often associated with loss or breakdown of social networks as it is with not living up to the ideals and standards of a "successful migration". The relational pathway into depression was perhaps not emphasized sufficiently in depression literature; depression in children, woman and immigrants from non-Western cultures brings this dimension more into prominence.

Both forms or clusters of psychopathology – relational and introjective – emerge from an accumulation of factors which may be located at various moments of development. In this sense, Blatt presents a complex model of developmental psychopathology. In Glazer we still find the idea that narcissistic depression occurs on the basis of problems during the period before the rapprochement crisis (*pre-rapprochement phase pathology*), while object-related depression occurs during the rapprochement crisis and/or later. Blatt does not make this distinction in developmental origin between the two types of depression, or certainly not in the same way. Although Blatt considers anaclitic depression as more primitive than introjective depression, he also refers to the idea of progression/regression and deferred action. In his theory, the subject is presented as vulnerable to anaclitic, sociotropic elements or to introjective, autonomous aspects. Various psycho-pathological syndromes are possible, based on this vulnerability on one of the two developmental lines. Within the framework of two (interacting) developmental lines, disturbances can be present at various levels: psychotic, borderline, neurotic.

For example, non-paranoid schizophrenia, hysterical borderline personality disorders, infantile ("narcissistic") personalities and anaclitic depressions are situated as deviations from the anaclitic developmental line. The introjective developmental line is concerned with paranoid schizophrenia, borderline persona-lity disorders with the emphasis on ideational problems, obsessional neurosis (obsessive-compulsive personalities), phallic-narcissistic problems (with an exaggerated involvement with the self) and introjective depression (see Blatt & Shichman, 1983; see also Chapter 3, this volume).

These various syndromes are not only closely linked within each dimension of psychopathology, they can also alternate through various kinds of regression and progression through time or occur in a mixed form at a well-defined moment. At the same time, restrictions are imposed (Blatt, 1995): both forms of schizophrenia are typical of difficulties which first occur on both developmental lines, specifically when in development object permanence emerges (*libidinal recognition constancy*). Both borderline conditions are then situated within the perspective of problems with object constancy (*evocative object constancy*), while the other syndromes are related to affect constancy (*post ambivalence constancy*). Using this division, schizophrenia and borderline conditions are preneurotic personality disorders – related to processes in pre-Oedipal development – while the other conditions (including both kinds of depression) are related to neurotic, intrapsychic Oedipal conflicts. Blatt therefore speaks not only of two developmental lines, but also of several developmental moments at which both developmental lines can be turned in the direction of various psychopathological syndromes.

This developmental psychopathological perspective fits in with the complexity of developmental lines and processes that contribute to a psychopathological outcome (Blatt & Homann, 1992). Yet, it still leaves questions unanswered. Firstly, although in theory Blatt's model links both kinds of depression to Oedipal development, it is still conceivable for introjective depression to be regarded as the most differentiated form of depression, while anaclitic depression could again be regarded as less differentiated (not triadic, but dyadic; not Oedipal but pre-Oedipal). The tendency to involve relational models in psychoanalysis, particularly for a better understanding of the first three – pre-Oedipal – years of life, while introjection in the classical sense is approached from an Oedipal perspective, certainly plays a role here. Object-relational models in psychoanalysis are closely linked to the discovery of the socio-emotional development in the first years of life, while superego formation in classical Freudian theory was associated with Oedipal development. It is hardly surprising then that the relational depressions can be linked to earlier developmental tracks more easily than the introjective depressions.

Secondly, although the various pathological syndromes linked to each of the two developmental lines can interact, each syndrome is linked to one developmental origin: pathology as a result of problems with object permanency, pathology as a result of problems with object constancy, or pathology as a result of problems with affect constancy. Without taking the complexity of Blatt's model well enough into consideration, the reader could inadvertently regard this again as a linear developmental model in psychoanalysis, a uniformity myth or single track model of which criticism is possible: "Psychoanalytic developmental models aim at a level of abstraction where there is a one-to-one relationship between a particular pattern of abnormality and a particular developmental cause" (Fonagy & Target, 2003, p. 10).

Thirdly, the various syndromes in both dimensions of psychopathology are linked to a developmental origin. But what exactly is meant by "origin"? Is the developmental line already deviating in the direction of depression at that critical moment in development, and how is this deviation expressed at these moments? Does vulnerability on a developmental line occur for the first time here? Is development under pressure, while resilience ensures that the developmental line still remains within the limits of normal variance? Does this pressure or risk factor then form a vulnerability which subsequently, in interaction with later developmental interferences, leads to deviance from the normal developmental line? In other words, how should we conceptualize continuity and discontinuity between early childhood risk or vulnerability, subsequent developmental interference and deviant developmental outcome? What interactions are conceivable between various influencing factors, from several developmental phases, in the emergence of psychopathology and, more specifically, depression? The phase specificity of the object tie of the child is a very important element to mention here. Winnicott (1964) stresses the importance of the father as a shield around the mother-child unit in the oral phase, enabling the mother and child to attune to one another and to make the first steps toward differentiation and individuation (see also Chapter 6, this volume). In the anal and Oedipal phases the father has another function for the child: helping the child with further ego-integration, personality structure building, gender identity, and psychosexual development. In the process of internalizing moral standards, the father also plays an important role. We do not want to suggest here that the mother-child tie is the only relational matrix, and the father-child relation the only introjective, structure-building matrix. Father and mother play an important part in both dimensions, but they do this in many different ways depending on the developmental phase the child is in.

The loss of a parent can also have differential effects on the relational and introjective dimension, depending on the developmental phase in which the loss is experienced. Whether a child is more vulnerable on the relational or the introjective dimension has to do with subjective aspects but perhaps also with the phase-specificity of the early experience of loss. Further research on the relational and introjective impact of childhood loss will be of great importance (e.g., Bravo, 2001; Dietrich & Shabab, 1989; Nagera, 1970).

Compared to the linear developmental models in psychoanalysis, Blatt's model has greater explanatory value but can still be reinforced in the aforementioned manner. It is a question of introducing further developmental differentiation within the concepts of "anaclitic" or "introjective" depression. Introjective problems within the context of dyadic relationships are not the same as introjective problems within triadic relationships; both may also possibly make a different contribution to the onset of depression and have a different influence on the progress of depression and the therapeutic process. The same applies to anaclitic problems which also emerge from different developmental phases: problems of relatedness in the pre-object phase, in the phase of dyadic relationships or in the phase of triadic relationships. It is no coincidence that Blatt and Spitz use the concept of "anaclitic depression" to refer to phenomena from widely varying developmental phases, Oedipal and pre-Oedipal. Moreover, greater developmental complexity will allow a more precise developmentally oriented therapeutic intervention.

It is therefore high time for psychoanalytic developmental psychopathology to discern how depression can assume different forms depending on whether aspects from various developmental phases are prominent (and, for example, are expressed subsequently during the various phases of a psychoanalytic process). Associated with this is the question of how anaclitic and introjective dimensions of depression differ in various clinical pictures which are thought to diverge at specific developmental moments – phase-specific – from normal development (in other words, what is anaclitic/introjective depression like in schizophrenia, in border-line conditions and in neurotic conflicts?). It is at this level that a developmental psychopathology perspective within psychoanalysis should be able to make progress. In the next section, we briefly discuss how a developmental model that would distinguish between three phases or moments in both the anaclitic and introjective developmental line might organize current and future research.

The term "anaclitic" is – under the influence of Spitz (1945, 1957) – spontaneously associated with very early pre-Oedipal, relationally determined depression. Introjective depression as a consequence of a certain perception of the gap between ideal and reality – is then spontaneously associated with later pre-Oedipal or Oedipal development.

Helplessness in the first months of life, therefore, is not so much the result of critical self-evaluation, but of contact problems or deficiencies in the earliest mother-child relation. The young child feels helpless, for example, because he cannot attain the necessary symbiosis with the mother: the child lost his mother or she is emotionally unavailable. This impossibility of making contact with the object or inability to remain in contact with a significant object forms an early developmental path to depression. Hermann (1936) and Szondi (1965) described this early contact dimension based on a double movement of "clinging to and going on search". Insufficient possibility to do this leads to relational depression, certain extreme forms of which are described in Spitz (1945, 1946): hospitalism and anaclitic depression.

Depression here is particularly related to difficulties in the earliest contact between the child and the outside world. Helplessness is therefore related to the impossibility of reaching the mother, of forming a symbiotic link with her, finding a self-object, encountering a safe relational matrix within which initial self-development can take place and from which the child can subsequently separate: *mothers have to be there to be left* (Furman, 1988). Fairbairn (1944/1952b) would argue that this is not depression because of aggression in love, but because of the feeling that one's own early love or binding impulses are not good enough. Winnicott (1963), in turn, would relate this kind of depression to the fact that the child's "*contributing in* (the first relationship) is not met". Tustin (1987) would refer to depression because of an inability to communicate early-childhood needs to the other either because that other is not there to be reached or because the child himself does not possess basal capacities for reaching out to the other. Her view is also interesting because she indicates that the relational dimension of depression has various levels: helplessness and depression in contact at the psychotic level, at the borderline level, at the neurotic level or in normal variation. The normal counterbalance to this early-childhood helplessness is a feeling of competence and agency of the child in relation to the other. Interestingly enough, Alvarez (1992) describes the need for *live company* and the echoes a deficiency in this company leads to in several levels of psychopathology.

Blatt indicates, not coincidentally, that we still do not know enough about this dimension of depression, certainly concerning the early, pre-Oedipal factors. Recent research in psychoanalysis addresses these early developmental phases and their importance for understanding depression and other psychopathological syndromes (e.g., Bravo, 2001; Cramer, 1987; Green, 1983; Kreisler, 1992; Meurs & Jullian, 2003; Stern, 1985; Vliegen, 2003).

To conclude our discussion of the anaclitic dimension, we should say that this object-relational dimension is also present in the later developmental phases, for example, in the fact that moral fear and guilt are not infrequently described in terms of fear of loss of the object, fear of loss of approval or love of the object, or fear of loss of approval by the internalized voice of the parental figures. In this sense – in the midst of moral reactions in the later pre-Oedipal and Oedipal phase – relational concerns and fears can occupy center stage.

The term "introjective" is used much more for the later moments in early childhood development because moral development or even the perception of the gap between ideal and reality requires some complexity in the structure of personality. Previously in this paper we have already extensively discussed authors who concentrated on this developmental line (see also Chapter 3 and 5, this volume).

A preferred angle of approach in describing this developmental line is the role of aggression in attachment and in love: the role of ambivalence in the emergence of introjective depression. As we have seen, two generations of ambivalence conflicts are described by Parens (1979): on the one hand, the ambivalence which is a normal part of a complex self-image (with positive and negative aspects), to which one can react with depressive moods; on the other hand, the ambivalence which is a normal part of love and hate toward both parents in the Oedipal constellation at a time when the child is more able to be aware of affective contradiction and the moral conflict in it, and also able to feel guilt more fully. By distinguishing these moments in moral development, specific developmental anchor points of introjective problems are suggested. The earliest revert to developmental phases that are often described as being relational in nature. In this way, the connection between relational-anaclitic and introjective-normative developmental lines is made clear.[5]

"Closed Doors and Landscapes in the Mist": Clinical Illustration of a Relational
Depression with Introjective Elements in a Grade-School Boy

In a short clinical vignette we will illustrate the way introjective and relational depressive themes are intertwined. Three fragments are extracted from a long-term

---

[5] Blatt clearly suggests that introjective depression (situated at the higher neurotic level) is associated with manifest ambivalence, this in contrast to the obsessional neurotic, in which aggression is clearly repressed/displaced. This perhaps suggests still another level of dealing with aggression, which is perhaps also more closely associated with narcissistic personality, the obsessional neurosis occupying a position between neurotic illness and preneurotic disturbances, thereby requiring a more extreme form of repression and isolation of aggression and ambivalence. At the same time, for constitutional or other reasons, in obsessional neurosis the aggression can be more pronounced; therefore a more extreme defense against aggression and some clear manifestations of strong ambivalence can be present simultaneously.

psychoanalytic child psychotherapy with a latency boy. These and other elements of this therapy have been published previously (see Meurs & Cluckers, 1999). In this chapter, we have chosen fragments from the therapy report that enable us to illustrate that a child seems to have a "preference" for one kind of depression but that the other depressive aspect comes into play after a while, leading to the situation that both depressive themes – relational and introjective – get connected in the clinical material.

Jan, a 9-year-old boy, was admitted to the paediatric wing of a local children's hospital with persistent stomach pain and nausea. An extensive somatic examination could find no adequate explanation for the symptoms, so Jan and his parents were referred to the child psychotherapist at the hospital. His father and stepmother admitted from the outset that things had been difficult at home with Jan for some time. Jan alternated between a high level of cooperation and sudden, violent aggression. At other times, the aggression assumed more covert forms. Jan agreed to everything, but just did not do what his stepmother asked him to do.

Jan's mother had a long history of depressive illness. After Jan's birth, however, she seemed to be improving; she was very excited about her boy. When Jan was one year old, however, she seemed to lose interest, a change that became very clear when Jan was a very active child in his rapprochement crisis. When Jan was 2 years old, his mother was admitted for long-term psychiatric care, due to depression that had become more severe. She had also had several psychotic episodes in the meantime. After a while, the mother broke off all contact with the family, and Jan had not seen her since he was 4 years old. At that point, Jan's mother was well aware of her mental problems; she even insisted that "when she goes too far", her husband should live his own life. Eventually, his father decided to go it alone. They were divorced when Jan was nearly 5 years old, and Jan continued to live with his father. The mother accepted the divorce but asked for a legal agreement about the possibility to have contact with Jan, especially when the boy would request it. She herself tended to withdraw from her family; on one occasion, when we spoke to her at the end of treatment, she said that in that period she was convinced that she would cause harm to her child by being with him in a such painful, depressive state.

When Jan was six years old, his father met his new partner and, when Jan was nearly 8, his father and his new partner moved in together. About a year later, Jan's mother unexpectedly renewed contact and asked to be able to visit Jan fairly regularly. This possibility had been left open at the time of divorce, but his mother had never taken it up. The occurrence of Jan's stomach complaints roughly coincided with his mother's request to re-establish contact.

Jan was diagnosed as suffering from childhood depression. He had serious doubts about himself and was never sure that he was doing well enough in contacts and tasks. Whenever he did something he thought of as being wrong, he wanted to make amends, yet at the same time feared it was never good enough. His father said that Jan frequently lost himself in contact with another: he would give everything away, just to be sure that the other would not lose interest in him.

The diagnostic examination took place while Jan was hospitalized for two weeks. After release, father and stepmother agreed to weekly child psychotherapy and parental guidance once every month. When Jan started visiting his mother, we also invited her to a parental guidance session. We spoke to her altogether three times over a period of eighteen months. Jan's psychotherapy lasted for two years.

At first, Jan was quite withdrawn in the play room. He played by himself, but whenever the therapist asked something about his play, Jan answered with an elaborate story. The therapist soon felt that the therapeutic alliance had been established; Jan seemed to be a very sensitive boy. In Session 8 Jan produced a drawing – "The landscape in the mist" - that was important for several reasons:

"There is a misty, gray landscape with all sorts of shapes and silhouettes. These figures (with no face) are lost in a wood and can no longer find one another. When the therapist asked what struck Jan most about his drawing, he said, 'They have no faces, they do not know if they can see or hear anything, a signal or something'".

The drawing evoked a certain vagueness that can occur in affective communication with a depressed person: Jan saw people as vague silhouettes without the sensory means to address one another affectively. People are no longer able to find one another; they even don't have the means to locate one another, to reach out to one another. Not being able to see, to reach out or to communicate: this is an expression of Jan's relational depression in the period when his mother had vanished after having had at first a meaningful and intense relationship; up till now he could not re-establish contact with her. The same anxieties seemed to play a role in the therapy room: after the first sessions, Jan became fearful about losing contact with his therapist. He was desperate about how to continue contact once it had been established. In the next sessions, he wanders around in the play room, not knowing what to do, repeating several times his question if he would be allowed to return to his therapist the next week. For one reason or another, he fears losing contact without having any control in this process. Grey colors in everything he draws accentuate this depressive impression. It is the contact dimension – the relational theme – that is at stake: joining the other, touching the other, approaching the other, keeping in touch.

In Session 20, after a period of despair for Jan – his first contact with his mother had been planned but also delayed; in the therapy room he was very difficult to reach – the therapist decided to intervene in the following way:

Th.: 'Jan, you have already led me to understand that people who want to be in contact with one another sometimes find it difficult. For some time now, I have felt that you were happy to come here. But you also have your doubts about how things will be between us from now on.'

Jan then produced another drawing: 'A house in the distance'. A child wants to visit the house. The inhabitants have left. The door is closed. The child wanted to go inside. Suddenly, Jan corrected this and said that the boy would certainly not try to go inside but would sit and wait at the door until somebody comes home. Nobody knew if and when they would return.

Th.: 'The boy knows that he wants to find someone there, but he feels that he is never certain whether and when somebody will be there for him.'

Jan nods in agreement. 'In any case, he will wait, then they cannot forget him when they come home.'

Th.: 'The boy thinks the only thing he can do is wait. He has the impression that everything else depends on the others. In any case, he makes sure that the others cannot get past him because he is waiting at the door.'

Jan: 'It might take a long time. They will probably not like him lying against the house. They would probably not let him in. The boy does not know how to do any good. Then he falls asleep.'

After having described a world where people can fade away (the relational depressive theme), Jan moves closer now to his own desire to make contact ("going to a house" and "wanting to go inside"). But this first longing for contact is connected with a sense of doing wrong. Jan's sudden correction could be understood as a defensive act (a kind of reaction formation or undoing), afterwards verbalized by saying "the boy does not know how to do any good". Anyhow, the door is closed: the residents have gone or they do not let the boy in. In reaction to this, the boy has a sense of acting in the wrong way and of being left behind. A first introjective (self-critical) theme comes into play: Is it my fault? Is the loss caused by my actions?

This combination of longing for relationships and fearing to drive away the longed-for other, now became much more important. In Session 41 Jan plays on "closed doors".

He pretends to be a boy waiting for a message from a distant world where the "earth mothers" live, deep underground. The boy sends various sound signals to this unknown world. This distant world and the world of the ordinary people in which the boy lives are separated by a wall. The world of the "earth mothers" is populated by motherly old women.

The sounds coming back from the world of the "earth mothers" come too quickly or become merged and confused in the very small opening in the wall through which the messages and sounds have to pass to reach the boy. This makes the message incomprehensible. Somewhere, there is a magic key that opens the closed door in the wall between the two worlds just enough to make the sounds and signals from the "earth mothers" comprehensible. The boy has the key. However, once he receives a signal from the "earth mothers", he cannot wait. He sets to work too quickly, so that the messages again become incomprehensible. The boy briefly notices an old man who knows how to use the key to understand the message better. But the boy wants to use the key to leave the wall behind and to go into or even merge with the world of the "earth mothers" as quickly as possible. The boy hesitates a little regarding the old man, but the man is eventually rejected with the words, "Do not take my key now".

Jan's desire for contact with a distant and sometimes incomprehensible mother becomes very clear now. After a period of being quite uncertain as to whether he was allowed to undertake any action to establish contact, he is now very much in contact with his relational desires. He is even very active at it, still in search of a good balance between activity and passivity. The symbolic play material of this session has an enormous complexity: the relational maternal theme – with a desire for merger – is connected to a paternal theme, with some fears of exclusion and/or castration. Fears of being overwhelmed by a "third" figure (the old man), of being unable to attune to messages from the earth world (the other world of the mothers) and of having been denied by the father figure the means (the key) to re-establish contact with the mother world, are different layers of this material. Specially with this last element, Jan moves closer to an introjective depressive fear: the boy can be punished for doing the wrong thing by acting upon his wish for contact (the punishment or exclusion is expressed in the following play themes: not being allowed to enter the house in Session 20, or, by being "castrated" for his desires and activities in Session 41).

The background still is Jan's fear of not getting connected (the relational depressive theme), but once he is in touch with his wish for contact, these relational themes and the associated activities become associated with introjective depressive themes ("due to what I am undertaking, I will lose contact or not be allowed to have contact or be punished"; "due to my activity, I will be judged as being wrong"). From now on, interpretations can focus on this complex weave of both core themes in depression: fears of relational loss, associated with one's activity (in the light of motivations, drives, desires, wishes) that is criticized by the superego.

Future Challenge: Formulating Complex Developmental Pathways and Reintegrating Psychoanalysis Into Mainstream Developmental Psychopathology

The widespread single-track model in psychoanalytic developmental psychopathology suggests that neurotic psychopathology can be regarded exclusively as a remnant of Oedipal concerns and conflicts (between the ages of 3 and 6). Personality disorders are then a remnant of deficient personality structuring in the second and third years of life, while psychoses are thought to go back to very earliest childhood:

"There is a tacit assumption of an isomorphism between pathology and development, which permits bi-directional causal inference between childhood and pathology. The assumption covers all psychopathology and all stages of development. (…) There is a single model for borderline personality disorder, narcissistic pathology, neurotic disorders, etc. Empirical studies, on the whole, are at odds with these accounts. (…) Developmental psychopathology research has demonstrated that developmental continuity is an empirically elusive and conceptually complex problem, and cannot be simply assumed, as psycho-analysts are wont to do" (Fonagy & Target, 2003, p. 5-10).

While the map of the first three years of life gradually has been drawn in much detail, the possibilities for clarifying the developmental origin of psychopatho-logical disorders increased. This provided enormous opportunities (better under-standing of pathological functioning based on some comparison with early develop-ment, detection of early risk factors in development) as well as disadvantages (reducing psychopathology to this early phase or deterministically thinking that difficult developmental phases would always lead to a certain type of pathology).

Among the advantages of psychoanalytic developmental psychopathology one could point to the thoughtful way of connecting psychopathological syndromes with crucial developmental phases. This has led to an enormous body of knowledge on the socio-emotional psychodynamics of the different developmental steps and complexes of childhood. These are understood and reconstructed from within the conflicts that are considered as reminiscences, later on in life, of these early childhood dynamics and complexes; at other moments, psychoanalysis hinted at domains that could be the object of childhood observation studies. Without psycho-analysis, Cicchetti & Cohen (1995) admit, these important normal developments (for example, the Oedipus complex, the separation-individuation process, the narcissistic and object-oriented phases, etc.) would not have been documented the way they are today. In these crucial processes the origins are found for vulnerabilit-ies that later in life lead to psychopathology: in these crucial childhood psycho-dynamics the crystal (personality) (Freud, 1932) receives its structure, with its strong aspects and with certain hidden ruptures. When later in life a stressor directly acts upon the hidden vulnerability, the crystal can break.

Another advantage is that in psychoanalysis a lot of knowledge is acquired about the pre-school phase; in mainstream developmental psychopathology this period of precursors of disturbances is the least well documented phase. Not surprisingly, in autism research, for example, psychoanalysis has a lot to say about the risks and vulnerabilities of this syndrome; in the same way psychoanalysis emphasizes the importance of problems with object constancy in children or adults with borderline characteristics and anti-social behavior or of problems with affect constancy in children with emotional disturbances or depression. Even in what we have been indicating as a low profile period for psychoanalytic developmental psychopath-ology (1975-1990), the developmental perspective within psychoanalysis became more important. Recently, under the influence of a wider acceptance of quantitative methodology in psychoanalysis and motivated by the success of mainstream developmental psychopathology, the developmental and the clinical model in psychoanalysis were brought in much stronger interaction again (Shapiro & Emde, 1995). This, in turn, has led to a revival of the developmental psychopathology project within psychoanalysis; in this revival a more complex model of developmental continuity is presented.[6]

We are in need of that complex model, since there are disadvantages to the psychoanalytic developmental model as it has been described above. The broader flow of developmental psychopathology represents a huge challenge to the dominant developmental model in psychoanalysis. The interaction of influences from various developmental phases is a complex matter. The same vulnerability in a certain developmental phase can produce widely varying forms of developmental trajectories (multifinality), while the same outcome can be achieved from widely varying lines of development (equifinality) (Von Bertalanffy, 1968; Cicchetti & Cohen, 1995; Cicchetti & Rogosch, 1996). These aspects are definitely exerting an influence on psychoanalysis, as is evident from the amount of research into pathways along which the internal representations of early experiences with care figures have an impact on the formation of subsequent relationships later in life (Emde, 1988; Fivaz-Depeursinge, 2004).

However, although authors like Shapiro and Emde (1991) have been working out this complexity in their developmental theories, we still regard this as a further challenge for future psychoanalytic developmental psychopathology. For the time being, insufficient clarity exists in psychoanalysis about the respective influences in the emergence of psychopathology of the three developmental moments in early childhood (distal antecedents) or of early childhood and subsequent school-age and adolescent development or adulthood (proximal antecedents) (Blatt, 2004). This complexity is recognized on a theoretical level, but has been seriously under-researched; we are still starting to work out a "complex-enough" developmental perspective on psychopathology that will exert a decisive influence on our clinical practice.

Mainstream developmental psychopathology teaches us that normal and pathological developmental lines emerge through a series of associated factors and mechanisms throughout all the phases of child development and life-span. Moreover, a more complex picture also allows us to predict that various clinical pictures will also have many shared aspects (for example, anaclitic or introjective features in depression and other psychopathological syndromes), while similar clinical pictures also have striking differences (for example, not all anaclitic or introjective psychopathology is equal).

If we regard these questions as future challenges for psychoanalysis, the specificity of its theories will increase. Crucial questions include, "What are examples of earlier and later developmental factors which contribute to

---

[6] American psychoanalysis, influenced by Hartmann's original empirical project, has probably been leading in this effort: it has always been closer to developmental psychology, the search for evidential basis for its theories and the reflection on complex developmental mechanisms such as differentiation, integration, continuity and transformation (see Shapiro & Emde, 1991) than most of European psychoanalytic thought.

depression?", "What is earlier and later anaclitic/introjective vulnerability and resilience?".

The challenge consists of sufficiently complicating the psychodynamic developmental perspective so that, within the broader flow of developmental psychopathology, it has its place. Psychoanalysis has always had a developmental perspective. Since a developmental perspective is not obvious in (child) psychiatry or clinical (child) psychology[7], or may even be lacking there, psychoanalysis has a huge advantage in this respect. After all, even in the broader flow of developmental psychopathology, a tendency remains to include "age" as an "empty variable" in research or to look at "development" as the evolution of incidence of psychopathology at different ages ("developmental epidemiology") or to limit it to cognitive micro processes (the development or the process of a pathological, depressive thought or of cognitive information processing). In response to these limitations, psychoanalysis possesses certain advantages: no other school of thought emphasizes to such an extent that developmental phases are well-rounded elements from a content point of view, with their own distinct processes, specific psychodynamics and conflicts. However, in order not to be drowned out in the broad field of psychiatry and psychology, the psychoanalytic researcher must also allow himself to draw inspiration from developmental psychopathology.

For depression research, this means that earliest development does not determine subsequent development; pathological functioning is not the same as early childhood functioning. The final clinical picture is the result of a pathway through many developmental phases and influenced by complex interactions of psychological, biological and contextual factors. Early developmental achievements are integrated in further developmental steps and phases; they support later developmental achievement, but do not guarantee them. Early developmental stressors reduce the probability of further adaptive development, but they do not rule it out altogether. This probabilistic, rather then deterministic, developmental reasoning shows that the ultimate outcome is the result of many developmental lines and several crucial influences at different moments on these developmental lines. Research should make this complexity easier to grasp; investigating the crucial determinants of adaptive and maladaptive development as well as their relative predictive power over the outcome (adaptive or maladaptive development) requires a complex model and well chosen statistical analyses within a quantitative methodological approach.

Clinically oriented psychoanalysts and their "developmental research-minded" colleagues will also be able to interact better: what Freud described as "deferred action" is after all a clinical way of thinking about how a certain outcome, whether pathological or not, comes about through a complex developmental pathway in which earlier "dynamic" impressions and experiences are continuing to work in

---

[7] "The impact of development on clinical dysfunction and how this information can be integrated into treatment may have important implications for conclusions about the effectiveness of treatment. Outcome research rarely considers features of development that may affect treatment. (…) Chronological age represents an empirical beginning. However, age, as a construct for research, is only seldom identified in specific processes (…) (e.g. attachment; moral, cognitive and socio-emotional development, etc.)" (Kazdin, 2004, p. 12)

later ones, attracted there by new similar experiences, reworked in the present and/or influencing the significance of present experience. The clinical concept of "deferred action" is much closer to a model of complex developmental pathways than to single track developmental models, as is illustrated by the following quote from three leading authors in the field of developmental psychopathology:

"It is also an error to assume that pathways between early and later development are relatively simple and straightforward (e.g., early depression predicts later depression). In fact, the way an individual responds to events is a function of past history or experience, as well as current experience. (…) Moreover, during development, an individual may move back and forth between pathways of adjustment and maladjustment, or show different constellations of problems at different ages. The assumptions of a pathway model provide a launching point for considering fundamental issues of continuity and discontinuity, (…) and the need to consider the stage or period of development" (Cummings, Davies, & Campbell, 2000, p. 18).

The expression of depression changes in childhood (see also Chapter 6, this volume). Early depression can lead to many different outcomes (from normal development to serious psychopathology), while late depression can arise at various times, both from previous normal development and psychopathology.

Conclusions

Certainly, there is work at hand for psychoanalytic developmental psychopathology. This observation, however, should not be a cause for pessimism. The blueprint we described contains a rich clinical realm and a sound developmental perspective. Usually, the two are not found together. However, in order to grow, psychoanalysis must be able to see over the wall of the psychoanalytic model and to answer questions posed from interaction with the broader flow of developmental psychopathology. Its integration, together with the use of various research methods, offers psychoanalysis new opportunities as well as the hope of a stronger position in interaction with other models.

In the meantime, we have reached the point where we have filled in important gaps in the relational-anaclitic and structural-introjective developmental lines of depression. Emde and colleagues (e.g., Emde, Polak, & Spitz, 1965; Emde, Johnson, & Easterbrooks, 1988) and Blatt (2004) – among others – are important authors presenting major models in psychoanalysis concerning depression, integrating drive, ego, object relational and self psychologies in a developmental perspective.

With the formulation of the separate anaclitic dimension of depression and the observation that pre-Oedipal and Oedipal elements as well as childhood and later developmental stages are important in both dimensions – the anaclitic and the introjective – the question of continuity and discontinuity throughout the entire course of development is clearly posed. Biological, psychological and contextual factors are sought which play a role in these different phases. At this level, progress is expected in the near future, both from carefully chosen case studies and from empirical research.

References

Abraham, K. (1953a). Contribution to the theory of the anal character. In K. Abraham (Ed.), *Selected papers on psychoanalysis* (pp. 370-392). New York: Basic Books. (Original work published 1921)

Abraham, K. (1953b). A short study of the development of the libido. In K. Abraham (Ed.), *Selected papers on psychoanalysis* (pp. 418-501). New York: Basic Books. (Original work published 1924)

Achenbach, T. (1974). *Developmental psychopathology.* New York: John Wiley & Sons.

Achenbach, T. (1991). *Manual for the Child Behavior Checklist/4-18 and 1991 Profile.* Burlington: University of Vermont, Department of Psychiatry Publications.

Alvarez, A. (1992). *Live company.* London: Karnac Books.

Antonovsky, A. M. (1991). Idealization and the holding of ideals. *Contemporary Psychoanalysis, 27,* 389-404.

Assoun, P.-L. (1981). L'archaïque chez Freud [The concept of 'the archaic' in Freud's work]. *Nouvelle Revue de Psychanalyse française, 26,* 11-44.

Barron, J. M., Eagle, M. N., & Wolitsky, D. L. (1992). *The interface of psychoanalysis and psychology.* Washington, DC: American Psychological Association.

Bibring, E. (1953). The mechanism of depression. In P. Greenacre (Ed.), *Affective disorders. Psychoanalytic contribution to their study* (pp. 13-48). New York: International Universities Press.

Bion, A. (1962). *Learning from experience.* London: Heinemann.

Blatt, S. J. (1974). Levels of object representation in anaclitic and introjective depression. *The Psychoanalytic Study of the Child, 29,* 107-157.

Blatt, S. J. (1995). Representational structures in psychopathology. In D. Cicchetti & S. L. Toth (Eds.), *Emotion, cognition, and representation (Rochester symposium on developmental psychopathology (*Vol. 6, pp. 1-33). New York: University of Rochester Press.

Blatt, S. J. (1998). Contributions of psychoanalysis to the understanding and treatment of depression. *Journal of the American Psychoanalytical Association, 46,* 722-752.

Blatt, S. J. (2004). *Experiences of depression. Theoretical, clinical, and research perspectives.* Washington, DC: American Psychological Association.

Blatt, S. J., D'Afflitti, J. P., & Quinlan, D. M. (1976). Experiences of depression in normal young adults. *Journal of Abnormal Psychology, 85,* 383-389.

Blatt, S. J., & Homann, E. (1992). Parent-child interaction in the etiology of dependent and self-critical depression. *Clinical Psychology Review, 12,* 47-91.

Blatt, S. J., & Shichman, S. (1983). Two primary configurations of psychopathology. *Psychoanalysis and Comtemporary Thought, 6,* 187-254.

Blatt, S. J., & Zuroff, D. C. (1992). Interpersonal relatedness and self-definition: Two prototypes for depression. *Clinical Psychology Review, 12,* 527-562.

Bowlby, J. (1981). *Attachment and Loss.* London: Hogarth Press.

Bravo, I. (2001). The impact of early loss on depression: Dynamic origins and empirical findings. In J. R.

Brandell (Ed.), *Psychoanalytic approaches to the treatment of children and adolescents* (pp. 47-69). New York: The Haworth Press.

Burlingham, D., & Freud, A. (1944). *Infants without families. The case for and against residential nurses.* London: George Allen & Unwin Ltd.

Cicchetti, D. (1984). The emergence of developmental psychopathology. *Child Development, 55,* 1-7.

Cicchetti, D. (1989). Developmental psychopathology: Some thoughts on its evolution. *Development and Psychopathology, 1,* 1-4.

Cicchetti, D., & Cohen, D.J. (1995). *Developmental psychopathology. Vol. I: Theory and methods.* New York: John Wiley & Sons.

Cicchetti, D., & Rogosch, F. A. (1996). Equifinality and multifinality in developmental psychopathology. *Development and Psychopathology, 8,* 597-600.

Cicchetti, D., & Toth, S. L. (1992). *Developmental perspectives on depression.* Rochester: University of Rochester Press.

Cramer, B. (1987). Objective and subjective aspects of parent-infant relations: An attempt at correlation between infant studies and clinical work. In J. Osofsky (Ed.), *Handbook of infant development* (pp. 1037-1057). New York: John Wiley & Sons.

Cummings, E. M., Davies, P. T., & Campbell, S. B. (2000). *Developmental psychopathology and family process. Theory, research, and clinical implications.* New York: Guilford Press.

Dietrich, D. R., & Shabad, P. C. (1989). *The problem of loss and mourning. Psychoanalytic perspectives.* Madison, CT: International Universities Press.

Emde, R. N. (1981). Changing models of infancy and the nature of early development: Remodelling the foundation. *Journal of the American Psychoanalytic Association, 29,* 179-219.

Emde, R. N. (1988). Development terminable and interminable. II: Recent psychoanalytic theory and therapeutic considerations. *International Journal of Psychoanalysis, 69,* 283-286.

Emde, R. N. (1999). Moving ahead: Integrating influences of affective processes for development and psychopathology. *International Journal of Psychoanalysis, 80,* 317-339.

Emde, R. N., Johnson, W. F., & Easterbrooks, M. A. (1988). The do's and don'ts of early moral development: Psychoanalytic tradition and current research. In J. Kagan & S. Lamb (Eds.), *The emergence of morality* (pp. 245-277). Chicago: University of Chicago Press.

Emde, R. N., Polak, P. R., & Spitz, R. A. (1965). Anaclitic depression in an infant raised in an institution. *Journal of the American Academy of Child Psychiatry, 4,* 545-553.

Fairbairn, R. (1952a). A revised psychopathology of the psychoses and psychoneurosis. In R. Fairbairn, *Psychoanalytic studies of personality* (pp. 28-38). London: Tavistock. (Original work published 1941)

Fairbairn, R. (1952b). Endopsychic structure considered in terms of object relationships. In R. Fairbairn, *Psychoanalytic studies of personality* (pp. 82-136). London: Tavistock. (Original work published 1944)

Fivaz-Depeursinge, E. (in press). *Attachment et intersubjectivité* [Attachment and intersubjectivity]. Lausanne: Unil.

Fonagy, P. (1995a). Psychoanalytic perspectives on developmental psychopathology. In D. Cicchetti & D. J. Cohen (Eds.), *Developmental psychopathology* (pp. 290-306). New York: John Wiley & Sons.

Fonagy, P. (1995b). Psychoanalytic and empirical approaches to developmental psychopathology: An object-relations perspective. In T. Shapiro & R. N. Emde (Eds.), *Research in psychoanalysis: Processes, development, outcome* (pp. 245-260). Madison, CT: International Universities Press.

Fonagy, P., & Target, M. (1997). Psychodynamic developmental theory for children: A contemporary application of child psychoanalysis. In E. D. Hibbs & P. S. Jensen (Eds.), *Psychosocial treatment research with children and adolescents* (pp. 53-77). Washington, DC: National Institute of Health and the American Psychological Association.

Fonagy, P., & Target, M. (2003). *Psychoanalytic theories: Perspectives from developmental psychopathology.* London/Philadelphia: Whurr Publications.

Freud, A. (1963). The concept of developmental lines. *The Psychoanalytic Study of the Child, 18,* 245-265.

Freud, A. (1966). Normality and pathology in childhood: Assessment of development. *The writings of Anna Freud* (Vol. 6, pp. 1-186). Harmondsworth: Penguin Books.

Freud, A. (1974). A psychoanalytic view of developmental psychopathology. *The writings of Anna Freud* (Vol. 8, pp. 57-74). Harmondsworth: Penguin Books.

Freud, A. (1981). The concept of developmental lines: Their diagnostic significance. *The Psychoanalytic Study of the Child, 36,* 129-136.

Freud, S. (1900). The interpretation of dreams. In J. Strachey (Ed. and Trans.), *The standard edition of the complete psychological works of Sigmund Freud* (Vol. 4 and 5, pp. 1-715). London: Hogarth Press.

Freud, S. (1905). Fragment of an analysis of a case of hysteria. In J. Strachey (Ed. and Trans.), *The standard edition of the complete psychological works of Sigmund Freud* (Vol. 7, pp. 7-122). London: Hogarth Press.

Freud, S. (1909a). Analysis of a phobia of a five-year-old boy. In J. Strachey (Ed. and Trans.), *The standard edition of the complete psychological works of Sigmund Freud* (Vol. 10, pp. 1-147). London: Hogarth Press.

Freud, S. (1909b). Notes upon a case of obsessional neurosis. In J. Strachey (Ed. and Trans.), *The standard edition of the complete psychological works of Sigmund Freud* (Vol. 10, pp. 153-320). London: Hogarth Press.

Freud, S. (1911). Psycho-analytic notes upon an autobiographical account of a case of paranoia (Dementia Paranoides). In J. Strachey (Ed. and Trans.), *The standard edition of the complete psychological works of Sigmund Freud* (Vol. 12, pp. 3-82). London: Hogarth Press.

Freud, S. (1917a). Mourning and melancholia. In J. Strachey (Ed. and Trans.), *The standard edition of the complete psychological works of Sigmund Freud* (Vol. 14, pp. 237-258). London: Hogarth Press.

Freud, S. (1917b). Introductory lectures on psycho-analysis. In J. Strachey (Ed. and Trans.), *The standard edition of the complete psychological works of Sigmund Freud* (Vol. 15, 16, 17). London: Hogarth Press.

Freud, S. (1920a). Beyond the pleasure principle. In J. Strachey (Ed. and Trans.), *The standard edition of the complete psychological works of Sigmund Freud* (Vol. 18, pp. 1-64). London: Hogarth Press.

Freud, S. (1922). Some neurotic mechanisms in jealousy, paranoia and homosexuality. In J. Strachey (Ed. and Trans.), *The standard edition of the complete psychological works of Sigmund Freud* (Vol. 18, pp. 225-230). London: Hogarth Press.

Freud, S. (1923). The ego and the id. In J. Strachey (Ed. and Trans.), *The standard edition of the complete psychological works of Sigmund Freud* (Vol. 19, pp. 1-59). London: Hogarth Press.

Freud, S. (1931). Female sexuality. In J. Strachey (Ed. and Trans.), *The standard edition of the complete psychological works of Sigmund Freud* (Vol. 21, pp. 221-246). London: Hogarth Press.

Freud, S. (1932). New introductory lectures on psychoanalysis. In J. Strachey (Ed. and Trans.), *The standard edition of the complete psychological works of Sigmund Freud* (Vol. 22, pp. 1-182). London: Hogarth Press.

Furman, E. (1988). Mothers have to be there to be left. *The Psychoanalytic Study of the Child, 43,* 345-367.

Glazer, M. W. (1979). Object-related vs. narcissistic depression. A theoretical and clinical study. *The Psychoanalytic Review, 66,* 323-337.

Green, A. (1983). The dead mother. In A. Green (Ed.), *On private madness* (pp. 48-58). London: Karnac Books.

Hartmann, H. (1939). *Ego-psychology and the problem of adaptation.* New York: International Universities Press.

Hermann, I. (1936). Sich anklammern – Auf Suche gehen [Clinging and searching]. *Internationale Zeitschrift für Psychoanalyse, 22,* 45-58.

Jacobson, E. (1953). The affects and their pleasure/unpleasure qualities in relation to the psychic discharge processes. In R. M. Loewenstein (Ed.), *Drives, affects and behavior* (pp. 38-66). New York: International Universities Press.

Jacobson, E. (1964). *The self and the object world.* New York: International Universities Press.

Jacobson, E. (1971). *Depression. Comparative studies of neurotic and psychotic conditions.* New York: International Universities Press.

Kareem, J. (1992). Ideas and experience in intercultural therapy: The Nafsiyat Intercultural Therapy Centre. In J. Kareem & R. Littlewood (Eds.), *Intercultural therapy: Themes, interpretations and practice* (pp. 14-37). Oxford: Blackwell.

Kazdin, A. E. (2004). Psychotherapy for children and adolescents. In M. J. Lambert (Ed.), *Bergin and Garfield's handbook of psychotherapy and behavior change* (5th ed.) (pp. 540-597). New York: John Wiley & Sons.

Kernberg, O. (1984). *Object relations theory and clinical psychoanalysis.* New York: Jason Aronson.

Klein, M. (1928). Early stages of the Oedipus complex. In M. Klein (Ed.), *The writings of Melanie Klein (Volume I): Love, guilt and reparation and other works 1921-1945* (pp. 186-198). London: Hogarth Press.

Klein, M. (1935). A contribution to the psychogenesis of manic-depressive states. In M. Klein (Ed.), *The writings of Melanie Klein (Volume I): Love, guilt and reparation and other works 1921-1945* (pp. 262-

289). London: Hogarth Press.

Klein, M. (1940). Mourning and its relation to manic-depressive states. In M. Klein (Ed.), *The writings of Melanie Klein (Volume I): Love, guilt and reparation and other works 1921-1945* (pp. 344-369). London: Hogarth Press.

Klein, M. (1945). The Oedipus complex in the light of early anxieties. In M. Klein (Ed.), *The writings of Melanie Klein (Volume I): Love, guilt and reparation and other works 1921-1945* (pp. 370-419). London: Hogarth Press.

Kleinman, A., & Good, B. (1985). *Culture and depression.* Berkeley: University of California Press.

Kortmann, F. A. M. (1995). Psychopathologie, cultuur en omgeving [Psychopathology, culture, and environment]. *Tijdschrift voor Psychiatrie, 37,* 3-14.

Kreisler, R. (1992). *Le nouvel enfant du désordre psychosomatique* [The new infant with psychosomatic symptoms]. Toulouse: Privat.

Littlewood, R. (2003). *Pathologies of the West. An anthropology of mental illness in Northern America and Europe.* London: Continuum.

Mahler, M. (1972). On the first three sub-phases of the separation-individuation process. *International Journal of Psycho-Analysis, 55,* 333-338.

Mahler, M., Pine, F., & Bergman, A. (1975). *The psychological birth of the human infant. Symbiosis and individuation.* New York: Basic Books.

Markus, H. R., & Kitayama, S. (1991). Culture and the self: Implications for cognition, emotion, and motivation. *Psychological Review, 98,* 224-253.

Meurs, P., & Cluckers, G. (1999). Psychosomatic symptoms, embodiment and affect. Weaving threads to the affectively experienced body in therapy with a neurotic and a borderline child. *Journal of Child Psychotherapy, 25,* 71-91.

Meurs, P., & Jullian, G. (2003). Cultuur sensitieve ontwikkelingsbegeleiding. Preventief werken aan veerkracht in de vroege ouder-kind interactie bij allochtone gezinnen in een kansarme wijk van Brussel [Culture sensitive developmental guidance. Preventive intervention and promoting resilience in early parent-child interaction in immigrant families in a disadvantaged urban quarter of Brussels], *Medische Antropologie, 15,* 221-236.

Nagera, H. (1970). Children's reactions to the death of important objects: A developmental approach. *The Psychoanalytic Study of the Child, 25,* 360-400.

Nagera, H. (1981). *The developmental approach to childhood psychopathology.* New York: Jason Aronson.

Parens, A. (1979). *The development of aggression in early childhood.* New York: Jason Aronson.

Parens, A. (1991). A view of the development of hostility in early life. In T. Shapiro & R. N. Emde (Eds.), *Affect: Psychoanalytic perspectives* (pp. 75-108). Madison, CT: International Universities Press.

Ricoeur, P. (1971). *Discours, communicatibilité et écriture* [Discours, communication, and writing]. Nijmegen: s.n.

Shapiro, T., & Emde, R. N. (1991). Developmental perspectives: Introduction. In T. Shapiro & R. N. Emde (Eds.), *Affect: Psychoanalytic perspectives* (pp. 3-5). Madison, CT: International Universities Press.

Shapiro, T., & Emde, R. N. (1995). *Research in psychoanalysis: Process, development, and outcome.* Madison, CT: International Universities Press.

Spitz, R. (1945). Hospitalism: An inquiry into the genesis of psychiatric conditions in early childhood. *The Psychoanalytic Study of the Child, 1,* 53-73.

Spitz, R. (1946). Anaclitic depression: An inquiry into the genesis of psychiatric conditions in early childhood. *The Psychoanalytic Study of the Child, 2,* 313-342.

Spitz, R. (1957). *No and yes: On the genesis of human communication.* New York: International Universities Press.

Spitz, R., & Cobliner G. (1965). *The first year of life.* New York: International Universities Press.

Sroufe, L. A., & Rutter, M. (1984). The domain of developmental psychopathology. *Child development, 55,* 17-29.

Stern, D. (1985). *The interpersonal world of the infant. A view from psychoanalysis and developmental psychology.* London: Karnac Books.

Szondi, L. (1965). *Schicksalsanalyse: Wahl in Liebe, Freundschaft, Beruf, Krankheit und Tod* [Analysis of destiny. Choice in love relations, friendship, profession, illness and death]. Basel: Schwabe.

Tustin, F. (1987). The rhythm of safety. *Winnicott Series, 2.*

Vliegen, N. (2003). *Affectieve communicatie en depressie in de moeder-kind dyade aan het einde van het eerste halfjaar* [Affective communication and depression in the mother-child dyad at the end of the first semester]. Unpublished manuscript, Department of Psychology, University of Leuven, Belgium.

von Bertalanffy, L. (1968). *General systems theory*. New York: Braziller.

Winnicott, D. W. (1958). Primitive emotional development. In D. W. Winnicott (Ed.), *Collected papers: Through paediatrics to psychoanalysis* (pp. 262-277). New York: Basic Books. (Original work published 1945)

Winnicott, D. W. (1963). The development of the capacity for concern. In D. W. Winnicott (Ed.), *The maturational processes and the facilitating environment: Studies in the theory of emotional development* (pp. 73-82). New York: International Universities Press.

Winnicott, D. W. (1964). What about father? In D. W. Winnicott (Ed.), *The child, the family, and the outside world* (pp. 113-118). London: Penguin.

Winnicott, D. W. (1984). Aggression, guilt, and reparation. In C. Winnicott, R. Shepherd & M. Davis (Eds.), *Deprivation and delinquency* (pp. 136-144). London: Tavistock. (Original work published 1960)

Yankelovitch, D., & Barrett, W. (1970). *Ego and instinct: The psychoanalytic view of human nature – revised.* New York: Random House.

Zetzel, E. (1965). Depression and the incapacity to bear it. In M. Schur (Ed.), *Drives, affects and behavior* (Vol. 2, pp. 243-274). New York: International Universities Press.

Chapter 8

Corticotropin-Releasing Factor (CRF)

and Major Depression: Towards an Integration

of Psychology and Neurobiology in Depression Research

Stephan J. Claes and Charles B. Nemeroff

Major depressive disorder (MDD), as defined by the Diagnostic and Statistical Manual of Mental Disorders, 4th edition (DSM-IV; APA, 1994), is a very common disorder as evidenced by the results of two large epidemiological studies, in which more than 10% and 16.2% of the population respectively were found to experience at least 1 MDD episode during their lifetime (Blazer et al., 1994; Kessler et al., 2003). The prevalence is higher in women compared to men, with a ratio approaching 2 to 1. It is a chronic disorder, with a high tendency for relapse in those who have recovered from a depressive episode (Frank et al., 1990). MDD is characterized by a variety of symptoms from different categories. Emotional dysregulation (low mood, instable mood, irritability, anxiety, emotional apathy) and cognitive dysfunction (concentration, memory) are accompanied by severe disturbances in fundamental biological systems such as sleep, appetite regulation, sexual drive and autonomic regulation. The disorder is also associated with an increased risk for a number of somatic disorders, such as osteoporosis and several cardiovascular diseases. This results in markedly increased morbidity and mortality in individuals with major depression, even if factors like smoking, diet and alcohol intake are corrected for (Vaillant, 1998). The Baltimore portion of the national Epidemiological Catchment Area (ECA) study revealed that major depression subsequently leads to a four- to fivefold increase in the risk for myocardial infarction (Pratt et al., 1996).

Psychosocial risk factors for developing major depression have been studied extensively. Life stress has been found to be an important risk factor, as well as the personality structure of the person undergoing the stressful experiences (see also Chapter 4, this volume). For this purpose, stress can be subdivided into three categories: acute stress, chronic stress and early life stress.

Acute stress, more specifically life events with a connotation of loss or humiliation, has been posited to be depressogenic. Kendler et al. (1999) reported that individuals reporting a major stressful life event in the last month had a large increase in the risk for the onset of major depression (Odds Ratio 5.64). However, the impact of life events on depression vulnerability is highly dependent on other factors such as gender and neuroticism (Kendler et al., 2004). At least equally important in the etiology of major depression is chronic stress (Tennant, 2002). In mice, chronic mild stress produces a number of signs and neurobiological alterations similar to the pathophysiology of major depression in humans (Grippo et al., 2003). Finally, early life stress (ELS) has recently been demonstrated to play an important role. Early life stress is a broad concept, of which physical and sexual child abuse are undoubtedly the most extreme forms. Several studies have shown that individuals exposed to severe ELS are particularly sensitive to develop major depressive disorder as adults. A study on almost 2,000 women linked a history of childhood abuse to an increase in depressive symptoms and suicide attempts (McCauley et al., 1997). Childhood abuse has also been associated with earlier onset and a more chronic course of depression (Heim & Nemeroff, 2001).

The personality structure of the individual confronted with stress is important as well. For instance, many studies have shown that anxiety-related personality traits increase the risk to develop major depression (Kendler et al., 2004).

Biological Factors in Depression

Genetic factors play an important role in the pathogenesis of major depression. Family studies show a high familial aggregation of the disorder: first degree family members of a patient with major depression have a risk that is 1.5-2 times higher than the general population (Jones et al., 2002). Twin and adoption studies have shown that a substantial part of this increased familial risk is genetic. The heritability of the disorder (defined as the extent to which individual genetic differences contribute to individual differences in observed behavior) is estimated at 40-50% (Jones et al., 2002).

Since the inception of the modern era of biological research in psychiatry, many hypotheses have been generated regarding the patho-etiology of depression. There is compelling evidence for a significant role of at least three different physiological systems: the monoamine neural circuits (serotonin, norepinephrine and dopamine), the immune system and the hypothalamic-pituitary-adrenal (HPA) axis. In those three areas, specific abnormal patterns have been shown to accompany the clinical phenotype of major depression. Because monoamine neurotransmission, immunity and the HPA axis are functionally interrelated at multiple levels, all these findings might reasonably be considered as different sides of the same coin.

In the 1950s, two classes of antidepressants, monoamine oxidase inhibitors (MAOIs) and tricyclic antidepressants (TCAs), were discovered serendipitously. These compounds were subsequently found to enhance neurotransmission by serotonin, norepinephrine and/or dopamine. For this reason, much biological research has focused on a potential role of these three monoamines in the pathogenesis of major depression. It is not the aim of this chapter to comprehensively review the massive data emanating from these studies. A large number of biochemical, challenge, imaging and post-mortem studies have demonstrated an abnormally reduced function of central serotonergic systems in major depression (Charney et al., 1981; Lopez et al., 1998, Drevets et al., 1999). Findings implicating dysfunction of norepinephrine and dopamine in the pathogenesis of major depression are also available (Mendels & Franzer, 1974; Meyers et al., 1999; Ressler & Nemeroff, 1999).

A second important field of biological research in major depression concerns the immune system. There is evidence that major depression is characterized by specific alterations in a number of important immune parameters. More specifically, the disorder is associated with activation of several aspects of cellular immunity, specifically the hypersecretion of proinflammatory cytokines (Kronfol, 2002; Musselman et al., 2003).

Finally, the most scrutiny has been directed towards the role of the hypothalamic – pituitary – adrenal axis (HPA axis) in major depression, which is the main focus of this chapter. The HPA axis plays a pre-eminent role in the endocrine, autonomic, immunological and behavioral response to stress. Evidence from multiple sources indicates that HPA axis hyperactivity is a common neurobiological feature of MDD. There is considerable evidence that this HPA axis hyperactivity is caused by a hypersecretion of the pre-eminent hormone which controls the activity of the axis, which is corticotropin releasing factor (CRF). Therefore, we focus on the physiology and pathophysiology of CRF in relation to affective disorders.

First, we describe the physiology of the HPA axis and of CRF, in both its endocrine and extra-endocrine role. Subsequently, the evidence summarizing alterations in CRF secretion and HPA axis function in major depression and in other stress-related psychiatric disorders is reviewed. How does such dysregulation arise? We describe how genetic factors, chronic stress and early life stress can all lead to chronic CRF hypersecretion. Finally, directions for further research integrating psychology and neurobiology are discussed in the last part of this chapter. This research integrates biological and psychological theories of the pathogenesis of major depression.

Physiological Functions of CRF

Vale and colleagues (1981) first elucidated the structure of a hypothalamic hormone, corticotropin releasing factor (CRF), which controls the activity of the HPA axis. In mammals, however, CRF has multiple extra-endocrine functions, including orchestrating the behavioral, immune and autonomic responses to stress.

The primary role of hypothalamic CRF, as noted above, is to control the activity of the HPA axis. The HPA axis plays a pivotal role in the response of the organism to stress, broadly defined as any change in the environment threatening homeostasis. Within seconds after exposure to stress, there is enhanced release of CRF from the median eminence in the hypothalamus. Arginine vasopressin (AVP) is a peptide hormone that augments the effect of CRF on the HPA axis, and that is cosecreted with CRF from parvocellular hypothalamic cells. CRF and AVP are transported by the portal vascular system to the anterior pituitary, where they stimulate the secretion of adrenocorticotropin (ACTH) from pituitary corticotrophs (Vale et al., 1981), leading in humans to the secretion of cortisol from the adrenal cortex. The HPA axis is schematically represented in Figure 1.

As is the case of many biological systems, the HPA axis contains its own negative feedback system, which regulates its activity, particularly after acute activation. Cortisol acts as a negative feedback regulator at both the hypothalamus and pituitary, decreasing the secretion of CRF and ACTH respectively (Swanson & Simmons, 1989), and also exerts a negative feedback function on the HPA axis via the hippocampus (Herman et al., 1989). Cortisol acts at both mineralocorticoid receptors (MR) and glucocorticoid receptors (GR). These two receptors differ in their affinity for cortisol and in their distribution in the CNS. Under physiological cortisol concentrations, negative feedback occurs mainly through the sensitive MR's in the hippocampus. Under stress and high cortisol concentrations, negative feedback is mainly achieved through GR's in the hippocampus, hypothalamus and pituitary.

In response to stress, the secretion of CRF is increased not only in the hypothalamus, but in the central nucleus of the amygdala as well. The amygdala plays a seminal role in the emotional response to stress, including anxiety (Davidson, 2002). The results of several studies have suggested that hypothalamic CRF secretion is quite sensitive to physiological stress, whereas CRF secretion from the amygdala is more reactive to psychological stress (Makino et al., 1999). Indeed, considerable evidence indicates that the amygdala plays a paramount role in the autonomic, endocrine and behavioural responses to stress (Davis, 1992).

CRF is found not only in the hypothalamus and the amygdala, but in many other brain regions, including the cerebral cortex, several limbic areas, and brainstem

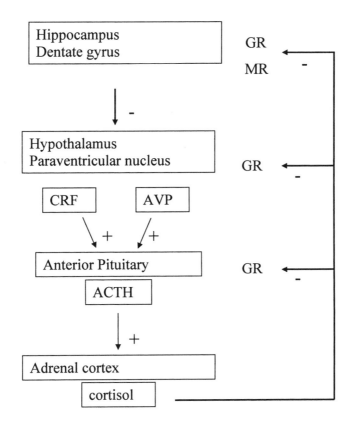

FIGURE 1.
Schematic representation of hypothalamus pituitary adrenal (HPA) axis function. Parvocellular neurons in the paraventricular nucleus of the hypothalamus cosecrete corticoptropin-releasing factor (CRF) and vasopressin (AVP), which stimulate the secretion of adrenocorticotrophin (ACTH) from the anterior pituitary into the blood. ACTH initiates the synthesis and secretion of cortisol from the adrenal cortex. Cortisol exerts a negative feedback control over the HPA axis. Under physiological cortisol concentrations, negative feedback occurs mainly through the sensitive mineralocorticoid receptors (MR) in the hippocampus. Under stress and high cortisol concentrations, negative feedback is mainly achieved through glucocorticoid receptors (GR) in the hippocampus, hypothalamus and pituitary.

nuclei, the latter responsible for autonomic function. A distinct population of CRF containing PVN hypothalamic neurons stimulates the locus coeruleus in the brainstem, leading to increased activity of noradrenergic neurons (Swanson et al., 1983) and of the sympathetic autonomous nervous system. CRF also acts as a neurotransmitter in the median and caudal dorsal raphe, suggesting a role in the regulation of serotonin systems (Austin et al., 2003). Finally, CRF is expressed in many peripheral tissues including the adrenal medulla, lymphocytes, pancreas, lung, liver, the gastrointestinal tract and skin (Orth, 1992).

The acute stress response, associated with a number of metabolic, neuro-endocrine and autonomic adaptations, is largely mediated by CRF. These adaptations include inhibition of sexual (Heinrichs et al., 1997) and ingestive behaviour (Heinrichs & Richard, 1999). It also inhibits growth hormone secretion (Raza et al., 1998) and the hypothalamic-pituitary-gonadal (HPG) axis (Nikolarakis et al., 1986). CRF-mediated secretion of cortisol from the adrenal cortex has numerous acute adaptive effects, while chronic HPA axis activation is associated with several adverse effects. Together with CRF, cortisol inhibits the growth hormone and reproductive axes. It also reduces the cellular immune system. Cortisol increases available energy by promoting gluconeogenesis, glycolysis and proteolysis, and augmenting insulin resistance. The activation of noradrenergic systems by CRF mediated activation of the locus coeruleus increases blood pressure, heart rate and blood sugar, and decreases gastro-intestinal bloodflow. All these adaptions allow the organism to react adequately to acute stressors and threats. This so-called "fight or flight reaction" has obvious and crucial importance in allowing the individual organism to respond adequately to acute threats, increasing chances of survival.

CRF in Depressive Disorders

Major depressive disorder. Beginning in the late 1960s, numerous studies reported cortisol hypersecretion in major depressive disorder (MDD), documented by elevated plasma corticosteroid concentration (Carpenter & Bunney, 1971), increased levels of cortisol metabolites (Sachar et al., 1970) and elevated 24-hour urinary free cortisol concentrations (McClure 1966; Carroll et al., 1976). In contrast to Cushing's disease, hypercortisolism may not occur every day in depressed patients. For example, urinary free cortisol excretion may be elevated for 21 days out of the month in depressed patients compared with 4–5 days out of the month for control subjects (Gold et al., 2002). Hypercortisolemia in MDD is considered to be a state marker, and not a trait marker, because it tends to normalize in most patients after clinical improvement. Postmortem studies revealed enlarged pituitary and adrenal glands in depressed patients, consistent with chronic HPA axis hyperactivity (Nemeroff et al., 1992).

Chronically elevated glucocorticoid levels have been shown to be associated with loss of neurons in the hippocampus of mammals including rats and monkeys (Sapolsky, 1990). Some investigations have found a decrease of hippocampal volume in MDD patients (Bremner et al., 2000), while others have not (Vakili et al., 2000). Posener et al. (2003), using high-resolution magnetic resonance imaging (MRI), obtained brain scans from 27 patients with MDD and 42 healthy comparison subjects. They found that MDD patients might have structural abnormalities of the hippocampus that can be detected by analysis of hippocampal shape but not volume, which might partly explain the conflicting earlier findings. Moreover, although hippocampal function seems to be disturbed after the first depression, hippocampal volume probably only decreases after multiple depressive episodes (McQueen et al., 2003). Finally, hippocampal volume reduction has been reported to be restricted to the specific subgroup of MDD patients with a history of early life trauma (Vythilingam et al., 2002).

The increased cortisol secretion in MDD has been associated with central CRF hypersecretion. Several studies reported elevated CRF concentrations in cerebrospinal fluid (CSF) of untreated MDD patients (Nemeroff et al., 1984; Banki et al., 1987; Risch et al., 1992). Indeed, Raadsheer et al. (1995) observed that CRF mRNA expression and CRF concentration in the PVN of depressed patients is markedly higher than those of comparison subjects. When the concentration of CRF is increased in the brain, downregulation of CRF receptors is to be expected. Nemeroff et al. (1988) found a marked (23%) reduction in the density of CRF receptor binding sites in the frontal cortex of suicide victims compared with controls, and these findings were recently confirmed (Merali et al., 2004). Another recent study found a shift in the ratio of the two known types of CRF receptors (CRF-R1/R2) in the pituitaries of suicide victims (Hiroi et al., 2001).

The hypersecretion of CRF clearly is not limited to the HPA axis, but is also present in other brain regions where CRF acts as a neurotransmitter. In a recent study, Austin et al. (2003) studied post-mortem brain material from 11 male suicide patients and 11 matched controls. They found that the level of CRF was increased by 30% in the locus coeruleus, 39% in the median raphe and 45% in the caudal dorsal raphe in depressed suicide subjects compared to controls. No difference in CRF was found in the dorsal tegmentum or medial parabrachial nucleus between the subject groups. These findings indicate that CRF availability is specifically increased in norepinephrine- and serotonin-containing pontine nuclei of depressed suicide men, and this is consistent with the hypothesis that CRF neurotransmission is elevated in extra-hypothalamic brain regions of depressed subjects. The specific involvement of the locus coeruleus and the raphe nuclei in this study provides a direct link between CRF hypersecretion and disturbances in the monoamine (noradrenaline and serotonin) systems which have long been posited to be integral in the pathophysiology of MDD.

In addition to the finding of hypercortisolemia and CRF hypersecretion in MDD, more sensitive provocative endocrine challenge tests such as the CRF stimulation test have been evaluated. Intravenous CRF administration provokes a marked increase of ACTH secretion from the pituitary gland in healthy control subjects. In MDD patients, ACTH response is blunted (Heim et al., 2001). This is at least in part secondary to downregulation of anterior pituitary CRF receptors, in response to CRF hypersecretion from the hypothalamus that is likely the primary cause of HPA axis dysfunction in MDD (Nemeroff, 1992; Heim & Nemeroff, 1999). Recently, Newport et al. (2003) reported that the magnitude of the blunted ACTH response to CRF is correlated with the patient's basal CRF concentrations in cerebrospinal fluid (CSF).

Other HPA axis functional studies included long term monitoring with the dexamethasone-suppression test (DST) in patients suffering from a depressive episode (Holsboer et al., 1988). The standard DST is composed of administration of a low dose (1–2 mg) of dexamethasone (DEX) at 23:00 h and the subsequent measurement of cortisol levels at one or more time points the following day. In healthy controls, the secretion of ACTH and cortisol is suppressed. In contrast, in depressed patients, the suppression of cortisol secretion by DEX is markedly reduced. Numerous studies contributed to the DST literature (for a review, see APA Task Force on Laboratory Tests in Psychiatry, 1987). The sensitivity of the DST (rate of a positive outcome, or non-suppression of cortisol) in MDD is modest (about 40-50%) but is higher (about 60-70%) in very severe, especially psychotic, affective disorders, including MDD with psychotic as well as melancholic features, mania, and schizoaffective disorder. The specificity (true negative outcome) of the DST in normal control subjects is above 90%, but it varies from less than 70% to more than 90% in psychiatric conditions that often need to be separated from major affective disorders. In addition, a number of medical conditions, including severe weight loss and use of alcohol and certain other drugs (barbiturates, anticonvulsants, and others) can produce false positive results. Early life trauma likely contributes to increased HPA axis activity (see also below). Therefore, the usefulness of the DST as a diagnostic tool is limited. It can be used as a predictive instrument, because failure to convert to normal suppression of cortisol with apparent symptomatic recovery from depression is associated with an increased risk for relapse into depression or suicidal behaviour (Ribeiro et al., 1993).

A considerably more sensitive test for HPA axis dysfunction is the combined Dex-CRF-challenge test (Dex-CRF test) (Holsboer-Trachsler et al., 1991). In healthy controls, the secretion of ACTH and cortisol is almost completely suppressed by DEX administration, even after IV administration of CRF. Depressed patients release significantly more cortisol and ACTH after DEX + CRF in comparison with age-matched controls. The sensitivity of the Dex-CRF test for MDD (about 80%) greatly exceeds that of the standard DST. Increased HPA axis activity as identified with the Dex-CRF test after clinical remission in depressed patients is a strong predictor of relapse (Zobel et al., 1999). Recently, Krieg et al. (2001) reported abnormal Dex-CRF test results in asymptomatic first-degree relatives of MDD patients.

Taken together, these studies provide convincing evidence of HPA axis abnormalities in MDD. The concatenation of data suggests increased cortisol concentrations in depressed patients, caused at least partly by CRF hypersecretion, which is not adequately suppressed by any negative feedback system.

Chronic HPA axis overactivity leads to a number of serious adverse effects on the organism (reviewed in Gold & Chrousos, 2002), including excessive fear and anxiety, increased atherosclerosis (through insulin resistance and visceral fat deposition), osteoporosis and decreased immune function. Remarkably, a number of these findings have been reported in major depression (Thakore et al., 1997). The increase in intra-abdominal fat likely contributes to the increased incidence of cardiovascular morbidity and mortality in depressed patients. Michelson et al. (1996) and Schweiger et al. (2000) showed that past or current depression in women is associated with decreased bone mineral density.

Recently, a preclinical study revealed that the mesolimbic dopaminergic (DA) system is suppressed by hypercortisolemia (Pacak et al., 2002). If confirmed this preliminary finding would provide a link between HPA axis overactivity and an impaired DA mediated reward system, possibly responsible for anhedonia (lack of the ability to experience pleasure), a core feature of major depression. This would add to the growing database supporting a role for DA circuit hypofunction in depression.

An important question is whether the neurobiological changes described here should be considered as concomitants, consequences, or causes of MDD. Most studies suggest that the HPA axis overactivity tends to normalize after clinical improvement (for a review, see Hatzinger, 2000). This seems compatible with the hypothesis that the HPA axis dysfunction is a consequence or concomitant of depression. However, in a subgroup of MDD patients, the function of the HPA axis does not return to normal after clinical remission (Zobel et al., 1999). Furthermore, in patients who fully recovered from bipolar depression, Watson et al. found that the Dex-CRF test was abnormal, even though the disturbance was smaller than in patients with current bipolar depression (Watson et al., 2004). Finally, Holsboer et al. (1995) reported that the abnormal Dex-CRF test results observed among patients with depression were also present in first-degree relatives of these patients, who had no history of psychiatric illness themselves. The most likely hypothesis is that a number of individuals show a chronic liability for HPA axis hyperactivity, which can be attributed to genetic factors or experiences of early abuse (see also below). This dysfunction aggravates during MDD, and falls back to basal, but not necessarily normal, levels after clinical remission.

Dysthymia. Dysthymia is a syndrome characterized by a prolonged period (at least 2 years) with unremitting depressive symptoms, not sufficient to continuously fulfil the criteria for MDD, but still very invalidating for the patient. Although dysthymia was once viewed as a prominent feature of personality disorders, and best treated with psychotherapy, it is now clear that the disorder also has biological underpinnings, and can respond to antidepressant pharmacotherapy. Studies regarding CRF and HPA axis function in dysthymia are scarce. Catalán et al. (1998) studied 10 dysthymia patients, together with 36 MDD patients, and found a comparable increase in serum CRF and cortisol concentrations in both groups. However, the many issues associated with the measurement of CRF in serum and its interpretation renders these findings preliminary. Oshima et al. (2000) tested 20 MDD patients, 8 dysthymia patients, and 12 healthy controls with the Dex-CRF test. In the MDD group, the ACTH increase to the Dex-CRF test was significantly increased compared to the controls. The dysthymia group exhibited ACTH levels intermediate between MDD patients and controls, but not significantly different from either groups; insufficient statistical power was available to test the hypothesis. These findings suggest that dysthymia may share similar HPA axis abnormalities compared to MDD, but further research is needed.

Atypical depression and seasonal affective disorder. Atypical depression is characterized by an inversion of the somatic symptoms seen in melancholic MDD. Patients show hypersomnia, hyperphagia, lethargy, fatigue, and relative apathy. Seasonal affective disorder (depression associated with a specific period of the year) is clinically similar to atypical depression. As the somatic symptoms in melancholic depression can be attributed to CRF hyperdrive, the symptoms in atypical depression have been posited to be due to a hypofunction of the CRF stress response system.

Casper et al. (1988) utilized the DST to measure cortisol levels in blood, CSF, and urine in 45 hospitalized male and female patients with primary major depressive disorder who reported hypersomnia or increase in appetite. They provided preliminary evidence that HPA activity in depression is diminished in the presence of hypersomnia and/or increased appetite. These findings were confirmed and extended by a study of Geracioti et al. (1997), who reported that in 10 patients with symptoms of atypical depression, CRF concentration in CSF and ACTH concentrations in plasma tended to be low, with normal plasma cortisol. Gold and Chrousos (2002) measured plasma ACTH and cortisol concentrations every three minutes for a 24 h period in 4 patients with atypical depression and 4 controls. Patients with atypical depression showed significant reductions in plasma ACTH secretion in the presence of normal cortisol concentrations, compatible with hypothalamic CRF hypoactivity. Although interesting, these studies are very small and should be considered preliminary.

CRF and other Stress-Related Psychiatric Disorders

Posttraumatic stress disorder. Experiences of overwhelming traumatic stress can lead to posttraumatic stress disorder (PTSD), a syndrome characterized by re-experiencing aspects of the traumatic experience and generalized arousal. Because of the seminal role of stress in the disorder, several studies have scrutinized HPA axis function in PTSD.

Similar to the findings in MDD, PTSD patients exhibit elevated CSF CRF concentrations (Bremner et al., 1997; Baker et al., 1999). The ACTH response to a standardized CRF stimulation test is diminished (Smith et al., 1989). One half of the PTSD patients also fulfilled criteria for MDD in this study.

However, unlike MDD, basal and stress-induced cortisol output is reportedly diminished in PTSD patients (For review, see Yehuda, 2001). Stein et al. (1997) studied 19 female survivors of childhood and/or adolescent sexual abuse. These women had significantly enhanced suppression of plasma cortisol in response to a low dose (0.5 mg) of DEX compared to women without an abuse history. These observations are consistent with findings in male veterans with combat-related PTSD (Yehuda et al., 1995; Kellner et al., 1997). This suggests that, in PTSD, the negative feedback of the HPA axis by cortisol is enhanced. Perhaps the low cortisol

236

secretion leads to an upregulation of glucocorticoid receptors (GR's), resulting in enhanced negative feedback of the system in response to a low dose of DEX. Upregulation of GR's was indeed observed in lymphocytes of PTSD patients (Yehuda et al., 1993).

In a recent study, Rinne et al. (2002) studied 39 patients with borderline personality disorder (BPD) with (n= 24) and without (n= 15) a history of childhood abuse and comorbid PTSD (n= 12) or MDD (n= 11) and 11 healthy control subjects. They observed super-suppression of cortisol and ACTH using the Dex-CRF test in the PTSD group.

Taken together, these data suggest that PTSD, like MDD, is characterized by central CRF hyperdrive, but that in contrast to MDD, the negative feedback of the HPA axis is enhanced in PTSD, resulting in a low cortisol output.

Chronic fatigue syndrome and fibromyalgia. Chronic fatigue syndrome (CFS) is characterized by persistent or relapsing debilitating fatigue for at least 6 months in the absence of any medical diagnosis that would explain the clinical presentation. CFS and fibromyalgia, two clinically related syndromes, are etiologically complex disorders. Infectious, immunological, neuroendocrine, sleep, and psychiatric mechanisms have been investigated; however, a unifying etiology has yet to emerge. Exposure to stress increases the vulnerability for CFS (Kang et al., 2003), and a recent comprehensive review of neuroendocrine studies reported an altered physiological response to stress (Parker, Wessely, & Cleare, 2001). Clinically, CFS shares some similar features with atypical depression. Neuroendocrinological studies suggest a disturbance of the HPA axis similar to that observed in atypical depression, characterized by CRF hyposecretion. Low basal cortisol values in plasma and low 24-hour urinary free cortisol excretion have been reported in CFS compared to healthy controls in some, but not all, studies (Demitrack et al., 1991). In a recent review, Parker et al. (2001) found that approximately one-third of the studies reported baseline cortisol secretion in CFS and fibromyalgia patients to be low, in approximately one-third of patients. Scott et al. (1999) found a volume reduction of over 50% of the adrenal glands in 8 CFS subjects with abnormal endocrine parameters (compared to 55 controls), indicative of significant adrenal atrophy. Similarly, 24-hour urinary free cortisol levels of patients with fibromyalgia tend to be in the lower part of the normal range. With respect to dynamic responsiveness of the HPA axis, the DST results are normal in CFS, but marked ACTH hypersecretion in response to severe acute stressors has been reported, perhaps indicative of chronic CRF hyposecretion and CRF receptor upregulation (Geenen et al., 2002).

There is clearly abundant data indicative of dysregulation of the CRF system in major depression, and in a number of other stress-related neuropsychiatric disorders. The next logical question is how such dysregulation arises. In the case of major depression, the question can be formulated more specifically: Are the biological and psychological factors that are known to increase the risk for major depression individually and collectively leading to a lasting disruption of the CRF and HPA axis system? In the next section, we scrutinize three well established risk factors for major depression, and evaluate their possible influence on the HPA axis: genetic factors, chronic stress and early life stress.

Genetic Factors

As stated earlier, family, twin and adoption studies have all shown that genetic factors play an important role in the vulnerability for major depression. The question here is whether genetic variations could contribute to persistent dysregulation of CRF secretion as well as HPA axis function, which would render such individuals more prone to depression.

Holsboer et al. (1995) reported that the HPA feedback disturbance observed among patients with depression was also present in otherwise healthy individuals who are at high risk for psychiatric disorders because they have a first-degree relative with an affective illness. Moreover, this disturbance was shown to be stable over a 5-year period (Modell et al., 1998). These data suggest that some individuals have a genetically determined vulnerability to develop chronic CRF hypersecretion and MDD. Whether they actually develop MDD probably depends on a number of factors such as early trauma experiences, chronic and acute stress.

It is not yet clear which genes underlie the individual susceptibility for such dysregulation. Several studies are currently underway examining the impact of a number of genes implicated in CRF and HPA axis regulation. In some cases, animal models have been developed that under- or overexpress these genes, and the stress coping and depression/anxiety-related behaviors of these transgenic animals have been evaluated. Other studies have searched for possible associations between polymorphisms of these genes and MDD (for a review, see Claes, 2004).

As stated earlier, CRF and AVP are the main neurohormones activating the HPA axis, and therefore genes coding for these hormones and their receptors are obvious functional candidate genes. There are 2 CRF receptor subtypes, CRF-R1 and CRF-R2, and the availability of CRF is further regulated by its binding to the CRF binding protein (CRF-BP). Preclinical studies have examined CRF-R1 gene "knockout" mice, transgenic mice in which both copies of the CRF-R1 gene have been inactivated by molecular genetic techniques. These animals exhibit HPA axis disruption and reduced anxiety, indicative of a key role for this gene in the development of a functional HPA axis (Timple et al., 1998). CRF-R2 knockout mice have been reported to be hypersensitive to stress, though discordant findings exist (Coste et al., 2000; Bale et al., 2000; Kishimoto et al., 2000). CRF-BP knockout mice exhibit increased anxiety on several behavioral measures (Seasholtz et al., 2001). In humans, there are no systematic studies looking at the association of the CRF-R1 gene with major depression. A preliminary genetic study revealed no association between CRF-R2 and major depression (Villafuerte et al., 2002). In contrast, the gene encoding for CRF-BP was associated with increased vulnerability for major depression in a Swedish population (Claes et al., 2003).

Because most patients with major depression show a deficient negative feedback of the HPA axis, and because this feedback is regulated through the GR, this represents another functional candidate gene. This is also true for the genes coding for the so-called chaperone molecules, proteins that interact functionally with the GR protein.

From animal models, a central role of the GR gene in stress coping seems plausible. Complete absence of functional GR is incompatible with life (Reichard, 1998). However, mice with functionally impaired GR have been studied, as well as mice with tissue-specific knockout of the GR gene. These animals show profound behavioral changes and elevated plasma corticotropin concentrations in response to stress. Treatment with moclobemide, a monoamine oxidase inhibitor antidepressant, reversed the behavioral deficits in this mouse model. Tronche et al. (1999) generated viable adult mice with loss of GR function in selected tissues. Loss of GR in the central nervous system (CNS) impaired regulation of the HPA axis, resulting in increased glucocorticoid plasma levels. Conditional mutagenesis of the GR in the CNS resulted in an impaired behavioral response to stress and reduced anxiety.

In humans, several genetic polymorphisms have been identified in the GR gene (De Rijk et al., 2002 for a review). Some of these influence the regulation of the HPA axis, and are associated with metabolic and cardiovascular alterations. Data on GR polymorphisms and psychiatric disorders are scarce. Five missense variants in the amino-terminal domain of the GR showed no association with puerperal psychosis or schizophrenia (Feng et al., 2000). An association analysis between GR polymorphisms and the vulnerability for MDD in two independent populations has been performed by one of us (SC) and no evidence for an association was observed (Van West et al., submitted).

Chronic Stress

In chronic stress, multiple mechanisms further activate the CRF system. These mechanisms have been described by Makino et al. (2002). In situations of chronic arousal, the glucocorticoid negative feedback system is less effective, possibly by downregulation of hippocampal GR. Furthermore, glucocorticoids upregulate CRF secretion in the amygdala and increase the expression of CRF receptors in the PVN (Rivest et al., 1995). These data perhaps explain why in some cases, chronic stress does not lead to HPA axis downregulation through the negative feedback effects of cortisol, but to sustained CRF hypersecretion, which likely contributes to MDD.

Early Life Stress

At birth, the stress response system is not fully mature. In rodents, the postnatal HPA axis is remarkably different from that of the adult, both in structure and function. The first 2 weeks postnatally are characterized by a "silent period" during which the developing animal is relatively hyporesponsive to stress (the so-called stress hyporesponsive period), followed by a new and unique phase of stress responsiveness when the animal fails to swiftly terminate glucocorticoid secretion (Vazquez, 1998). Increasing evidence from animal and human studies has revealed a critical period postnatally when sustained stress (trauma) disrupts the normal development of the stress response system. We will review the available data in three different species: rats, non-human primates and humans. A comprehensive review on this topic has recently been published (Heim et al., 2004).

Rats. Plotsky et al. (1993) studied rat pups 2-14 days of age, that were exposed daily to handling (H) (15 min of separation from mother and home cage), maternal separation (MS; 180 min of comparable separation), or were left entirely undisturbed (non-handled; NH). As adults, MS rats showed increased hypothalamic CRF mRNA expression compared with NH rats. CRF mRNA expression in H rats were significantly lower than either MS or NH animals. Hypothalamic CRF concentration under basal conditions exhibited the same pattern as CRF mRNA expression. Restraint stress produced significantly greater increases in plasma corticosterone in MS and NH animals than in H animals. In a subsequent experiment, Ladd et al. (1996) found that adult male rats previously isolated for 6 hours daily during postnatal days 2-20 exhibited an increase in both basal and stress-induced serum ACTH concentrations. Moreover, these rats exhibited a 125% increase in immunoreactive CRF concentrations in the median eminence and a reduction in the density of CRF receptor binding in the anterior pituitary. Alterations in extrahypothalamic CRF systems were also apparent: these animals showed a 59% increase in the number of CRF receptor 1 - binding sites in the raphe nucleus. Marked increases in CRF mRNA expression and concentration in the central nucleus of the amygdala, the bed nucleus of the stria terminalis and the locus coeruleus of the adult exposed to ELS were also observed. These results indicate that maternal deprivation before weaning in male rats produces effects on CRF neural systems throughout the central nervous system and pituitary that are apparent several months later and are associated with persistent alterations in behavior. In a recent study, Huot et al. (2002) confirmed the persistent HPA axis changes in maternally deprived rats, and found that maternal separation and subsequent reunion with the dam resulted in elevated plasma corticosterone levels at a time when rat pups are normally hyporesponsive to stressors and show limited pituitary-adrenal responses. Structural studies in these traumatized rats showed decreased mossy fiber density in the stratum oriens region of the hippocampus. These changes may be the result of neonatal exposure to elevated glucocorticoids and/or changes in other signaling systems in response to maternal separation. Overall the results suggest that repeated, daily, 3 h maternal separations during critical periods of hippocampal development can disrupt hippocampal cytoarchitecture in a stable manner. The resulting change in morphology may contribute to the subtle but consistent learning deficit and overall stress hyper-responsive phenotype observed in these animals.

Primates. Similar to the studies in rodents, several investigators have evaluated the effects of prolonged deprivation or repeated separations of infant non-human primates from their mothers or peers. Evidently, primates are more valid models for human behavior compared to rats. Monkey and human infants indeed demonstrate similar acute behavioral and physiological reactions to separations (Sanchez et al., 2001). When tested as adults, non-human primates exposed to prolonged periods of maternal or social deprivation exhibit marked behavioral, physiological, and neurobiological changes. These include increased fearfulness and anxiety, social dysfunction, aggression, aberrant stereotypic and self-directed behaviors, altered ingestion and anhedonia, as well as altered neurochemical, immune, and autonomic function (reviewed in Sanchez et al., 2001; Pryce et al., 2002; Gilmer & McKinney, 2003).

Two studies on squirrel and marmoset monkeys respectively, showed lowered basal and stress induced cortisol excretion and stronger negative feedback of the HPA axis in monkeys exposed to separation stress early in life (Lyons et al., 1999, 2000; Dettling et al., 2002). Infant bonnet macaques raised by mothers foraging under unpredictable conditions exhibited persistently elevated cerebrospinal fluid (CSF) concentrations of CRF as adults, compared to monkeys reared by mothers foraging under predictable conditions (Coplan et al., 1996). Summarizing, these studies suggest that monkeys with early adverse experiences show hyperactivity of CNS CRF systems, a strong negative feedback and a reduced cortisol output, similar to what is seen in human individuals with PTSD.

Humans. More recently, studies in humans have become available. The most common forms of ELS in humans are sexual, physical, and emotional maltreatment, as well as parental loss. Other forms of ELS include accidents, surgeries and chronic illness, natural disasters, war and terrorism-related events. Heim et al. (2000) studied women with a history of childhood abuse, some of which fulfilled criteria for major depression. Traumatized women exhibited increased pituitary-adrenal and autonomic responses to stress compared with controls. This effect was particularly robust in women with current major depression. Indeed, women with a history of childhood abuse and a current major depression diagnosis exhibited a more than 6-fold increase in ACTH response to stress.

In a subsequent study by the same group (Vythilingham et al., 2002), hippocampal volume was measured using MRI. A smaller hippocampal volume in adult women with major depressive disorder was found only in the group with a history of severe and prolonged physical and/or sexual abuse in childhood. Taken together, the data in humans, although preliminary, seem comparable to the observations in rodents and primates: specific stressors early in life can cause structural changes in the limbic system (hippocampus and probably other structures) and permanently dysregulate the stress response system.

It is probable that the lifelong disturbance of HPA axis function induced by early life trauma is dependent on several factors: the critical time-window, the nature of the stressor, the presence or absence of a supportive environment and the genetic liability of the individual. Elucidation of these factors is an important target for subsequent research.

It is important to be aware of the limitations in comparing animal and human studies. In animal studies, the paradigm used is a model of maternal neglect, which differs from the abuse experiences studied in humans. Whether maternal neglect and abuse lead to similar neurobiological consequences, also needs to be established in further research.

Outlook: Integrative Research

In CRF and HPA axis research, integration of psychological and neurobiological parameters of major depression has already begun. The most obvious example is our growing understanding of the neurobiology of early life stress. The concept of early physical or sexual abuse leading to lifelong disturbances in stress resilience, and to an increased vulnerability for stress-related disorders such as major depression will sound familiar to psychodynamic psychotherapists. Many questions remain to be answered in this area. Which specific early life stressors are most disruptive of the neurobiology of the stress response system? Looking more closely at the specific model of early life stress in rats, the neurobiological consequences are not solely due to the effect of being taken away from the dam for three hours a day, but also a response to the way these pups are treated by the dam once they are returned to the nest.

It is generally believed that there is a critical time window, stretching from infancy to puberty, in which abuse experiences are particularly deleterious, but we have only scarce scientific data to support this assumption. We don't know whether this is one homogenous period, or whether it should be subdivided into different periods, each having a unique sensitivity for HPA axis and CRF circuit disruption by specific stressors.

A number of factors are thought to protect children against the negative effects of early life stress: attachment to trustworthy important others and certain personality traits. Whether these factors can mitigate the negative effect of early life trauma on the function of the HPA axis, is unknown.

Another clinical observation is that there are clearly individual differences in the response to the deleterious effects of early abuse. In some families, several children will undergo important early life stress, but not all of them will develop psychiatric disorders. Genetic factors most probably play some role in such individual differences, but more research is needed to identify which genes are involved.

Future studies should further evaluate whether ELS associated alterations in the HPA axis and the other demonstrated biological alterations, normalize in response to different treatment regimens in depression. Indeed, little is known in clinical populations as to whether certain treatments can alter or reverse the neurobiological consequences of ELS. In rat models, SSRI's such as paroxetine reversed the effects of maternal separation (Huot et al., 2001).

If childhood trauma leads to disruptions in HPA axis function in genetically sensitive individuals, would pharmacotherapy or psychotherapy prevent the development of psychiatric disorders such as major depression in these individuals? If so, which form of psychotherapy or pharmacotherapy should be utilized and for how long? One recent study showed that treatment with fluvoxamine, an SSRI, reversed HPA axis hyper-responsiveness in the dexamethasone/CRF test, particularly in those borderline personality disordered patients who reported sustained histories of child abuse, independent of symptomatic status (Rinne et al., 2003). In order to improve the treatment response in depression, it is likely that new treatment strategies directly target the underlying pathophysiology. These treatments that directly target the neuronal circuits and mechanisms that are modified by ELS, such as CRF receptor antagonists, might be particularly effective in the treatment or prevention of depression related to ELS.

However promising, this type of integrative research is fraught with difficulties. First, it is labor intensive, requiring collaboration between experienced clinicians and neurobiologists. One of the key problems is gathering retrospective information about early childhood experiences, and linking this to sensitive functional tests of the HPA axis. As Sigmund Freud already discovered, gathering retrospective information about abuse experiences in childhood is notoriously difficult.

In order to address complex questions such as the interaction between genetic liability and specific early life stressors, very large samples of traumatized patients and healthy control persons will be needed. For all these reasons, it would be inappropriate to assume that these questions can be solved rapidly. However, the importance of this type of integrative research cannot be overstated.

Many of these factors are also relevant when assessing the impact of chronic life stress on the HPA axis and subsequent vulnerability to stress related psychiatric disorders. We have solid data linking chronic stress to chronic CRF hypersecretion, but many questions remain. Which forms of chronic stress are most relevant? How do they interact with genetic factors to lead to chronic CRF hypersecretion? What is the role of personality in this matter? Which factors protect an individual against HPA axis disruption by chronic stress?

In terms of the question of specificity of stressors, the available data are simply too discordant to come to any firm conclusions and we must await additional data. It is known that physical stressors such as blood volume loss and psychological stressors such as fear elicit clearly distinct neurobiological responses. Neurobiological and neuroendocrinological responses to different psychosocial stressors also likely exist but it is premature to draw any firm conclusions in this area.

These and related questions represent a fascinating challenge for psycho-therapists, psychiatrists and neurobiologists alike, and these groups will need to collaborate in order to achieve progress. Alterations in HPA axis activity have been reported in several different psychiatric disorders. As expected, these endocrine alterations are not limited to specific DSM-IV diagnostic entities. The central CRF hyperdrive seen in MDD is, for example, similar to what is seen in anorexia nervosa and end stage Alzheimer's disease. The data in atypical depression, chronic fatigue syndrome and fibromyalgia, although preliminary, seem more compatible with a CRF hypofunction, characterized by low cortisol secretion. PTSD is characterized by central CRF hyperdrive and reduced cortisol secretion possibly due to strong negative feedback associated with an upregulation of glucocorticoid receptors. These data suggest the existence of specific HPA axis dysfunctional phenotypes that transcend DSM-IV diagnostic boundaries. For that reason, future research efforts should emphasize the link between early adverse experiences, genetic factors, specific types of HPA axis function and clinical symptoms, regardless of the DSM category in which these symptoms occur. Such an approach should lead to a disease classification system with increased etiological and neurobiological validity, compared to the current DSM-IV classification.

Conclusion

CRF circuits play a major role in the physiological adaptations to acute and chronic stress. CRF is the main regulator of the HPA axis, but also acts as a neurotransmitter in numerous brain regions. Whether or not this stress response system functions adequately is probably determined by the interplay of genetic factors and environmental events. A growing body of evidence from preclinical and human studies indicates that adverse experiences during a critical period in childhood can lead to persisting dysfunctions of CRF and HPA axis function throughout adult life. These findings are changing the face of psychiatry, because they make the link between neurobiological and psychological factors underlying psychiatric disorders.

Numerous studies have revealed HPA axis abnormalities in MDD, and data are also accumulating for other psychiatric disorders. Based on these findings, an integrative view of the pathogenesis of MDD can be formulated. This is graphically demonstrated in figure 2. Genetic factors and adverse early experiences can lead to a stable vulnerability pattern of increased sensitivity to stress, CRF hyperdrive in response to stress, and hippocampal shrinkage. When individuals with this phenotype are confronted with acute or chronic stress, further CRF hyperdrive and HPA axis dysregulation occur, leading to the clinical phenotype of MDD, possibly involving changes in monoamine neurotransmitter and immune function.

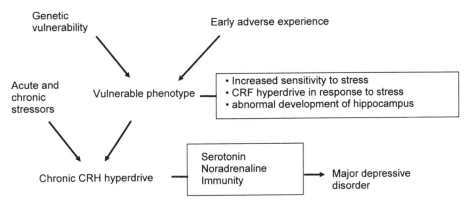

FIGURE 2.

An integrative model. Genetic vulnerability and early life stress (or the interaction between both) lead to persistent dysregulations of the HPA axis, characterized by increased stress sensitivity, CRF hyperdrive and neuronal damage in the hippocampus (and possible other brain areas). When individuals with this vulnerable phenotype are confronted with chronic stress or negative life events, the system is prone to further dysregulation and CRF hyperdrive. This will in turn cause changes in other neurobiological systems such as the immune system and neurotransmission by serotonin and norepinephrine. The combination of these neurobiological changes leads to the development of clinical psychiatric disorders such as major depression or other stress related disorders.

The central CRF hyperdrive seen in MDD is probably very similar to what is seen in dysthymia. The data in atypical depression, chronic fatigue syndrome and fibromyalgia, though preliminary, seem more compatible with CRF hypoactivity, characterized by low cortisol secretion. In PTSD, central CRF hyperdrive goes together with a strong negative feedback and low cortisol output.

These data suggest the existence of specific HPA axis dysfunctional phenotypes irrespective of DSM diagnostic borders. The available evidence indicates that several stress-related psychiatric disorders are characterized by similar patterns of CRF circuit abnormalities. This challenges the borders DSM has defined between disorders on the basis of clinical criteria. In future DSM editions, clinical entities that have been separated might be reunited based on a common neurobiological background.

It is possible that the finding of central CRF hyperdrive in MDD is in fact restricted to a (large) proportion of MDD patients: those with a history of childhood abuse (Nemeroff, 2003). This is also compatible with the study of Rinne et al. (2002), who found CRF hyperdrive in borderline personality patients with childhood abuse, regardless of whether they were depressed or not.

These data suggest the existence of a specific vulnerability phenotype, caused by sustained childhood abuse, and characterized by hyperreactivity to stress, central CRF hyperdrive, hypersecretion of cortisol and impaired function and decreased volume of the hippocampus (Nemeroff, 2003). Whether this phenotype leads to MDD or other stress related psychiatric diseases in a particular individual, would then depend on other, yet unknown, genetic and environmental factors.

A large and fascinating field for research integrating psychological and neurobiological factors in psychiatry lies open before us. It seems appropriate to warn against undue optimism however: This research will require large numbers of patients being investigated by experienced clinicians, neurobiologists and geneticists, and will therefore be laborious, time consuming and expensive. Nevertheless, it is only this kind of scientific approach that can do justice to the complex nature of psychiatric disorders, and will undoubtedly lead to better treatments for our patients.

Acknowledgements

The authors are supported by the following grants: NIH MH-92088 (CBN), MH-39415 (CBN), MH-58922 (CBN).

References

APA Task Force on Laboratory Tests in Psychiatry (1987). The dexamethasone suppression test: An overview of its current status in psychiatry. *American Journal of Psychiatry*, *144*, 1253-1262.

American Psychiatric Association (1994). *Diagnostic and statistical manual of mental disorders* (4th ed.). Washington, DC: Author.

Austin, M. C., Janosky, J. E., & Murphy, H. A. (2003). Increased corticotropin-releasing hormone immuno-reactivity in monoamine-containing pontine nuclei of depressed suicide men. *Molecular Psychiatry*, *8*, 324-332.

Baker, D. G., West, S. A., Nicholson, W. E., Ekhator, N. N., Kasckow, J. W., Hill, K. K., Bruce, A. B., Orth, D. N., & Geracioti, T. D., Jr. (1999). Serial CSF corticotropin-releasing hormone levels and adrenocortical activity in combat veterans with posttraumatic stress disorder. *American Journal of Psychiatry*, *156*, 585-588.

Bale, T. L., Contarino, A., Smith, G. W., Chan, R., Gold, L. H., Sawchenko, P. E., Koob, G. F., Vale, W. W., & Lee, K. F. (2000). Mice deficient for corticotropin-releasing hormone receptor-2 display anxiety-like behaviour and are hypersensitive to stress. *Nature Genetics*, *24*, 410-414.

Banki, C. M., Bissette, G., Arato, M., O'Connor, L., & Nemeroff, C. B. (1987). CSF corticotropin-releasing factor-like immunoreactivity in depression and schizophrenia. *American Journal of Psychiatry*, *144*, 873-877.

Blazer, D. G., Kessler, R. C., McGonagle, K. A., & Swartz, M. S. (1994). The prevalence and distribution of major depression in a national community sample: The National Comorbidity Survey. *American Journal of Psychiatry*, *151*, 979-986.

Bremner, J. D., Licinio, J., Darnell, A., Krystal, J. H., Owens, M. J., Southwick, S. M., Nemeroff, C. B., & Charney, D. S. (1997). Elevated CSF corticotropin-releasing factor concentrations in posttraumatic stress disorder. *American Journal of Psychiatry*, *154*, 624-629.

Bremner, J. D., Narayan, M., Anderson, E. R., Staib, L. H., Miller, H. L., & Charney, D. S. (2000). Hippocampal volume reduction in major depression. *American Journal of Psychiatry*, *157*, 115-118.

Carpenter, W. T. Jr., & Bunney, W. E. Jr. (1971). Adrenal cortical activity in depressive illness. *American Journal of Psychiatry*, *128*, 31-40.

Carroll, B. J., Curtis, G. C., Davies, B. M., Mendels, J., & Sugerman, A. A. (1976). Urinary free cortisol excretion in depression. *Psychological Medicine, 6*, 43-50.

Casper, R. C., Kocsis, J., Dysken, M., Stokes, P., Croughan, J., & Maas J. (1988). Cortisol measures in primary major depressive disorder with hypersomnia or appetite increase. *Journal of Affective Disorders, 15*, 131-140.

Catalán, R., Gallarta, J. M., Castellanosa, J. M., & Galarda, R. (1998). Plasma corticotropin-releasing factor in depressive disorders. *Biological Psychiatry, 44*, 15-20.

Charney, D. S., Menkes, D. B., & Heninger, G. R. (1981). Receptor sensitivity and the mechanism of action of antidepressant treatment. Implications for the etiology and therapy of depression. *Archives of General Psychiatry, 38*, 1160-1180.

Claes, S. J. (2004). CRH, stress, and major depression: A psychobiological interplay. *Vitamins and Hormones, 69*, 117-150.

Claes, S., Villafuerte, S., Forsgren, T., Sluijs, S., Del-Favero, J., Adolfsson, R., & Van Broeckhoven, C. (2003). The CRF binding protein is associated with major depression in a population from Northern Sweden. *Biological Psychiatry, 54*, 867-872.

Coplan, J. D., Andrews, M. W., Rosenblum, L. A., Owens, M. J., Friedman, S., Gorman, J. M., & Nemeroff, C. B. (1996). Persistent elevations of cerebrospinal fluid concentrations of corticotropin-releasing factor in adult nonhuman primates exposed to early-life stressors: Implications for the pathophysiology of mood and anxiety disorders. *Proceedings of the National Academy of Sciences of the United States of America, 93*, 1619-1623.

Coste, S. C., Kesterson, R. A., Heldwein, K. A., Stevens, S. L., Heard, A. D., Hollis, J. H., Murray, S. E., Hill, J. K., Pantely, G. A., Hohimer, A. R., Hatton, D. C., Phillips, T. J., Finn, D. A., Low, M. J., Rittenberg, M. B., Stenzel, P., & Stenzel-Poore, M. P. (2000). Abnormal adaptations to stress and impaired cardiovascular function in mice lacking corticotropin-releasing hormone receptor-2. *Nature Genetics, 24*, 403-409.

Davidson, R. J. (2002). Anxiety and affective style: Role of prefrontal cortex and amygdala. *Biological Psychiatry, 51*, 68-80.

Davis, M. (1992). The role of the amygdala in conditioned fear. In J. P. Aggleton (Ed.), *The amygdala* (pp. 255-306). New York: Wiley.

Demitrack, M. A., Dale, J. K., Straus, S. E., Laue, L., Listwak, S. J., Kruesi, M. J., Chrousos, G. P., & Gold, P. W. (1991). Evidence for impaired activation of the hypothalamic-pituitary-adrenal axis in patients with chronic fatigue syndrome. *The Journal of Clinical Endocrinology and Metabolism, 73*, 1224-1234.

DeRijk, R. H., Schaaf, M., & de Kloet, E.R. (2002). Glucocorticoid receptor variants: Clinical implications. *Journal of Steroid Biochemistry and Molecular Biology, 81*, 103-122.

Dettling, A. C., Feldon, J., & Pryce, C. R. (2002). Repeated parental deprivation in the infant common marmoset (Callithrix jacchus, primates) and analysis of its effects on early development. *Biological Psychiatry, 52*, 1037–1046.

Drevets, W. C., Frank, E., Price, J. C., Kupfer, D. J., Holt, D., Greer, P. J., Huang, Y., Gautier, C., & Mathis, C. (1999). PET imaging of serotonin 1A receptor binding in depression. *Biological Psychiatry, 46*, 1375-1387.

Feng, J., Zheng, J., Bennett, W. P., Heston, L. L., Jones, I. R., Craddock, N., & Sommer, S. S. (2000). Five missense variants in the amino-terminal domain of the glucocorticoid receptor: No association with puerperal psychosis or schizophrenia. *American Journal of Medical Genetics, 96*, 412-417.

Frank, E., Kupfer, D. J., Perel, J. M., Cornes, C., Jarrett, D. B., Mallinger, A. G., Thase, M. E., McEachran, A. B., & Grochocinski, V. J. (1990). Three-year outcomes for maintenance therapies in recurrent depression. *Archives of General Psychiatry, 47*, 1093-1099.

Geenen, R., Jacobs, J. W., & Bijlsma, J. W. (2002). Evaluation and management of endocrine dysfunction in fibromyalgia. *Rheumatic Disease Clinics of North America, 28*, 389-404.

Geracioti, T. D. Jr., Loosen, P. T., & Orth, D. N. (1997). Low cerebrospinal fluid corticotropin-releasing hormone concentrations in eucortisolemic depression. *Biological Psychiatry, 42*, 165-174.

Gilmer, W. S., & McKinney, W. T. (2003). Early experience and depressive disorders: Human and non-human primate studies. *Journal of Affective Disorders, 75*, 97-113.

Gold, P. W., & Chrousos, G. P. (2002). Organization of the stress system and its dysregulation in melancholic and atypical depression: High vs low CRF/NE states. *Molecular Psychiatry, 7*, 254-275.

Gold, P. W., Drevets, W. C., & Charney, D. S. (2002). New insights into the role of cortisol and the glucocorticoid receptor in severe depression. *Biological Psychiatry, 52*, 381-385.

Grippo, A. J., Beltz, T. G., & Johnson, A. K (2003). Behavioral and cardiovascular changes in the chronic mild stress model of depression. *Physiology & Behavior*, *78*, 703-710.

Hatzinger, M. (2000). Neuropeptides and the hypothalamic-pituitary-adrenocortical (HPA) system: Review of recent research strategies in depression. *World Journal of Biological Psychiatry*, *1*, 105-111.

Heim, C., & Nemeroff, C. B. (1999). The impact of early adverse experiences on brain systems involved in the pathophysiology of anxiety and affective disorders. *Biological Psychiatry*, *46*, 1509-1522.

Heim, C., & Nemeroff, C. B. (2001). The role of childhood trauma in the neurobiology of mood and anxiety disorders: Preclinical and clinical studies. *Biological Psychiatry*, *49*, 1023-1039.

Heim, C., Newport, D. J., Bonsall, R., Miller, A. H., & Nemeroff, C. B. (2001). Altered pituitary-adrenal axis responses to provocative challenge tests in adult survivors of childhood abuse. *American Journal of Psychiatry*, *158*, 575-581.

Heim, C., Newport, D. J., Heit, S., Graham, Y. P., Wilcox, M., Bonsall, R., Miller, A. H., & Nemeroff, C. B. (2000). Pituitary-adrenal and autonomic responses to stress in women after sexual and physical abuse in childhood. *Journal of the American Medical Association*, *284*, 592-597.

Heim, C., Plotsky, P. M., & Nemeroff, C. B. (2004). Importance of studying the contributions of early adverse experience to neurobiological findings in depression. *Neuropsychopharmacology*, *29*, 641-648.

Heinrichs, S. C., Min, H., Tamraz, S., Carmouche, M., Boehme, S. A., & Vale, W. W. (1997). Anti-sexual and anxiogenic behavioral consequences of corticotropin-releasing factor overexpression are centrally mediated. *Psychoneuroendocrinology*, *22*, 215-224.

Heinrichs, S. C., & Richard, D. (1999). The role of corticotropin-releasing factor and urocortin in the modulation of ingestive behavior. *Neuropeptides*, *33*, 350-359.

Herman, J. P., Schafer, M. K., Young, E. A., Thompson, R., Douglass, J., Akil, H., & Watson, S. J. (1989). Evidence for hippocampal regulation of neuroendocrine neurons of the hypothalamo-pituitary-adrenocortical axis. *Journal of Neuroscience*, *9*, 3072-3082.

Hiroi, N., Wong, M. L., Licinio, J., Park, C., Young, M., Gold, P. W., Chrousos, G. P., & Bornstein, S. R. (2001). Expression of corticotropin releasing hormone receptors type I and type II mRNA in suicide victims and controls. *Molecular Psychiatry*, *6*, 540-546.

Holsboer, F., Lauer, C. J., Schreiber, W., & Krieg, J. C. (1995). Altered hypothalamic-pituitary-adrenocortical regulation in healthy subjects at high familial risk for affective disorders. *Neuroendocrinology*, *62*, 340-347.

Holsboer, F., Liebl, R., & Hofschuster, E. (1988). Repeated dexamethasone suppression test during depressive illness. *Journal of Affective Disorders*, *4*, 93-101.

Holsboer-Trachsler, E., Stohler, R., & Hatzinger, M. (1991). Repeated administration of the combined dexamethasone-human corticotropin releasing hormone stimulation test during treatment of depression. *Psychiatry Research*, *38*, 163-171.

Huot, R. L., Plotsky, P. M., Lenox, R. H., & McNamara, R. K. (2002). Neonatal maternal separation reduces hippocampal mossy fibre density in adult Long Evans rats. *Brain Research*, *950*, 52-63.

Huot, R. L., Thrivikraman, K. V., Meaney, M. J., & Plotsky, P. M. (2001). Development of adult ethanol preference and anxiety as a consequence of neonatal maternal separation in Long Evans rats and reversal with antidepressant treatment. *Psychopharmacology*, *158*, 366-373.

Jones, I., Kent, L., & Craddock, N. (2002). Genetics of affective disorders. In P. McGuffin, M. J. Owen & I. I. Gottesman (Eds.), *Psychiatric genetics and genomics* (pp. 211-246). Oxford: Oxford University Press.

Kang, H. K., Natelson, B. H., Mahan, C. M., Lee, K. Y., & Murphy, F. M. (2003). Post-traumatic stress disorder and chronic fatigue syndrome-like illness among Gulf War veterans: A population-based survey of 30,000 veterans. *American Journal of Epidemiology*, *157*, 141-148.

Kellner, M., Baker, D. G., & Yehuda, R. (1997). Salivary cortisol in Operation Desert Storm returnees. *Biological Psychiatry*, *42*, 849-850.

Kendler, K. S., Karkowski, L. M., & Prescott, C. A. (1999). Causal relationship between stressful life events and the onset of major depression. *American Journal of Psychiatry*, *156*, 837-841.

Kendler, K. S., Kuhn, J., & Prescott, C. A. (2004). The interrelationship of neuroticism, sex, and stressful life events in the prediction of episodes of major depression. *American Journal of Psychiatry*, *161*, 631-636.

Kessler, R. C., Berglund, P., Demler, O., Jin, R., Koretz, D., Merikangas, K. R., Rush, A. J., Walters, E. E., & Wang, P. S. (2003). National Comorbidity Survey Replication. The epidemiology of major depressive disorder: Results from the National Comorbidity Survey Replication (NCS-R). *Journal of the American Medical Association*, *289*, 3095-3105.

Kishimoto, T., Radulovic, J., Radulovic, M., Lin, C. R., Schrick, C., Hooshmand, F., Hermanson, O.,

Rosenfeld, M. G., & Spiess, J. (2000). Deletion of crhr2 reveals an anxiolytic role for corticotropin-releasing hormone receptor-2. *Nature Genetics, 24*, 415-419.

Krieg, J. C., Lauer, C. J., Schreiber, W., Modell, S., & Holsboer, F. (2001). Neuroendocrine, polysomnographic and psychometric observations in healthy subjects at high familial risk for affective disorders: The current state of the 'Munich vulnerability study'. *Journal of Affective Disorders, 62*, 33-37.

Kronfol, Z. (2002). Immune dysregulation in major depression: A critical review of existing evidence. *International Journal of Neuropsychopharmacology, 5*, 333-343.

Ladd, C. O., Owens, M. J., & Nemeroff, C. B. (1996). Persistent changes in corticotropin-releasing factor neuronal systems induced by maternal deprivation. *Endocrinology, 137*, 1212-1218.

Lopez, J. F., Chalmers, D. T., Little, K. Y., & Watson, S. J. (1998). A. E. Bennett Research Award. Regulation of serotonin1A, glucocorticoid, and mineralocorticoid receptor in rat and human hippocampus: implications for the neurobiology of depression. *Biological Psychiatry, 43*, 547-573.

Lyons, D. M., Martel, F. L., Levine, S., Risch, N. J., & Schatzberg, A. F. (1999). Postnatal experiences and genetic effects on squirrel monkey social affinities and emotional distress. *Hormones and Behavior, 36*, 266–275.

Makino, S., Hashimoto, K., & Gold, P. W. (2002). Multiple feedback mechanisms activating corticotropin-releasing hormone system in the brain during stress. *Pharmacology, Biochemistry and Behavior, 73*, 147-158.

Makino, S., Shibasaki, T., Yamauchi, N., Nishioka, T., Mimoto, T., Wakabayashi, I., Gold, P. W., & Hashimoto, K. (1999). Psychological stress increased corticotropin-releasing hormone mRNA and content in the central nucleus of the amygdala but not in the hypothalamic paraventricular nucleus in the rat. *Brain Research, 850*, 136-143.

McCauley, J., Kern, D. E., Kolodner, K., Dill, L., Schroeder, A. F., DeChant, H. K., Ryden, J., Derogatis, L. R., & Bass, E. B. (1997). Clinical characteristics of women with a history of childhood abuse: Unhealed wounds. *Journal of the American Medical Association, 277*, 1362-1368.

McClure, D. J. (1966). The diurnal variation of plasma cortisol levels in depression. *Journal of Psychosomatic Research, 10*, 189-195.

McQueen, G. M., Campbell, S., McEwen, B. S., Macdonald, K., Amano, S., Joffe, R. T., Nahmias, C., & Young, L. T. (2003). Course of illness, hippocampal function, and hippocampal volume in major depression. *Proceedings of the National Academy of Sciences of the United States of America, 100*, 1387-1392.

Mendels, J., & Frazer, A. (1974). Brain biogenic amine depletion and mood. *Archives of General Psychiatry, 30*, 447-451.

Merali, Z., Du, L., Hrdina, P., Palkovits, M., Faludi, G., Poulter, M. O., & Anisman, H. (2004). Dysregulation in the suicide brain: mRNA expression of corticotropin-releasing hormone receptors and GABA(A) receptor subunits in frontal cortical brain region. *Journal of Neuroscience, 24*, 1478-1485.

Meyers, B. S., Alexopoulos, G. S., Kakuma, T., Tirumalasetti, F., Gabriele, M., Alpert, S., Bowden, C., & Meltzer, H. Y. (1999). Decreased dopamine beta-hydroxylase activity in unipolar geriatric delusional depression. *Biological Psychiatry, 45*, 448-452.

Michelson, D., Stratakis, C., Hill, L., Reynolds, J., Galliven, E., Chrousos, G., & Gold, P. (1996). Bone mineral density in women with depression. *New England Journal of Medicine, 335*, 1176-1181.

Modell, S., Lauer, C. J., Schreiber, W., Huber, J., Krieg, J. C., & Holsboer, F. (1998). Hormonal response pattern in the combined DEX-CRF test is stable over time in subjects at high familial risk for affective disorders. *Neuropsychopharmacology, 18*, 253-262.

Musselman, D. L., Miller, A. H., Porter, M. R., Manatunga, A., Gao, F., Penna, S., Pearce, B. D., Landry, J., Glover, S., McDaniel, J. S., & Nemeroff, C. B. (2001). Patients with depression: Preliminary findings. *American Journal of Psychiatry, 158*, 1252-1257.

Nemeroff, C. B. (1992). New vistas in neuropeptide research in neuropsychiatry: Focus on corticotropin-releasing factor. *Neuropsychopharmacology, 6*, 69-75.

Nemeroff, C. B. (2003). *The neurobiological consequences of childhood abuse.* Presentation at the 2003 meeting of the American Psychiatric Association, San Francisco, CA, May 17-22, 2003.

Nemeroff, C. B., Krishnan, K. R., Reed, D., Leder, R., Beam, C., & Dunnick, N. R. (1992). Adrenal gland enlargement in major depression: A computed tomographic study. *Archives of General Psychiatry, 49*, 384-387.

Nemeroff, C. B., Owens, M. J., Bissette, G., Andorn, A. C., & Stanley, M. (1988). Reduced corticotropin releasing factor binding sites in the frontal cortex of suicide victims. *Archives of General Psychiatry,*

45, 577-579.

Nemeroff, C. B., Widerlov, E., Bissette, G., Walleus, H., Karlsson, I., Eklund, K., et al. (1984). Elevated concentrations of CSF corticotropin-releasing factor-like immunoreactivity in depressed patients. *Science, 226*, 1342-1344.

Newport, D. J., Heim, C., Owens, M. J., Ritchie, J. C., Ramsey, C. H., Bonsall, R., et al. (2003). Cerebrospinal fluid corticotropin-releasing factor (CRF) and vasopressin concentrations predict pituitary response in the CRF stimulation test: A multiple regression analysis. *Neuropsychopharmacology, 28*, 569-576.

Nikolarakis, K. E., Almeida, O. F., & Herz, A. (1986). Corticotropin-releasing factor (CRF) inhibits gonadotropin-releasing hormone (GnRH) release from superfused rat hypothalami in vitro. *Brain Research, 377*, 388-390.

Orth, D. N. (1992). Corticotropin-releasing hormone in humans. *Endocrine Reviews, 13*, 164-191.

Oshima, A., Yamashita, S., Owashi, T., Murata, T., Tadokoro, C., Miyaoka, H., Kamijima, K., & Higuchi, T. (2000). The differential ACTH responses to combined dexamethasone/CRF administration in major depressive and dysthymic disorders. *Journal of Psychiatric Research, 34*, 325-328.

Pacak, K., Tjurmina, O., Palkovits, M., Goldstein, D. S., Koch, C. A., Hoff, T., & Chrousos, G. P. (2002). Chronic hypercortisolemia inhibits dopamine synthesis and turnover in the nucleus accumbens: An in vivo microdialysis study. *Neuroendocrinology, 76*, 148-157.

Parker, A. J., Wessely, S., & Cleare, A. J. (2001). The neuroendocrinology of chronic fatigue syndrome and fibromyalgia. *Psychological Medicine, 31*, 1331-1345.

Plotsky, P. M., & Meaney, M. J. (1993). Early, postnatal experience alters hypothalamic corticotropin-releasing factor (CRF) mRNA, median eminence CRF content and stress-induced release in adult rats. *Brain Research. Molecular Brain Research, 18*, 195-200.

Posener, J. A., Wang, L., Price, J. L., Gado, M. H., Province, M. A., Miller, M. I., Babb, C. M., & Csernansky, J. G. (2003). High-dimensional mapping of the hippocampus in depression. *American Journal of Psychiatry, 160*, 83-89.

Pratt, L. A., Ford, D. E., Crum, R. M., Armenian, H. K., Gallo, J. J., & Eaton, W. W. (1996). Depression, psychotropic medication, and risk of myocardial infarction. Prospective data from the Baltimore ECA follow-up. *Circulation, 94*, 3123-3129.

Pryce, C. R., Ruedi-Bettschen, D., Dettling, A. C., & Feldon, J. (2002). Early life stress: Long-term physiological impact in rodents and primates. *News in Physiological Sciences, 17*, 150–155.

Raadsheer, F. C., van Heerikhuize, J. J., Lucassen, P. J., Hoogendijk, W. J., Tilders, F. J., & Swaab, D. F. (1995). Corticotropin-releasing hormone mRNA levels in the paraventricular nucleus of patients with Alzheimer's disease and depression. *American Journal of Psychiatry, 152*, 1372-1376.

Raza, J., Massoud, A. F., Hindmarsh, P. C., Robinson, I. C., & Brook, C. G. (1998). Direct effects of corticotrophin-releasing hormone on stimulated growth hormone secretion. *Clinical Endocrinology, 48*, 217-222.

Reichardt, H. M., Kaestner, K. H., Tuckermann, J., Kretz, O., Wessely, O., Bock, R., Gass, P., Schmid, W., Herrlich, P., Angel, P., & Schutz, G. (1998). DNA binding of the glucocorticoid receptor is not essential for survival. *Cell, 93*, 531-541.

Ressler, K. J., & Nemeroff, C. B. (1999). Role of norepinephrine in the pathophysiology and treatment of mood disorders. *Biological Psychiatry, 46*, 1219-1233.

Ribeiro, S. C., Tandon, R., Grunhaus, L., & Greden, J. F. (1993). The DST as a predictor of outcome in depression: A meta-analysis. *American Journal of Psychiatry, 150*, 1618-1629.

Rinne, T., de Kloet, R., Wouters, L., Goekoop, J. G., DeRijk, R. H., & van den Brink, W. (2002). Hyperresponsiveness of hypothalamic-pituitary-adrenal axis to combined dexamethasone/corticotropin-releasing hormone challenge in female borderline personality disorder subjects with a history of sustained childhood abuse. *Biological Psychiatry, 52*, 1102-1112.

Risch, S. C., Lewine, R. J., Kalin, N. H., Jewart, R. D., Risby, E. D., Caudle, J. M., Stipetic, M., Turner, J., Eccard, M. B., & Pollard, W.E. (1992). Limbic-hypothalamic-pituitary-adrenal axis activity and ventricular-to-brain ratio studies in affective illness and schizophrenia. *Neuropsychopharmacology, 6*, 95-100.

Rivest, S., Laflamme, N., & Nappi, R. E. (1995). Immune challenge and immobilization stress induce transcription of the gene encoding the CRF receptor in selective nuclei of the rat hypothalamus. *Journal of Neuroscience, 15*, 2680-2695.

Sachar, E. J., Hellman, L., Fukushima, D. K., & Gallagher, T. F. (1970). Cortisol production in depressive illness. A clinical and biochemical clarification. *Archives of General Psychiatry, 23*, 289-298.

Sanchez, M. M., Ladd, C. O., & Plotsky, P. M. (2001). Early adverse experience as a developmental risk factor for later psychopathology: Evidence from rodent and primate models. *Developmental Psychopathology, 13*, 419–449.

Sapolsky, R. M. (1990). Glucocorticoids, hippocampal damage and the glutamatergic synapse. *Progress in Brain Research, 86*, 13-23.

Schweiger, U., Weber, B., Deuschle, M., & Heuser, I. (2000). Lumbar bone mineral density in patients with major depression: Evidence of increased bone loss at follow-up. *American Journal of Psychiatry, 157*, 118-120.

Scott, L. V., Teh, J., Reznek, R., Martin, A., Sohaib, A., & Dinan, T. G. (1999). Small adrenal glands in chronic fatigue syndrome: A preliminary computer tomography study. *Psychoneuroendocrinology, 24*, 759-768.

Seasholtz, A. F., Burrows, H. L., Karolyi, I. J., & Camper, S. A. (2001). Mouse models of altered CRH-binding protein expression. *Peptides, 22*, 743-751.

Smith, M. A., Davidson, J., Ritchie, J. C., Kudler, H., Lipper, S., Chappell, P., & Nemeroff, C. B. (1989). The corticotropin-releasing hormone test in patients with posttraumatic stress disorder. *Biological Psychiatry, 26*, 349-355.

Stein, M. B., Yehuda, R., Koverola, C., & Hanna, C. (1997). Enhanced dexamethasone suppression of plasma cortisol in adult women traumatized by childhood sexual abuse. *Biological Psychiatry, 42*, 680-686.

Swanson, L. W., Sawchenko, P. E., Rivier, J., & Vale, W. W. (1983). Organization of ovine corticotropin-releasing factor immunoreactive cells and fibers in the rat brain: An immunohistochemical study. *Neuroendocrinology, 36*, 165-186.

Swanson, L. W., & Simmons, D. M. (1989). Differential steroid hormone and neural influences on peptide mRNA levels in CRF cells of the paraventricular nucleus: A hybridization histochemical study in the rat. *Journal of Comparative Neurology, 285*, 413-435.

Tennant, C. (2002). Life events, stress and depression: A review of recent findings. *Australian and New Zealand Journal of Psychiatry, 36*, 173-182.

Thakore, J. H., Richards, P. J., Reznek, R. H., Martin, A., & Dinan, T. G. (1997). Increased intra-abdominal fat deposition in patients with major depressive illness as measured by computed tomography. *Biological Psychiatry, 41*, 1140-1142.

Timpl, P., Spanagel, R., Sillaber, I., Kresse, A., Reul, J. M. H. M., Stalla, G. K., Blanquet, V., Steckler, T., Holsboer, F., & Wurst, W. (1998). Impaired stress response and reduced anxiety in mice lacking a functional corticotropin-releasing hormone receptor 1. *Nature Genetics, 19*, 162-166.

Tronche, F., Kellendonk, C., Kretz, O., Gass, P., Anlag, K., Orban, P. C., Bock, R., Klein, R., & Schutz, G. (1999). Disruption of the glucocorticoid receptor gene in the nervous system results in reduced anxiety. *Nature Genetics, 23*, 99-103.

Vaillant, G. E. (1998). Natural history of male psychological health, XIV: Relationship of mood disorder vulnerability to physical health. *American Journal of Psychiatry, 155*, 184-191.

Vakili, K., Pillay, S. S., Lafer, B., Fava, M., Renshaw, P. F., Bonello-Cintron, C. M., & Yurgelun-Todd, D. A. (2000). Hippocampal volume in primary unipolar major depression: A magnetic resonance imaging study. *Biological Psychiatry, 47*, 1087-1090.

Vale, W., Spiess, J., Rivier, C., & Rivier, J. (1981). Characterization of a 41-residue ovine hypothalamic peptide that stimulates secretion of corticotropin and beta-endorphin. *Science, 213*, 1394-1397.

Vazquez, D. M. (1998). Stress and the developing limbic-hypothalamic-pituitary-adrenal axis. *Psychoneuroendocrinology, 23*, 663-700.

Villafuerte, S. M., Del-Favero, J., Adolfsson, R., Souery, D., Massat, I., Mendlewicz, J., Van Broeckhoven, C., & Claes, S. (2002). Gene-based SNP genetic association study of the corticotropin-releasing hormone receptor-2 (CRFR2) in major depression. *American Journal of Medical Genetics, 114*, 222-226.

Vythilingam, M., Heim, C., Newport, J., Miller, A. H., Anderson, E., Bronen, R., Brummer, M., Staib, L., Vermetten, E., Charney, D. S., Nemeroff, C. B., & Bremner, J. D. (2002). Childhood trauma associated with smaller hippocampal volume in women with major depression. *American Journal of Psychiatry, 159*, 2072-2080.

Watson, S., Gallagher, P., Ritchie, J. C., Ferrier, I. N., & Young, A. H. (2004). Hypothalamic-pituitary-adrenal axis function in patients with bipolar disorder. *British Journal of Psychiatry, 184*, 496-502.

Yehuda, R. (2001). Biology of posttraumatic stress disorder. *Journal of Clinical Psychiatry, 62 (Suppl 17)*, 41-46.

Yehuda, R., Boisoneau, D., Lowy, M. T., & Giller, E. L., Jr. (1995). Dose-response changes in plasma cortisol and lymphocyte glucocorticoid receptors following dexamethasone administration in combat veterans with and without posttraumatic stress disorder. *Archives of General Psychiatry, 52,* 583-593.

Yehuda, R., Boisoneau, D., Mason, J. W., & Giller, E. L. (1993). Glucocorticoid receptor number and cortisol excretion in mood, anxiety, and psychotic disorders. *Biological Psychiatry, 34,* 18-25.

Zobel, A. W., Nickel, T., Künzel, H. E., Ackl, N., Sonntag, A., Ising, M., & Holsboer, F. (2000). Effects of the high-affinity corticotropin-releasing hormone receptor 1 antagonist R121919 in major depression: The first 20 patients treated. *Journal of Psychiatry Research, 34,* 171-181.

Zobel, A. W., Yassouridis, A., Friesboer, R. M., & Holsboer, F. (1999). Prediction of medium-term outcome by cortisol response to the combined Dexamethasone-CRF test in patients with remitted depression. *American Journal of Psychiatry, 156,* 949-951.

Epilogue

Towards Integration in the Theory and Treatment of Depression?

The Time is Now

Patrick Luyten, Sidney J. Blatt, & Jozef Corveleyn

The chapters in this book represent a wide diversity of approaches to research on depression, including epidemiological, cognitive-behavioral, psychodynamic, developmental psychopathological, and neurobiological approaches. Some readers may wonder whether there is any common ground between these approaches. We believe and hope to demonstrate that there is.

In what follows, we will first discuss what we believe to be five major common themes that come to the fore in many, if not most, chapters of this volume. These are: (1) a general dissatisfaction with the DSM approach of depression, (2) a focus on personality dimensions and on mental representations or cognitive-affective structures, (3) the importance of interpersonal and (4) environmental factors, and finally (5) the need for a developmental perspective on depression. One of the primary goals of this discussion is to foster a dialogue that attempts to stimulate integration among various theoretical and methodological approaches to research on depression. Along the way, we will also propose an etiologically-based, transdiagnostic dynamic interactionism model as an alternative for the DSM view of depression. In this model, we will emphasize the centrality of maladaptive mental representations of self and other in both the development as well as the treatment of depression and other disorders. Although our focus will primarily be on psychodynamic, cognitive-behavioral and neurobiological approaches, we will attempt to integrate aspects from other approaches as well, including psychiatric genetics, developmental psychopathology, social cognition, and attachment theory. Finally, we will consider future research tasks and the clinical implications that follow from the proposed dynamic interactionism model.

Avenues For Further Integration

Dissatisfaction with the DSM: Plea for a Transdiagnostic Perspective

Dissatisfaction with DSM. Most frequently emphasized in the various chapters and perhaps the most important finding of this book, is the general *dissatisfaction with the categorical view of depression in the DSM.* Time and again, research from perspectives as diverse as epidemiology, cognitive-behavioral and psychodynamic models of depression, developmental psychopathology, and neurobiology, point to serious problems with the DSM taxonomic approach. These issues with DSM are of central concern because the development of a valid taxonomic system is central to all research on psychopathology, including depression.

First, DSM distinguishes several categories of depression (e.g., major depression versus minor depression or dysthymia) mainly on the basis of differences in severity. Research, however, shows that a dimensional view, which conceptualizes depression as situated on a continuum from mild dysphoria to full-blown clinical depression, is more valid and useful than the DSM categorical view (see Demyttenaere, Van Oudenhove, & De Fruyt, Chapter 1, this volume). DSM appears not to "carve nature at its joints" but rather introduces sharp distinctions where they do not, in reality, exist (Kendler & Gardner, 1998; Solomon, Haaga, & Arnow, 2001). This reliance on a weak categorical system seriously impedes all research efforts. One of the many negative consequences of the creation of these "pseudo-entities" (Parker, 1999, p. 102) is the underestimation of the importance of "subclinical" depressive symptoms and syndromes (such as minor depression, subthreshold depression) (Kessler et al., 2003). Recent research has clearly demonstrated both the clinical importance of such subclinical mood disturbances in predicting later psychopathology and severe psychosocial impairment (e.g., Kessler et al., 2003; Judd, Akiskal, & Paulus, 1997), as well as identifying the continuity between biopsychosocial factors implied in both "subclinical" and "clinical" mood disturbances (e.g., Ormel, Oldehinkel, & Brilman, 2001).

Second, under the influence of the DSM, depression has been increasingly considered as a disease with a specific etiology and pathogenesis, and as a state which is clearly distinct from "normality", from normal sadness and from other psychiatric disorders. This has had serious unfortunate consequences. Research has been overly focused on trying to establish the "unique" etiology and characteristics of depression (see also Van Praag, de Kloet, & van Os, 2004). From a treatment perspective, psychiatrists and clinical psychologists have started treating disorders and their symptoms instead of individuals. This is further amplified by the DSM assumption that Axis I disorders and personality characteristics are completely independent because DSM assumes that Axis I and Axis II are orthogonal and thus independent. This view has led to an increasingly confusing literature on the comorbidity of depression (and other Axis I disorders) and Axis II disorders. If there is one conclusion that can be drawn about this literature, apart from the fact that Axis II itself suffers from serious validity problems (Shedler & Westen, 2004), is that depression and personality (disorders) are closely associated and even causally linked. Thus, the DSM view that depression and personality are orthogonal is clearly incorrect. Moreover, apart from this issue of the relation of personality disorders to depression, the DSM approach has contributed to investigators underestimating the importance of *subclinical* personality problems (e.g., enduring problems concerning intimacy and relatedness), which are present in many if not most depressed patients (Blatt, 2004; Morrison, Bradley, & Westen, 2003). As reviewed in Chapter 4, research has for example clearly identified the causal relationship between the personality dimensions of Dependency/Sociotropy and Self-Critical Perfectionism/Autonomy and depression. These cognitive-affective styles appear to be relatively unresponsive to brief treatments, and probably require more intensive treatment (Blatt, 2004; see also Chapter 4, this volume).

DSM has also promoted the view that individuals with Axis I disorders such as depression are "hosts" for a certain "pathogen". Yet, as Westen and Shedler (2000) have pointed out, while this disease analogy might be appropriate for some forms of psychopathology (e.g., Posttraumatic Stress Disorder after severe trauma), for many difficulties it is clearly not. Congruent with research findings reviewed in this book this "analogy quickly breaks down because 'host' and 'pathogen' are not so neatly distinguishable in the psychological realm. Humans often seek, evoke, or elicit the environmental pathogens to which they are then exposed" (Westen & Shedler, 2000, p. 113; see also Blatt & Zuroff, 1992). In sum, DSM has introduced an arbitrary and unproductive distinction between axis I and II, thereby neglecting the important role of personality factors in psychopathology. Both in diagnosis and in treatment, much is to be gained by a person rather than a symptom focus — that it is important to evaluate the life experiences and the meaning structures that determine how people experience their world, both in normal as well as in disrupted functioning.

A person focus is also consistent with the conceptualization of depression in this volume as a deviation of "normal" development, which can vary in intensity (e.g., see Chapters 3, 5, 7, and 8 in this volume). Depression, according to this view, is a more or less "normal" phenomenon that is intimately tied to the human condition and not so much a disease that is present in those unfortunate individuals who have a particular, although as yet unknown, (biological) vulnerability. The ubiquity of depression has been demonstrated, for example, by Monroe and Simons (1991). These investigators have shown that while the risk of becoming clinically depressed after one severe negative life event is relatively small, the likelihood of becoming depressed rises considerably with each new negative life event until, under increasing stress, almost everyone becomes clinically depressed. In fact, perhaps with the exception of some extremely resilient individuals (Bonnano, 2004), after experiencing three or more severe negative life events in a one year period almost everyone becomes depressed (Monroe & Simons, 1991). Findings such as these seriously challenge the view that depression is a disease that is only present in some unfortunate few. Instead, these findings favor the view that depression is a disorder that is intrinsically associated with human development and life experiences (see also Chapters 3 and 7, this volume).

Third, the DSM promotes a disease model of depression that defines depression by a number of symptoms, and the outcome of treatment with an almost exclusive focus on symptom reduction. It has become increasingly clear, however, that treatments that focus on symptom reduction alone are insufficient. On average, two thirds of patients relapse after brief, symptom-focused treatments of depression (Westen & Morrison, 2001; Westen, Novotny, & Thompson-Brenner, 2004a; Zuroff & Blatt, 2002). Moreover, as we will discuss in detail below, although depressive symptoms may quickly disappear in symptom focused treatments, underlying vulnerabilities, including impaired and disrupted interpersonal relationships, are likely to persist. Hence, treatment needs to focus on underlying vulnerability factors to prevent future relapse, a theme that is echoed in many chapters in this volume.

Fourth, one of the major limitations of DSM is its focus on manifest symptomatology to define psychopathology. This is particularly true concerning the diagnosis of major depression, the main depression category in DSM, which can be diagnosed based on almost any combination of a number of symptoms. Because of this a-etiological view, individuals who receive a DSM diagnosis such as major depression are a very heterogeneous group in terms of etiology and pathogenesis (Parker, 2000). This is detrimental for both research as well as clinical practice (Van Praag et al., 2004). For example, often a world of difference exists between someone who becomes depressed after losing a partner in a car accident, versus an overly dependent individual that becomes depressed after his or her partner ends their relationship after twenty long years of relational conflicts, struggles, and frustrations. Although both would receive a DSM diagnosis major depressive disorder, first episode, it is very likely that the course and prognosis in both individuals will be markedly different. Moreover, congruent with findings that depression, personality, and environmental factors reciprocally influence one another, it is also important to take into account the active role of individuals in creating their own "depressogenic" environment, as well as both intrapersonal and interpersonal changes as a consequence of being depressed (see Chapter 4 and Chapter 5, this volume).

An alternative: An etiologically-based, dynamic interactionism approach. To summarize, although the DSM approach to mood disorders has led to important insights and discoveries, it is clearly limited. Despite much dissatisfaction with this approach in clinicians and researchers, the DSM approach continues to dominate both research and treatment guidelines. However, the time appears ripe for developing a more valid, etiologically-based diagnostic system (Blatt & Levy, 1998) that takes into account the dynamic interactionism between person, environment, and depression (Blatt, 2004; Kendler, Kuhn, & Prescott, 2004; Zuroff, Mongrain, & Santor, 2004), and that considers depression as a disorder that is linked to normal development (Blatt & Levy, 1998). Ideally, such a diagnostic system would consist of several components or axes:

(1) We believe that assessment should start with a detailed *descriptive diagnosis* that documents depressive symptoms as well as their severity. This enables the clinician to appreciate the nature of a patient's complaints, as well as their influence on daily functioning. Moreover, a descriptive diagnosis should also contain important leads concerning etiological and pathogenetic factors. Although historically many unsuccessful attempts have been made to identify distinct depressive subtypes based on symptoms, future research might identify distinct clusters of symptoms that delineate specific depressive disorders. For example, there is increasing evidence for the existence of a melancholic subtype of depression, which is mainly characterized by pronounced psychomotor retardation (Parker, 2000; Pier, Hulstijn, & Sabbe, 2004). Likewise, anxious and hostile or irritable subgroups of non-melancholic depression may exist, which are presumably linked to temperament and personality features (Parker et al., 1998, 1999a, 1999b) such as Dependency/Sociotropy versus Self-Critical Perfectionism/ Autonomy respectively. Next, future studies should investigate whether these subtypes, if they exist, are associated with a different course, prognosis, etiology, pathogenesis, and treatment responsivity. For instance, evidence suggests that the melancholic subtype of depression (and psychomotor retardation in particular) is associated with a positive response to antidepressant treatment (Pier et al., 2004) and electroconvulsive therapy (Parker, 2000). In addition, both clinicians and researchers as well as insurance companies might find it often more convenient to speak in terms of categories (see also Chapter 1, this volume). Furthermore, the fact that depression generally is situated on a continuum does not necessarily exclude the existence of some discrete categories of depression (such as the melancholic subtype) (see also Parker, 2000). The (methodological) challenge for future research might lie in integrating continuous/dimensional and categorical viewpoints with the hope that this would improve the validity of diagnostic distinctions.

(2) The next step in diagnosis should consist of a consideration of depression from a *dimensional perspective*. From a clinical point of view, many patients present with depressive problems that warrant clinical attention, but cannot be adequately diagnosed by DSM. Many of these patients receive diagnoses such as "minor depression, "subclinical depression", "subthreshold depression", or "depression not otherwise specified". As reviewed in Chapter 1, no real "cut-off" exists between these "subclinical" syndromes and clinical depression. While some distinct symptom-defined subtypes of depression, qualitatively different from each other and/or from "subclinical" depression or dysphoria may exist, as stated before, depression appears to be best situated on a continuum going from mild dysphoria to full-blown clinical depression (Blatt, 1974, 2004). In addition, as stated earlier, the biopsychosocial processes implied in the etiology and pathogenesis of "normal"

257

(e.g., normal sadness), "subclinical" (often referred to as distress) and "clinical" depression are essentially the same. Hence it is important to assess mood and mood fluctuations across the life span. For example, when did the first signs of mood change appear? Are we dealing with a person who has suffered from continuous bouts of depression? Or are depressive moods always associated with severe events, and, if so, what is the nature of these events? Consideration of such issues almost automatically leads to a third component in the process of diagnosing – the factors involved in the etiology and pathogenesis.

(3) The next step is thus to consider factors involved in the *etiology* and *pathogenesis*. It is very unlikely that clinical symptoms alone are sufficient to identify etiological and pathogenetical factors implied in subclinical and clinical depression (Blatt, 2004; Parker, 2000). And it is likely that several etiological and pathogenetic pathways exist towards subclinical and clinical depression. As various chapters in this book emphasize, careful attention should be given to environmental factors such as parental style, early life stress, life events, chronic stress, and daily hassles, and cognitive-affective schemas or personality styles such as Dependency/Sociotropy and Self-Critical Perfectionism/Autonomy. In addition, the interaction between these factors in the developmental history of the individual should be carefully mapped (see Chapter 4 and Chapter 5, this volume; Ormel et al., 2001). Furthermore, apart from the identification of vulnerabilities, strengths or resilience should be taken into account, as they provide important clues with regard to both biological and psychosocial processes implied in depression (e.g., Bonnano, 2004; Charney, 2004). Moreover, for too long, diagnosis has been exclusively aimed at documenting deficits, and neglecting strengths and possibilities.

These considerations concerning etiology and pathogenesis are likely to lead to a more relativistic view of diagnosis because the psychosocial (e.g., Chapters 3 and 6, this volume) and biological (e.g., Chapter 6, this volume) processes implied in depression are likely to be related to many other disorders. Hence, we believe that a *transdiagnostic perspective* should be adopted in diagnosing different forms of psychopathology including depression. In contrast to DSM, research findings suggest that it is very unlikely that each psychopathological disorder has its unique and specific etiology and pathogenesis. The same holds for what is now currently considered as subthreshold psychiatric conditions (e.g., Lewinsohn, Shankman, Gau, & Klein, 2004). For example, the effects of early life stress on HPA axis functioning are likely to play a role in several psychopathological (e.g., depression, PTSD), functional (e.g., Chronic Fatigue Syndrome), as well as medical disorders (see Chapter 8, this volume; see also Segerstrom & Miller, 2004; Van Houdenhove & Egle, 2004). Likewise, there appear to be few life events that specifically predict depression (Paykel, 2003). And finally, personality factors such as Dependency/ Sociotropy and Self-Critical Perfectionism/Autonomy have been shown to play a role in various other disorders than depression (e.g., Blatt, 2004; Blatt & Shichman, 1983; Shafran & Mansell, 2001), and may explain the high comorbidity between various Axis I and Axis II disorders (Bieling, Summerfeldt, Israeli, & Antony, 2004; Blatt & Levy, 1998).

Hence, research and assessment should concentrate on charting the various biopsychosocial processes implied in normal development, and in deviations from normal development, and how these deviations can be expressed in various (clusters of) disorders (Blatt, 1995; Blatt & Levy, 1998; Blatt & Shichman, 1983). Here, the developmental psychopathological principles of equifinality and multifinality may assist in clarifying this argument (Cicchetti & Cohen, 1995). The principle of equifinality, rather than assuming that one single etiology exists for a disorder, as is currently implied by DSM, holds that various etiological pathways are possible towards one disorder. In contrast, the principle of multifinality refers to the fact that the same etiological factors may result, depending on other influences, in a variety of disorders. Thus, various etiological pathways may exist towards depression, as suggested by recent psychodynamic and cognitive-behavioral formulations (see Chapter 3, this volume), whereas the same etiological factors may results in various disorders, as suggested by neurobiological research on stress and the HPA axis (see Chapter 8, this volume). Hence, patients with the same clinical presentation may have a very different etiological background and patients with similar etiological backgrounds, depending on other factors, may express their problems in different ways. Thus, assessment should not be solely aimed at diagnosing a particular *disorder at a particular moment in time*, but should include a developmental assessment of the underlying vulnerabilities as well as strengths of an *individual*, which should then inform treatment options *for that individual*. Much can be gained, in our view, from this person, rather than symptom or disorder-focused approach.

For example, early in adolescence, because of emotional neglect and abuse, a young boy may start to experience problems in relating to peers, teachers, and parents. As is often the case, he may express these difficulties primarily in school and conduct problems. Later on, he may start experimenting with drugs to compensate for his feelings of emptiness. Then, faced with the realities of adult life, he may start to show the first signs of a mixed anxious/depressed condition, which is subdued when he believes he has met the girl of his life. However, because he is overly dependent on her, he is very jealous and clinging, and she ends the relationship, and he becomes severely depressed. From a DSM perspective, this individual would have had several clinical and subclinical diagnoses. Although perhaps correct from a descriptive perspective, it would be incorrect to assume that he has several "diseases" (e.g., conduct disorder, substance abuse disorder, dysthymia), each associated with a particular vulnerability, and each needing a different treatment approach. Rather, at various points in life, his problems, influenced by many psychosocial and biological variables, are expressed in different ways (see also Harrington, 2001). At various points in life, his life could have taken different paths (e.g., what if a teacher or an athletic coach had taken a particular interest in him, or if he had met another girl, or moved to another part of the country, or had found a job that gave him some satisfaction and recognition?).

Ample evidence supports the principles of equifinality and multifinality in the development of psychological disturbances (Cicchetti & Cohen, 1995). Concerning depression, several studies have shown that etiological and pathogenetic factors implied in depression are also found in a variety of other disorders (multifinality), which is reflected in the high comorbidity between depression and other Axis I, such as anxiety disorders (Nemeroff, 2002) and Axis II disorders. On the other hand, there are several etiological and pathogenetic pathways to depression (equifinality) (e.g., Blatt, 2004; Claes, 2003; Gilmer & McKinney, 2003; Kasen et al., 2001; Klein, Lewinsohn, Seeley, & Rohde, 2001; Lewinsohn, Rohde, Seeley, Klein, & Gotlib, 2003; Weissman et al., 1999a, 1999b).

(4) Finally, descriptive/categorical, dimensional and etiological/pathogenetic considerations should be combined in making a systematic statement concerning the *likely course* and *prognosis* of the disorder, as well as the *treatment possibilities*. We will return to this issue further below.

Although such a transdiagnostic, multiaxial dynamic interactionist model of diagnosing depression is not currently used in mainstream research, many important aspects of this interactional model have been fairly clearly documented by research over recent decades, as discussed in the various chapters in this volume. For example, research has clearly shown how cognitive-affective styles such as Dependency/Sociotropy and Self-Critical Perfectionism/Autonomy interact with (congruent) life events in predicting depression (see Chapter 4 and 5, this volume). Likewise, the role of early adversity, and its impact on both neurobiological and psychosocial factors implied in depression, has now been clearly established (see Chapter 8, this volume). Other pieces of the puzzle (e.g., how genetic factors determine temperament and subsequent personality development, and how these factors interact with specific parental styles) can be, at least in principle, investigated (see also Van Praag et al., 2004). Moreover, in clinical practice, regardless of theoretical orientation, many clinicians (implicitly) use such an etiologically-based diagnostic model, as both common sense and research suggests (e.g., Morrison et al., 2003). Yet, as long as the DSM categorical disease view continues to dominate depression research and treatment guidelines, and research funding continues to depend largely on the adoption of this approach, there is little reason to believe that research programs including treatment research will seek to develop an alternative diagnostic system (Westen et al., 2004a).

Personality and Mental Representations or Cognitive-Affective Schemas

A second area of convergence in this volume concerns the emphasis on personality and mental representations or cognitive-affective schemas and depression. This appears to be a particularly fruitful area for dialogue and integration among the various approaches to depression because the notion of mental representation or cognitive-affective schema is a central construct not only in psychodynamic object-relational and cognitive-behavioral formulations, but also in cognitive science, social psychology, developmental psychopathology, and attachment theory (Blatt, Auerbach, & Levy, 1997), and thus may provide a common language for many investigators and clinicians.

Research from various theoretical perspectives has contributed to our knowledge concerning how mental representations of self and others develop throughout life from the early infant-caregiver relationship to senescence, and how they organize, shape and guide our cognitions, affects, and behaviors (Blatt et al., 1997). Moreover, our knowledge of both adaptive and maladaptive pathways in the development of mental representations has increased substantially, particularly with the advent of object-relational psychoanalytic theory, attachment theory, and developmental psychopathology. It has now become clear that specific forms or clusters of psychopathology are associated with specific disturbances in the content and/or structure of mental representations (Blatt, 1995; Blatt et al., 1997). For instance, various psychodynamic (e.g., Blatt, 1974, 1995, 2004; Westen, 2002) and cognitive-behavioral (Beck, 1999; Linehan, 1993; Young, 1999) investigators link psychopathology with specific disturbances in the content and/or structure of mental representations. In fact, it can be argued that all major psychological theories of depression focus on aspects of mental representations as a major factor in depression and a major factor in the treatment process (Blatt, 2004; Blatt, Stayner, Auerbach, & Behrends, 1996). Most theorists, like Beck (1999), focus on the content of these representations, while psychodynamic formulations often focus more on the structural (cognitive or developmental) organizations of these representations (e.g., Blatt, 1995; Blatt et al., 1996; Westen, 2002) because these reflect more implicit or procedural aspects of these cognitive structures as well as important developmental characteristics.

It is interesting to note that theoretical formulations have increasingly linked these disturbances in mental representations with broader personality dimensions. This is not only the case in psychodynamic formulations, but also in cognitive-behavioral theory, as is exemplified by the work of Beck (1999), Linehan (1993), and Young (1999). As Beck (1999) explains, considerations concerning personality and personality structure once were considered to be typical of psychodynamic formulations but cognitive-behavioral approaches have shifted from an exclusive focus on the symptomatic expressions of depression to considerations concerning personality and personality structure as vital to an understanding of psychopathology (Beck, 1999). Despite symptomatic improvement, many patients, particularly those with personality disorders, relapse because of continuing vulnerability associated with often highly resistant cognitive-affective schemas that are deeply embedded in the personality of an individual. This turn towards personality in cognitive-behavioral research has resulted primarily from the disappointing results of "traditional" cognitive-behavior therapy with many patients, and the realization that treatment should not be exclusively aimed at "surface" cognitions and symptom relief, but at reducing underlying vulnerabilities such as rather stable and relatively resistance cognitive-affective schemas to prevent relapse. Interestingly, this change has also been accompanied by the growing importance of developmental considerations within the cognitive-behavioral movement. Young (1999), for example, has been a strong advocate of introducing the notion of "Early Maladaptive Schemas" (EMS), i.e., maladaptive schemas that develop early in life, into cognitive-behavioral theory.

Thus, the construct of mental representations may provide a bridge between clinicians and investigators from various theoretical orientations. What these various theoretical formulations concerning mental representations have in common, is that they not only propose that representations of self and other are relatively stable characteristics that organize and guide the individual's affects, cognitions, and behaviors, but that treatment can be seen as a process aimed at changing the content and/or structure of these representations (Bateman & Fonagy, 2004; Blatt et al., 1996; Blatt et al., 1997). An important question for further research will be whether these mental representations or cognitive-affective schemas can be changed (that is, become developmentally more mature and adaptive) via cognitive suggestions that focus on the content of representations (e.g., to think differently about yourself and others) or whether changes in these cognitive-affective schemas can most effectively occur, with strength and stability, primarily as they are experienced in an intense interpersonal relationship such as the therapeutic relationship, where one begins to relinquish prior maladaptive, inappropriate, and developmentally more primitive representations through experiencing and becoming aware of their repetitive distortion of life experiences, and replacing these impaired representations with new, more adaptive representations of self and others as they are experienced in the intensity of the therapeutic relationship, implying a focus on both content and structural characteristics (Blatt et al., 1996).

Furthermore, a change in mental representations can range from the micro-level (e.g., targeting overgeneral autobiographical memories, see Chapter 2, this volume), traditionally the level at which cognitive-behavior therapy is aimed, to the macro-level (e.g., discussing broader issues concerning personality or cognitive-affective schemas associated with Dependency/Sociotropy and Self-Critical Perfectionism/Autonomy (Blatt, 1974; see Chapter 3, this volume), traditionally the level on which psychodynamic psychotherapy focuses (Westen, 2000). Hence, the concept of mental representation may link micro- and macro-processes in psychopathology and foster further dialogue between treatment strategies that are mainly directed at micro-processes (e.g., CBT) versus macro-processes (e.g., psychodynamic psychotherapy). In addition, because various theoretical formulations concerning mental representations include a developmental perspective (e.g., cognitive developmental psychology, attachment theory, object-relational psychodynamic formulations), these concepts may also foster integration with developmentally based assessment and treatment (see also Chapter 7, this volume).

Research on mental representations may also provide a bridge between different areas of research. In Chapter 2, Hermans, Raes and Eelen, for example, illustrate how theoretical and methodological approaches in cognitive science may inform clinical research on the role of (autobiographical) memory in depression. They show how mental representations in depressed patients tend to be overgeneral and how memory tends to be selective, resulting in a rapid onset and the eventual deepening of depressed mood. Investigation of relations between these memory disturbances in depression and broad cognitive-affective schemas associated with Dependency/Sociotropy and Self-Critical Perfectionism/Autonomy (e.g., Blatt, 1974; Blatt, Wein, Chevron, & Quinlan, 1979; Moore & Blackburn, 1993; Nunn, Mathews, & Trower, 1997), could foster the interchange between cognitive science and clinical research.

Finally, an important issue for further research is the neurobiology of mental representations. As Herman et al. suggest in Chapter 2, new techniques such as brain imaging are likely to play a vital role in furthering our knowledge of the relationship between the psychology and neurobiology of mental representations (Beutel, Stern, & Silbersweig, 2003; Goldapple et al., 2004; Laakso et al., 2003).

A Focus on the Interpersonal Context of Depression

Psychological formulations concerning depression often debate the question whether depression has mainly intrapsychic versus interpersonal origins. It is clear from the various contributions to this volume that this is unproductive. Both theoretical formulations and empirical research demonstrate that intrapsychic and interpersonal factors are intertwined (e.g., Joiner, 2001; Shahar, Blatt, Zuroff, Krupnick, & Sotsky, 2004; see also Chapter 3, this volume), and that both are often two sides of the same coin. Again, a focus on mental representations may help bridge the intrapersonal-interpersonal gap, because developmental research has clearly shown how interactions with significant others, from early on, form the basis of representations of self and other – the building blocks of relatively stable cognitive-affective schemas or internal working models that organize and guide the individual (Blatt, 1991, 1995; Blatt et al., 1997; Bowlby, 1988; Main, Kaplan, & Cassidy, 1985; Stern, 1985).

Aside from these theoretical considerations, research reviewed in this volume (e.g., see Chapter 4, 5 and 8, this volume) clearly shows the central importance of interpersonal processes in the pathogenesis, etiology, maintenance, relapse, and treatment of depression (see also Beach, 2001; Brown & Harris, 1978; Coyne, Burchill, & Stiles, 1991; Joiner, Metalsky, Katz, & Beach, 1999; Segrin, 2000; Tse & Bond, 2004). Depression is not just a "personal pathology", but also a "relational pathology" (Hammen, 2003). Again, these findings caution against considering depression as a disease that should be treated by a symptom-focused approach. Moreover, the individual is not merely a host to a pathogen, to which he or she passively responds. To the contrary, as reviewed in Chapter 4 and 5, specific interpersonal styles not only play a role in the etiology and pathogenesis of depression, but being depressed also leads to further relational problems (e.g., lowered social skills, contempt and rejection by others, etc.), leading to a vicious cycle (Wachtel, 1997), so that after the depression has remitted, a "depressogenic" interpersonal style, with its associated conflicts, may persist. Consider, for example, an overly dependent woman who is admitted to hospital because of severe depression after her husband left her. Although she may be feeling much better after a couple of weeks, when she returns home she is not only faced with the fact that she probably lost her husband, and therefore has to re-arrange her life completely, but others in her environment have not forgotten how depressed she was and how she, for instance, has threatened to kill herself in front of her children. Perhaps her children are now afraid of her, and prefer to live with their father. In addition, although she may be feeling better, her dependent, clinging relational style may persist. Thus, often, the individual remains at considerable risk for relapse, particularly because such vicious cycles, resulting from a dysfunctional transactional style (see Chapter 4, this volume), are easily activated because of the bias in the encoding and perception typical of depressed patients. As Hermans et al. argue in Chapter 2, for depressed individuals "everything seems to come back" very quickly, in part because of their biased perception and underlying fears which they tend to confirm by their interpersonal style (see Chapter 4, this volume).

Thus, an important area for future research is the integration of current formulations concerning interpersonal processes in depression, including psychodynamic (e.g., Blatt, 2004) and cognitive-behavioral (e.g., Beck, 1983; Safran & Segal, 1990), with approaches such as systems and family approaches (see Beach, 2001). From a clinical perspective, the central importance of interpersonal processes in the etiology and pathogenesis of depression suggests an urgent need to incorporate interventions more explicitly aimed at relational processes in the treatment of depression (Hammen, 2003) as expressed in Interpersonal Therapy (IPT), a treatment that focuses on contemporary interpersonal relationships, and, more generally, in a relational emphasis in individual psychotherapy as expressed in understanding transference enactments of repetitive interpersonal patterns. In particular, the therapeutic relationship provides the basis for the patient to observe, revise, and eventually relinquish maladaptive representations of self and other, and begin to build and internalize more mature, integrated, and adaptive representations of self and others (e.g., Blatt et al., 1996). Despite growing evidence for the efficacy of couple and family approaches in the treatment of depression (e.g., Denton, Golden, & Walsh, 2003), this area is often neglected, particularly in existing guidelines for the treatment of depressed patients (e.g., American Psychiatric Association, 2000). Again, treatment guidelines appear to lag behind the findings of empirical research. In this context, much may also be gained from the experiential perspective which has long emphasized the importance of the therapeutic alliance and interpersonal factors in treating depressed individuals. The increasing dialogue between experiential, cognitive (Ottens & Hanna, 1998), and psychodynamic (e.g., Greenberg & Watson, 1998) approaches is a step in the right direction, but much more needs to be done in this effort.

Environmental Factors and the Nature versus Nurture Debate

Historically, research on depression has long been dominated by the question whether there are two subtypes of depression, one more biological in origin (e.g., endogenous depression), the other one more environmentally determined (e.g., reactive or neurotic depression). This discussion reflects the familiar issue of nature versus nurture. It has become clear, however, that the nature versus nurture debate is unproductive, especially given the increasing evidence for gene-environment correlations and interactions (Kendler, 2001; Rutter, 2002; Rutter et al., 1997; Van Praag et al., 2004), and recursive interactions between biological and psychosocial factors (Raison & Miller, 2003; Tsigos & Chrousos, 2002; Uchino, Cacioppo, & Kiecolt-Glaser, 1996).

Gene-environment correlations in the context of depression refer to the notion that genes may affect the exposure to certain environmental stressors (or vice versa) associated with depression, while gene-environment interactions refer to the synergistic interaction of genes and environment in predicting depression (e.g., a certain gene may increase the sensitivity for life stressors). Again, the construct of cognitive-affective schemas (or personality) may play a central role here, as temperament and personality factors are currently viewed as the most likely crucial factors that mediate the effect of genes on environment (e.g., Kendler & Karkowski-Shuman, 1997; Saudino, Pedersen, Lichtenstein, McClearn, & Plomin, 1997). Broad personality traits such as neuroticism, for example, have shown to be associated with the occurrence of dependent (fateful) life events, thus increasing the risk of depression (e.g., Kendler, Gardner, & Prescott, 2003; Kendler et al., 2004; Kendler, Neale, Kessler, Heath, & Eaves, 1993; Ormel et al., 2001; Ormel, Stewart, & Sanderman, 1989; Van Os & Jones, 1999; Van Os, Park, & Jones, 2001). Also, evidence for gene-environment interactions suggests that certain genes may lead to increased sensitivity to life stress associated with depression (e.g., Caspi et al., 2003).

Unfortunately, most research has not yet investigated recursive interactions between genes, individuals, their environment, and depression, and has mainly focused on broad personality traits such as neuroticism which may be less informative.[1] As discussed in Chapter 3, theoretical formulations concerning gene-environment correlations and interactions are congruent with our proposed dynamic interactionism model. Future studies should adopt a full dynamic interactionism perspective, focusing on more specific personality dimensions such as Dependency/Sociotropy and Self-Critical Perfectionism/Autonomy and their interactions with congruent events (see Chapter 4 and Chapter 5, this volume), and try to take into account the complex recursive interactions between individuals, their environment, and depression. These studies are likely to transform current treatment strategies for depression because they clearly emphasize the importance of the patient's (social) environment when treating depression (Zuroff & Blatt, 2002). Again, we believe that systems and family approaches may have much to offer in this context as well as intensive, non-symptom focused, individual psychotherapy in which the patient-therapist relationship is a foremost factor in the therapeutic process.

---

[1] This research has also been complicated by the fact that although there is clear evidence for the role of family transmission in depression, no genes have been definitely associated with depression (Van Praag et al., 2004). In addition, although the human genome project may lead to the identification of certain genes associated with depression, we consider it unlikely that one particular gene or set of genes will be associated with depression. Rather, congruent with our transdiagnostic dynamic interactionism view, we expect that particular genes might be involved in the etiology of several disorders, particularly through the effects they have on temperamental and personality factors (see also Kendler, 2001 and Chapter 8, this volume).

In addition, evidence has increasingly indicated the importance of recursive interactions between psychosocial and neurobiological processes implied in various disorders, including depression (Claes, 2003; Gold & Chrousos, 2003). As reviewed in Chapter 8 by Claes and Nemeroff, research, particularly on the effects of early adversity on the psychobiological reactions to stress, is rapidly increasing our knowledge concerning interactions between neurobiological and psychosocial factors. As Claes and Nemeroff point out, research on the HPA axis, in particular, might play a vital role in bridging the gap between biological and psychological approaches. Although Claes and Nemeroff indicate that this integrative research has already begun, truly interdisciplinary and integrative research is still a rarity, although several theoretical models have been proposed in this area (e.g., Kandel, 1999; Cloninger, Svrakic, & Przybeck, 1993).

To summarize, the nature-nuture debate in depression (what part of depression is genetically or environmentally determined) has become obsolete. The time has come to give up the outmoded Cartesian dualism that characterizes much of the literature on life stress and depression, and depression in general. For example, estimates of heritability of what is often considered to be a purely "environmental" factor such as social support have ranged between 40% and 80% (e.g., Henderson, 1998; Kendler, 1997). Again, personality dimensions such as Neuroticism and Dependency/Sociotropy and Self-Critical Perfectionism/Autonomy are likely mediators in the relationship between genetic factors and social support (Kendler, 1997). In this context, Kendler (2001) distinguishes between "within-the-skin" physiological pathways (i.e., the direct effect of genes on attitudes, affects, and behaviors), and "outside-the-skin" behavioral pathways (i.e., the effects of genes on the [social] environment, such as exposure to stress or social support) (see also Silberg et al., 1999; Thapar, Harold, & McGuffin, 1998). According to Kendler (2001, p. 1005), studies of both pathways provide "an important complement to and context for current efforts to localize individual susceptibility genes". In general, based on a meta-analysis (Sullivan, Neale, & Kendler, 2000), the heritability of depression is estimated at 30-40%. How much of this heritability is due to a "within-the-skin" or "outside-the-skin" effect is largely unknown, and may differ depending on environmental factors. What is clear, however, is that research is moving beyond the old dichotomies such as the nature versus nurture dichotomy (Rose, 2001) to more complex models that emphasize dynamic, recursive interactions between biological and psychosocial factors, and between genes and environment. As Rose (2001, p. 3) has put it: "Organisms are in constant interaction with their environment: that is, organisms select environments just as environments select organisms. Like organisms, environments evolve and are homeodynamic rather than homeostatic; both 'genome' and 'envirome' are abstractions from this continuous dialectic". One of the great challenges of future research will be to model and unravel these dialectic interactions. This brings us to our last point, namely the need to consider depression from a developmental perspective.

Strikingly, all chapters in this volume emphasize the importance of a developmental perspective. In Chapter 1 and 6, epidemiological research is cited that clearly shows that depression is not a static and isolated disorder, but a highly recurrent condition, which has its onset more often than not in childhood or adolescence. In Chapter 2, Hermans and colleagues link disturbances in autobiographical memory from a cognitive perspective to (early) trauma, thereby implying a developmental perspective in the etiology of depression. In addition, psychodynamic and cognitive-behavioral (see Chapter 3, 4, 5, and 7, this volume), as well as neurobiological research (see Chapter 8, this volume), suggest that an understanding of developmental factors is crucial to an understanding of depression. This emphasis on developmental factors is striking because, as we noted in the introduction of this volume, until recently many even doubted whether depression in childhood even existed.

Congruent with the proposed etiologically-based, transdiagnostic alternative to the DSM symptom-based categorization of depression and psychopathology in general, these findings strongly suggest that research on the assessment and treatment of depression should be based on a thorough knowledge of developmental pathways that lead to expressions of depression (see also Ormel & de Jong, 1999). Stated otherwise: the classification, assessment, and treatment of psychopathology should be linked to normal developmental processes and to disruptions in these processes (Blatt & Homann, 1992; Blatt & Levy, 1998). Such a developmental perspective could provide a strong theoretical foundation and a basis for integrating many of the issues that various approaches to depression, and psychopathology more generally, have in common. Briefly, future research should investigate how personal genetic predispositions correlate and interact with and shape environmental events and how these interactions result in the construction of mental representations of self and other in both normal and pathological development. Psychopathology can then be conceptualized as disturbances in the process of the development of representations of self and other (Blatt, 1995), such that these representational structures become locked in relatively immature forms that are relatively ineffective in later phases of the life cycle. These impairments of developmental processes forestall subsequent development in some individuals and thus these individuals need constructive reparative interpersonal experiences (e.g., in psychotherapy) that enable them to recognize the repetitive and maladaptive nature of their mode of experiencing their interpersonal world and to be able to revise this mode, based on experiences with a constructive caring other.

Unfortunately, as reviewed in detail in Chapter 6, few longitudinal studies exist that have studied developmental pathways towards depression. In addition, these studies have mostly concentrated on the relationship between DSM diagnoses, and between these diagnoses and clinical variables, rather than on theoretically derived hypotheses about possible etiological pathways. However, as illustrated in Chapter 6, 7, and 8, several interesting and promising areas of research exist, such as research on care giving patterns of non-clinical and depressed parents and the attachment styles of the children of these parents, and the role of early life stress on neurobiological factors implied in depression and other disorders.

Although currently few truly interdisciplinary developmental studies of depression exist, a true dialogue and integration between psychosocial and biological approaches of depression may develop under the influence of developmental psychopathological research (Rutter, 2002). For example, theoretical notions such as gene- and person-environment correlations and interactions are broad enough to accommodate many different theoretical approaches, while at the same time being specific enough to lead to clear and testable hypotheses concerning the complex, recursive interactions between nature and nurture, between psyche and soma. In addition, with the continuing development and growing availability of complex statistical analyses methods such as Structural Equation Modeling (SEM), survival analysis, and growth-curve modeling, we may be able to begin to answer complex questions concerning the multiple intertwining of the biopsychosocial factors implied in depression and other disorders.

The Limits of Dialogue and Integration

Before discussing research and clinical implications of the emerging dialogue in depression research, it would be well to pause and ask if we have not overestimated the possibilities for further dialogue and integration. And indeed, we believe that some cautionary caveats are needed.

First, whereas many recognize limitations of DSM, there is no reason to believe that the next edition of DSM will be fundamentally different. Plans for DSM-V, to be published in 2012, mention no fundamental changes in the DSM approach to mood disorders. In addition, although the recent Strategic Plan for Mood Disorders Research by the National Institute of Mental Health (NIMH, 2003) recognizes some limitations of DSM, and aims at funding interdisciplinary research on depression, it has no plans to fund alternative research programs that aim at developing an etiology-based classification of mood disorders.

Second, it must be clear that, despite considerable common ground, differences do exist between various theoretical approaches of depression. These differences are not only limited to differences concerning the DSM approach of depression, but, as noted in Chapter 3, they often involve differences in their concept of human nature that are not easily surmounted, particularly because these views are not always based on empirical data, but also on ideological preferences.

Third, although dialogue and integration should ideally lead to more comprehensive theories and ultimately more effective treatments, it is unlikely that dialogue and integration have only advantages. In this context, one should carefully distinguish between various forms of integration (Arkowitz, 1997). On a first level, dialogue and integration often begins, and also but unfortunately ends, with *technical* integration (i.e., incorporating techniques used in other theoretical approaches). Hence, technical integration should be accompanied by *theoretical* integration – by changes in theoretical formulations. Otherwise, the result could be an "empty" eclecticism, without a firm grounding in overarching, comprehensive theories. Messer (1986), for example, proposes the notion of "assimilative integrationism", which refers to the fact that concepts, hypotheses, and therapeutic techniques borrowed from other theoretical orientations are assimilated in a theoretically meaningful way in an existing theoretical framework.

Finally, we believe that a certain tension between theoretical orientations is healthy and even vital for further development in the field. Theoretical and methodological pluralism often prevent monolithic thinking, which always risks creating a one-sided, false sense of certainty. Hence, tension among various approaches may be constructive, leading to new discoveries and paradigms.

But, as indicated in the various chapters in this volume, there appears to be much common ground between various approaches of depression which should limit the often artificial separation and competition between different theoretical approaches. In addition, in clinical practice there is often much more similarity in clinical approaches than is suggested by theoretical writings. For instance, Morrison, Bradley and Westen (2003), studying a group of randomly selected psychiatrists and clinical psychologists, found that the average clinician, regardless of theoretical orientation (including CBT and IPT), treated depressed patients much longer than is currently suggested in treatment guidelines. More importantly, they found, regardless of theoretical orientation, that more than two thirds of the clinicians indicated that the depressed patient they were describing had clinically significant problems with relatedness or commitment in relationships, and with the expression of anger, that needed treatment. Thus, most clinicians, regardless of theoretical orientation, attend to similar issues. Likewise, in another study of patients with eating disorders, Thompson-Brenner and Westen (2004) found that clinicians, regardless of theoretical orientation, used more structured or more open clinical interventions, depending on circumstances. For example, in patients with comorbid (personality) pathology, clinicians, including cognitive-behavioral clinicians, used more typical psychodynamic interventions. Ablon and Jones (2002), consistent with these findings, found that treatment process in both IPT and CBT in the NIMH Treatment of Depression Collaborative Research Program actually resembled most the prototype for CBT, a surprising finding given that these therapists received considerable training and supervision to adhere as closely as possible to their therapeutic orientation.

Recommendations for Future Research

As Ingram and Price (2001, p. ix) have noted, after an era in which research was mainly focused on diagnosis and symptoms, "there is little doubt that the future of clinical research and treatment efforts lies in the study of vulnerability processes." This is particularly true for depression research. Moreover, given the high relapse figures associated with depression, even when treated with so-called Empirically Supported Treatments (ESTs) (Westen et al., 2004a), an additional area of increasing importance is the study of the different biopsychosocial factors influencing relapse, particularly in first versus subsequent episodes of depression (see Chapter 1, this volume).

Thus, a refinement of diathesis-stress theories is clearly needed (Coyne & Whiffen, 1995; Monroe & Simons, 1991). The lack of more comprehensive and integrated theoretical models is currently one of the main impediments to further dialogue and fuller integration of research findings concerning depression. Ultimately, the integration of research findings should provide the basis for an etiologically-based diagnostic alternative to the current a-theoretical approach of DSM.

Methodological pluralism holds considerable promise to articulate and test comprehensive, integrative theories. Using various methodologies, ranging from $N=1$ designs, to experimental and naturalistic studies in both animals and humans, to epidemiological studies of representative community samples as well as studies of high-risk samples (e.g., children of depressed mothers) should provide the basis for more comprehensive theoretical formulations. In particular, we need inter-disciplinary, developmentally informed, multiwave research programs to study theoretically derived hypotheses concerning the dynamic interactions between various biopsychosocial factors in normal and psychopathological development (including depression). One of the most urgent problems in such studies is the need to operationalize the construct of depression. As stated above, depression research is currently divided over whether there are only quantitative or also qualitative differences between normal dysphoria and clinical depression, although increasingly the bulk of the evidence seems to support a continuum view. New statistical analyses methods may help to settle this issue (Solomon et al., 2001).

Concerning treatment research, we believe that it is also time for a paradigm change, both theoretically and methodologically (Beutler, Clarkin, & Bongar, 2000; Guthrie, 2000; Westen et al., 2004a). As Blatt, Shahar and Zuroff (2002) and Westen et al. (2004a) have argued, it is time to move beyond the dichotomous judgment concerning *treatments* (or treatment packages) of depression as supported versus unsupported, as is currently the case in the treatment guidelines for identifying empirically supported treatments (e.g., APA, 2000), to identifying the mechanisms of therapeutic change (Blatt et al., 2002) and testing of specific *theories of change* which then can be subsequently integrated in *empirically informed treatments* (Westen et al., 2004a). This will also necessitate the use of research designs other than the randomized clinical trial (Blatt, Berman, Cook, & Ford, 1998; Blatt & Zuroff, 2004).

As we noted in the Introduction to this volume, meta-analytic reviews of so-called ESTs provide a much more nuanced and often more pessimistic view concerning the efficacy of these treatments (Westen et al., 2004a). Concerning depression, response rates in the short run are about 50%, with many patients remaining symptomatic (Westen & Morrison, 2001). The few available studies on the long term effects of ESTs for depression show that at best only about one third of the patients remain improved after two years. In addition, as noted in the Introduction to this volume, solid evidence for theoretically hypothesized effects of ESTs for depression is largely lacking (e.g., Parker, Roy, & Evers, 2003).

Faced with these disappointing results, more extended forms of CBT and IPT have been developed to provide continuation and/or maintenance treatment. Although continuation and maintenance treatments have been shown to be effective in reducing relapse, Westen et al. (2004a) have correctly argued that this approach, that is, extending brief treatments, may be highly problematic. In fact, it is ironic to note that current guidelines for the treatment of depression now tend to promote *long-term* versions of *brief* treatments. As Westen et al. (2004a) suggest (see also Blatt & Shahar, 2004; Blatt et al., 2002), perhaps it is time to change our strategy, and to ask ourselves from the start which patients need what kinds of treatment (e.g., brief versus long-term). Hence, what is needed is the identification of treatment relevant patient dimensions (Beutler et al., 2001). This also implies that more research is needed on the efficacy and effectiveness of other, often long-term, currently practiced treatments for depression, besides the brief treatments that are currently included in lists of ESTs, especially in view of the growing research literature that documents the effectiveness and efficacy as well as necessity of long-term treatments such as experiential (Elliott, Greenberg, & Lietaer, 2004) and psychodynamic psychotherapies (Bateman & Fonagy, 2001; Blatt, 1992; Blatt & Shahar, 2004; Blomberg, Lazar, & Sandell, 2001; Leichsenring & Leibling, 2003). Since the NIMH Strategic Plan for Mood Disorders Research (NIMH, 2003) includes plans for funding outcome research of long-term treatments, more information on the efficacy and effectiveness of these treatments should become available in the near future.

Furthermore, we need methodological pluralism in treatment research. The randomized clinical trial (RCT) is clearly not the only gold that glitters in outcome research (Blatt & Zuroff, 2004; Slade & Priebe, 2001; Westen et al., 2004a). For example, because of strict exclusion criteria, it is often unknown how results from RCTs can be translated to our daily clinical practice. More importantly, Westen et al. (2004a) have shown that RCTs, currently considered by many as the "gold standard", are often inadequate for outcome research because many of the methodological assumptions of RCTs (e.g., that psychopathology is highly malleable, that most patients have only one diagnosis or disorder, etc.) are violated in the treatment of various disorders. For example, RCTs are based on the assumption that a patient typically has only one disorder, and can therefore be treated for that one disorder with a manualized treatment. However, most patients show high rates of comorbidity between Axis I disorders and between Axis I and Axis II disorders, violating this assumption. For research on depression, most assumptions of RCTs appear to be violated, and thus alternative designs should be used or developed (for a detailed discussion, see Westen et al., 2004a).

From the various contributions to this volume, it also becomes clear that interdisciplinary outcome research is needed that not only includes carefully chosen symptomatic measures, but also broader outcome measures, including personality vulnerabilities, level of psychosocial functioning, and the capacity to cope with new life stressors ("resilience"; Blatt & Zuroff, 2004; Westen et al., 2004a; Zuroff, Blatt, Krupnick, & Sotsky, 2003). In addition, such studies should include multiwave, clinically meaningful, follow-up intervals (e.g., from 2 to 5 years) to assess the impact of treatment (Zuroff & Blatt, 2002; Westen et al., 2004a). Given the high relapse rates associated with brief treatments for depression, future psychotherapy research should also investigate which patients need longer treatment and should differentiate between patients who may be more responsive to supportive interventions and patients who may be more responsive to exploration and interpretation (Blatt, 1992; Blatt & Shahar, 2004). In addition, studies have shown that (brief) treatment of depression may only temporarily *deactivate* maladaptive cognitive-affective schemas. Hence, psychotherapy studies should include measures that tap into latent vulnerabilities, including Dependency/Sociotropy and Self-Critical Perfectionism/Autonomy, that influence the onset and/or relapse of depression. Studies need to address the role of these personality vulnerabilities in the etiology, clinical course, and treatment of depression (Blatt et al., 2002; Widiger & Anderson, 2003). Finally, outcome research should routinely include both psycho-social and biological outcome measures to unravel the relationship between process and outcome at both the biological and the psychosocial level. The work of Kandel (1999) suggests that psychosocial interventions may not only lead to neurobiological changes, but also to changes in the expression of certain genes. Hence, a truly interactive model also implies that psychosocial interventions may lead to lasting biological changes, and that biological treatment may influence either directly or indirectly the psychosocial factors implicated in depression (see also Fonagy, Gergely, Jurist, & Target, 2004; Gabbard, 2000).

As Westen, Novotny and Thompson-Brenner (2004b) argue, this will necessitate funding research that is not restricted to categorical DSM diagnoses and research that is more closely in touch with clinical interventions as they are practiced in the community. For example, research teams as well as research funding organizations should include practicing clinicians in their review panels in efforts to reduce the current gap between research and clinical practice.

Clinical Implications: Bridging the Gap between Research and Clinical Practice

With the consideration of the clinical implications of the emerging dialogue in depression research, we have come full circle. As noted in the Introduction to this volume, the efficacy and effectiveness of so-called ESTs for depression is quite limited, and much remains unknown about the long term effects of currently practiced ESTs and other forms of treatment for depression. Not surprisingly, therefore, many clinicians are dissatisfied with current guidelines for the treatment of depression. They have the feeling that these guidelines are simplistic and do not do justice to the complexities of clinical practice. In fact, the study by Morrison et al. (2003) clearly demonstrates that clinicians, including clinicians using CBT and

IPT, treat the average patient at least twice as long as prescribed by current guidelines. In addition, most clinicians are of the opinion that the majority of depressed patients need also treatment for clinical or subclinical personality problems. And as Blatt and colleagues (Blatt, Sanislow, Zuroff, & Pilkonis, 1996) demonstrated, more effective therapists believe that depressed patients need longer treatment, primarily treatment that has a psychosocial focus. Thus, many clinicians experience a wide gap between clinical guidelines promulgated by government agencies and HMOs and what they encounter in their clinical practice.

The chapters in this volume clarify aspects of this gap between theory and research on the one hand and clinical practice on the other. Let us recapitulate briefly how this gap developed, and what should be done to close this gap. Initially, it was believed that depression was a relatively benign disorder, which was expected to respond well to brief pharmacological and psychosocial treatments. In the meantime, epidemiological research, however, has pointed out that depression is a highly recurrent disorder, which often has its onset in childhood or adolescence (see Chapter 1 and Chapter 6, this volume). Moreover, depression shows high comorbidity with other Axis I disorders (particularly anxiety disorders) and many Axis II disorders. Many depressed patients also show subclinical personality problems, such as problems concerning autonomy and identity, and intimacy and relatedness (Blatt, 2004; Morrison et al., 2003). Also, depressed individuals often continue to experience a range of subclinical personality and interpersonal problems after brief treatment because of underlying, relatively stable and treatment resistant, maladaptive cognitive-affective schemas or personality dimensions, such as Dependency/Sociotropy and Self-Critical Perfectionism/Autonomy. Therefore, they often remain vulnerable to future episodes, in part because of their distinct cognitive biases (see Chapter 2, this volume) that lead them to generate their own "depressogenic" environment (see Chapter 3, 4 and 5, this volume). In addition, vulnerability associated with depression is probably also embedded in relatively stable neurobiological disturbances, such as disturbances in HPA axis functioning (Gutman & Nemeroff, 2003; see also Chapter 8, this volume). Not surprisingly, therefore, brief treatments for depression have been relatively ineffective.

The first response to these issues was to extend brief treatments into maintenance and continuation treatments. This approach certainly has its merits because it results in much lower relapse rates. Another approach has been to develop alternative treatments, particularly concerned about changing underlying maladaptive cognitive-affective schemas or personality dimensions (e.g., Beck, 1983, 1999; Blatt, 1974, 2004; McCullough, 2003; Linehan, 1993; Segal, Williams, & Teasdale, 2002; Young, 1999). Not surprisingly, many of these approaches originated from experiences with the treatment of personality disorders (e.g., Beck, 1999; Linehan, 1993; Young, 1999), and often involve treatments that are considerable longer than the typical 16-sessions of "traditional" CBT or IPT. This should not be surprising. In fact, a general consensus has emerged that indicates that pharmacological treatment for depression needs to be extended in many patients up to 6 months or even a year or more (Geddes, Carney, Davies, Furukawa, Kupfer, Frank, & Goodwin, 2003; Kupfer & Frank, 2001). Thus, perhaps the pendulum is starting to swing in the other direction, after an era in which the predominant view was that brief treatments were effective for all patients. Also, studies have been done and are underway to determine which depressed patients benefit most from what kinds of treatment (e.g., Blatt, 1992; Blatt & Shahar, 2004; Beutler et al., 2000).

Where does this leave the clinician? Until more data become available, research reviewed in this volume suggests the following preliminary guidelines, guidelines that reflect our belief that assessment and treatment should be intrinsically linked with each other and with basic research.

Assessment of depression. In accordance with the proposed dynamic inter-actionism model of depression discussed earlier, assessment of the depressed patient should consist of:

(1) Detailed assessment of depressive symptoms and the severity of depression
(2) A consideration of depression from a dimensional view, preferably including a life-span perspective
(3) Charting of etiological and pathogenetic factors involved, with special attention for the interaction between genetic factors (such as temperament), parental styles, early adversity, subclinical (e.g., Dependency/Sociotropy and Self-Critical Perfectionism/Autonomy) and clinical (personality disorders) personality problems, and life stress. For example, course and treatment prospects will look dramatically different when one is dealing with a depressed patient functioning at the neurotic level, versus a depressed patient with borderline features. However, current guidelines hardly account even such obvious distinctions.
(4) A systematic statement concerning likely course and prognosis, together with assessment of treatment possibilities for the patient. This should also include an assessment of the patient's treatment preferences. Here the question is: what treatment, if any treatment is needed, is likely to be most effective for which patient? For example, recent research clearly suggests that dependent/socio-tropic and self-critical/autonomous patients need a different therapeutic approach that focuses on relatedness versus autonomy and self-definition, respectively (Blatt, 1992; Blatt et al., 2002; Blatt & Shahar, 2004). In addition, self-critical/autonomous patients typically need more intensive treatment. More research on the influence of these and other personality dimensions on process and outcome in the treatment of depressed patients is needed. In particular, congruent with our dynamic interactionism model, we believe that a crucial factor in treatment is addressing the structural organization, content, and development of maladaptive and often rigid cognitive-affective structures in the context of the therapeutic relationship.

Several instruments are available to document more objectively steps one to three listed above. Concerning step four, the clinician has currently precious little information, precisely because etiological factors are often excluded in outcome research. However, recent work is increasingly filling this gap (e.g., Beutler et al., 2000; Blatt, 1992; Blatt & Shahar, 2004).

Treatment of depression. In general, clinicians should benefit from a growing dialogue and integration between various theoretical approaches. It is clear that earlier exaggerated differences among various forms of psychotherapy are starting to diminish. For example, psychodynamic approaches of depression are becoming more flexible and directive and are incorporating techniques from other approaches, while cognitive-behavioral approaches incorporate several techniques and conceptualizations from other theoretical approaches, including a fuller appreciation of childhood experiences and the interpersonal dimensions of the treatment process, mainly from the psychodynamic and experiential tradition (Bemporad, 1995; Blatt, 2004; Bateman & Fonagy, 2004; Jones & Pulos, 1993; Kwon, 1999).

Cognitive-behavioral approaches are not only increasingly focusing on underlying cognitive-affective schemas, but also are beginning to consider therapist competence (Shaw et al., 1999), and the therapeutic relationship and transference in particular as an important source of information and vehicle for interventions (e.g., Linehan, 1993; Waddington, 2002). Mindfulness Based Cognitive Therapy (MBCT; Segal et al., 2002; Teasdale et al., 2000), a treatment package specifically aimed at reducing relapse in depression, in turn, focuses on developing a meta-perspective in depressed patients, which entails patients observing their own (ruminative) thoughts without judging or suppressing them (see also Chapter 2, this volume). This comes very close to the psychoanalytic emphasis on exploration, free association, and interpretation, and particularly to the notion of mentalization or reflective functioning, which is the basis of Mentalization Based Treatment (MBT), a psychoanalytic, evidence-based long-term treatment for borderline personality disorder (Bateman & Fonagy, 2004). As Hermans and colleagues note in Chapter 2, mindfulness based treatment is about "providing patients with life-long skills for adequately dealing with negative emotion in the future". In psychodynamic terms, this refers to the internalization of the "analytic function", i.e., the capacity for insight and mentalization (Blatt & Behrends, 1987). Interestingly, patients treated with MBT continued to improve during an 18-month follow-up (Bateman & Fonagy, 2001), which is dramatically different than the typical high relapse rates after brief treatments for most disorders. Findings such as these not only illustrate the need for long-term follow-up in outcome research, but at the same time they also illustrate that longer treatment may result in substantial and sustained change.

These integrative trends in psychosocial treatments clearly reflect the fact that brief treatments, which focus on "surface" cognitions and symptoms, are ineffective in many patients. Instead, the focus has shifted towards underlying relatively stable cognitive-affective schemas, or personality dimensions, in order to prevent relapse. Further dialogue and integration concerning the treatment of depression could be achieved by focusing on the five areas of convergence earlier discussed, i.e., (1) taking into account etiological and pathogenetic factors in the classification of mental disorders, (2) focusing on mental representations and underlying cognitive-affective schemas or personality dimensions, (3) taking into account the interpersonal dimensions of depression, and (4) more generally, the role of environmental factors and their interaction with depression and cognitive-affective schemas, and (5) focusing on developmental factors implied in depression.

Concerning treatment more specifically, findings reviewed in this volume point to the fact that current guidelines for the treatment of depression have the following limitations:

(1) They underestimate the recurrent nature of depression
(2) They largely neglect patient, therapist, and therapeutic alliance factors in favor of specific techniques, and
(3) They overemphasize the importance of symptoms to the neglect of the role of etiological and pathogenetic factors implied in depression (see Blatt, 2004).

It is clear that these issues are linked to the fact that current guidelines are closely linked to the DSM approach of depression. If, from a DSM perspective, depression is a relatively benign Axis I disorder (a state disorder, unrelated to personality), that can be diagnosed and treated based on an assessment of symptoms, one can develop and manualize, analogous to the development of a medication for a disease, a treatment package specifically designed for this particular "disease". When symptoms disappear, the disease has been "cured". The disease model and the drug metaphor of the DSM (e.g., see Stiles & Shapiro, 1989; Wampold, 1997) has clearly impacted on the current guidelines for the treatment of depression. As the findings reviewed in this volume illustrate, all these DSM assumptions have been refuted by empirical research (Blatt & Zuroff, 2004). Therefore, until more data become available, clinicians should attend particularly to the following issues when treating depressed patients:

(1) *Depression is often a highly recurrent disorder, and should be seen as a distortion of normal development.* Many patients treated for depression have had several episodes of depression and experience significant psychosocial difficulties, often beginning in childhood or adolescence. Because many depressed patients also have considerable subclinical or clinical personality problems, most often reflected in interpersonal difficulties (e.g., problems concerning relatedness), it is extremely unlikely that such lifelong difficulties will be solved, or even diminished, by focusing on symptoms alone. While long-term treatment may not be indicated for many patients, all treatments should be concerned about reducing relapse. This may be achieved by different means, ranging from psycho-education, to using treatment packages that are specifically aimed at reducing relapse (e.g., Segal et al., 2002), to more extended treatment (Blatt et al., 2002). Because personality dimensions or cognitive-affective structures play a central role in the development of depression, as stated above, treatment should focus on the development of the structural organization and content of these cognitive-affective structures in the context of the therapeutic relationship. Moreover, because the importance of relational factors in depression, both as an antecedent and as a consequence, treatment should also pay particularly attention to interpersonal issues, both in the focus of the treatment and in the consideration of the need for couple and/or family therapy.

(2) *More weight should be given to patient, therapist, and alliance factors* (Beutler et al., 2001; Blatt & Zuroff, 2004; Lambert & Ogles, 2004). As stated before (see also Chapter 4, this volume), it is ironic that current guidelines for the treatment of depressed patients have almost exclusively focused on particular therapeutic techniques or treatment packages given the fact that more than four decades of psychotherapy research have pointed to the importance of patient (Blatt, 2004; Clarkin & Levy, 2004), and therapist (Beutler et al., 2004) variables, as well as the therapeutic alliance (Blatt & Zuroff, 2004; Division 29 Task Force on Empirically Supported Therapy Relationships, 2002). This neglect of personality and interpersonal factors in the therapeutic process is all the more ironic given the fact that, with some important exceptions, for many disorders different forms of treatment appear to have similar effects (the famous "Dodo bird verdict"). Therefore, we would like to make a strong plea to include consideration of patient, therapist, and alliance factors in establishing guidelines for the treatment of depressed patients.

(3) *Etiological and pathogenetic factors should inform treatment.* Depressed patients are a heterogeneous group from an etiological and pathogenetic perspective. Current guidelines, however, treat depressed patients as uniformly responsive to a variety of psychosocial (e.g., CBT, IPT) and pharmacological treatments. This assumption of uniformity is clearly incorrect. Again, because these treatment guidelines were not informed by basic science (i.e., research on etiological pathways to depression), the influence of etiological factors on treatment response has not been given sufficient attention. Therefore, considerations concerning etiological and pathogenetic factors should be included in developing treatment guidelines. In particular, special attention should be given to the role of genetic factors, which can exert their influence both "inside" and "outside" the skin (Kendler, 2001), neurobiological disturbances associated with HPA axis functioning, and their interaction with psychosocial factors such as parental style, early adversity, life stress, and relatively stable personality dimensions or cognitive-affective schemas.

Conclusions

Our work on this volume has made us acutely aware of the increasing opportunities of further dialogue and integration in depression research. In particular, an etiologically-based, dynamic interactionism view of depression, emphasizing interactions among genetics, early adversity, current life stress, and relatively stable cognitive-affective schemas or personality dimensions, emerges as a model that may facilitate the integration of various theoretical, methodological, and clinical approaches to depression. At the same time, much work remains to be done. The future of research on depression therefore promises to be exciting and will undoubtedly lead to many new advances in our knowledge of this disabling disorder. It is our sincere belief that ultimately the quality of clinical services will benefit from these advances. In particular, the proposed etiologically-based dynamic interactionism model not only promises to lead to important theoretical insights in depression that can subsequently inform treatment of depression, but it may also assist in developing theory-driven and empirically-based prevention programs that are aimed at etiological and pathogenetic factors implied in depression.

In closing, we would like to re-emphasize in this context the importance of maladaptive representations in the development and treatment of depression, that is, how maladaptive representations of self and other, that have developed starting in early life as a result of interactions between biological and psychosocial factors, make certain individuals vulnerable to particular depressive experiences and other, related subclinical and clinical problems, such as anxiety, substance abuse, and perhaps also somatic and functional disorders. Hence, the notion of mental representations may not only build bridges between various approaches towards the etiology and pathogenesis of depression, it may also provide a unified view on the treatment of depression. A focus on mental representations implies, regardless of theoretical orientation, that the treatment of depression should primarily consist in making these individuals aware of their maladaptive representations and help them to build and internalize more adaptive representations of self and others.

References

Ablon, J. S., & Jones, E. E. (2002). Validity of controlled clinical trials of psychotherapy: Findings from the NIMH Treatment of Depression Collaborative Research Program. *American Journal of Psychiatry, 159,* 775-783.

American Psychiatric Association (2000). *Practice guidelines for the treatment of patients with major depression.* Retrieved September 3, 2004, from http://www.psych.org/psych_pract/treatg/pg/Depression2e.book.cfm

Arkowitz, H. (1997). Integrative theories of therapy. In P. Wachtel & S. Messer (Eds.), *Theories of psychotherapy: Origins and evolution* (pp. 227-288). Washington, DC: American Psychological Association Press.

Bateman, A., & Fonagy, P. (2001). Treatment of borderline personality disorder with psychoanalytically oriented partial hospitalisation: An 18-month follow-up. *American Journal of Psychiatry, 158,* 36-42.

Bateman, A., & Fonagy, P. (2004). *Psychotherapy for borderline personality disorder. Mentalization-based treatment.* Oxford: Oxford University Press.

Beach, S. R. H. (Ed). (2001). *Marital and family processes in depression. A scientific foundation for clinical practice.* Washington, DC: American Psychological Association.

Beck, A. T. (1983). Cognitive therapy of depression: New perspectives. In P. J. Clayton & J. E. Barrett (Eds.), *Treatment of depression: Old controversies and new approaches* (pp. 265-290). New York: Raven Press.

Beck, A. T. (1999). Cognitive aspects of personality disorders and their relation to syndromal disorders: A psychoevolutionary approach. In C. R. Cloninger (Ed.), *Personality and psychopathology* (pp. 411-429). Washington, DC/London: American Psychiatric Press.

Bemporad, J. R. (1995). Long-term analytic treatment of depression. In E. E. Beckham & W. R. Leber (Eds.), *Handbook of depression* (2nd ed.) (pp. 391-403). New York: Guilford Press.

Beutel, M. E., Stern, E., & Silbersweig, D. A. (2003). The emerging dialogue between psychoanalysis and neuroscience: Neuroimaging perspectives. *Journal of the American Psychoanalytic Association, 51,* 773-801.

Beutler, L. E., Clarkin, J. F., & Bongar, B. (2000). *Guidelines for the systematic treatment of the depressed patient*. New York/Oxford: Oxford University Press.

Beutler, L. E., Malik, M., Alimohamed, S., Harwood, T. M., Talebi, H., Noble, S., & Wong, E. (2004). Therapist variables. In M. J. Lambert (Ed.), *Bergin and Garfield's handbook of psychotherapy and behavior change* (5th ed.) (pp. 227-306). New York: John Wiley & Sons.

Bieling, P. J., Summerfeldt, L. J., Israeli, A. L., & Antony, M. M. (2004). Perfectionism as an explanatory construct in comorbidity of Axis I disorders. *Journal of Psychopathology and Behavioral Assessment, 26*, 193-201.

Blatt, S. J. (1974). Levels of object representation in anaclitic and introjective depression. *The Psychoanalytic Study of the Child, 29*, 107-157.

Blatt, S. J. (1991). Depression and destructive risk-taking behavior in adolescence. In L. P. Lipsitt & L. L. Mitnick (Eds.), *Self-regulatory behavior and risk-taking: Causes and consequences* (pp. 285-309). Norwood, NJ: Ablex Press.

Blatt, S. J. (1992). The differential effect of psychotherapy and psychoanalysis with anaclitic and introjective patients: The Menninger psychotherapy research project revisited. *Journal of the American Psychoanalytic Association, 40*, 691-724.

Blatt, S. J. (1995). Representational structures in psychopathology. In D. Cicchetti & S. L. Toth (Eds.), *Emotion, cognition, and representation (Rochester Symposium on developmenal psychopathology Vol. 6)* (pp. 1-33). New York: University of Rochester Press.

Blatt, S. J. (2004). *Experiences of depression: Theoretical, clinical and research perspectives*. Washington, DC: American Psychological Association.

Blatt, S. J., Auerbach, J. S., & Levy, K. N. (1997). Mental representation in personality development, psychopathology, and the therapeutic process. *Review of General Psychology, 1*, 351-374.

Blatt, S. J., & Behrends, R. S. (1987). Internalization, separation-individuation, and the nature of therapeutic action. *International Journal of Psycho-Analysis, 68*, 279-297.

Blatt, S. J., Berman, W. H., Cook, B., & Ford, R. Q. (1998). Effectiveness of long-term, intensive, inpatient treatment for seriously disturbed young adults: A reply to Bein. *Psychotherapy Research, 8*, 42-53.

Blatt, S. J., & Homann, E. (1992). Parent-child interaction in the etiology of dependent and self-critical depression. *Clinical Psychology Review, 12*, 47-91.

Blatt, S. J., & Levy, K. N. (1998). A psychodynamic approach to the diagnosis of psychopathology. In J. W. Baron (Ed.), *Making diagnosis meaningful. Enhancing evaluation and treatment of psychological disorders* (pp. 73-109). Washington, DC: American Psychological Association.

Blatt, S. J., Sanislow, C. A., Zuroff, D. C., & Pilkonis, P. A. (1996). Characteristics of effective therapists: Further analyses of data from the NIMH TDCRP. *Journal of Consulting and Clinical Psychology, 64*, 1276-1284.

Blatt, S. J., & Shahar, G. (2004). Psychoanalysis: With whom, for what, and how? Comparisons with psychotherapy. *Journal of the American Psychoanalytic Association, 52*, 393-447.

Blatt, S. J., Shahar, G., & Zuroff, D. C. (2002). Anaclitic/Sociotropic and Introjective/Autonomous dimensions. In J. C. Norcross (Ed.), *Psychotherapy relationships that work. Therapist contributions and responsiveness to patients* (pp. 315-333). Oxford: Oxford University Press.

Blatt, S. J., & Shichman, S. (1983). Two primary configurations of psychopathology. *Psychoanalysis and Contemporary Thought, 6*, 187-254.

Blatt, S. J., Stayner, D., Auerbach, J. S., & Behrends, R. S. (1996). Change in object and self representations in long-term, intensive, inpatient treatment of seriously disturbed adolescents and young adults. *Psychiatry: Interpersonal and Biological Processes, 59*, 82-107.

Blatt, S. J., Wein, S. J., Chevron, E., & Quinlan, D. M. (1979). Parental representations and depression in normal young adults. *Journal of Abnormal Psychology, 88*, 388-397.

Blatt, S. J., & Zuroff, D. C. (1992). Interpersonal relatedness and self-definition: Two prototypes for depression. *Clinical Psychology Review, 12*, 527-562.

Blatt, S. J., & Zuroff, D. C. (2004). *Empirical evaluation of the assumptions in identifying evidence-based treatments in mental health*. Manuscript submitted for publication.

Blomberg, J., Lazar, A., & Sandell, R. (2001). Long-term outcome of long-term psychoanalytically oriented therapies: First findings of the Stockholm Outcome of Psychotherapy and Psychoanalysis Study. *Psychotherapy Research, 11*, 361-382.

Bonanno, G. A. (2004). Loss, trauma, and human resilience. Have we underestimated the human capacity to thrive after extremely aversive events? *American Psychologist, 59*, 20-28.

Bowlby, J. (1988). *A secure base: Clinical applications of attachment theory*. London: Routledge.

Brown, G. W., & Harris, T. O. (1978). *Social origins of depression*. Routledge: London.

Caspi, A., Sugden, K., Moffitt, T. E., Taylor, A., Craig, I. W., Harrington, H., McClay, J., Mill, J., Martin, J., Braithwaite, A., & Poulton, R. (2003). Influence of life stress on depression: Moderation by a polymorphism in the 5-HTT gene. *Science, 301*, 386-389.

Charney, D. S. (2004). Psychobiological mechanisms of resilience and vulnerability: Implications for successful adaptation to extreme stress. *American Journal of Psychiatry, 161*, 195-216.

Cicchetti, D., & Cohen, D. J. (1995). Perspectives on developmental psychopathology. In D. Cicchetti & J. Cohen (Eds.), *Developmental psychopathology* (pp. 3-20). New York: Wiley.

Claes, S. (2003). Corticotropin-releasing hormone (CRH) in psychiatry: From stress to psychopathology. *Annals of Medicine, 35*, 1-12.

Clarkin, J., & Levy, K. N. (2004). The influence of client variables on psychotherapy. In M. J. Lambert (Ed.), *Bergin and Garfield's handbook of psychotherapy and behavior change* (5th ed.) (pp. 194-226). New York: John Wiley & Sons.

Cloninger, C. R., Svrakic, D. K., & Przybeck, T. R. (1993). A psychobiological model of temperament and character. *Archives of General Psychiatry, 50*, 975-990.

Coyne, J. C., Burchill, S. A. L., & Stiles, W. B. (1991). An interactional perspective on depression. In C. R. Snyder & D. O. Forsyth (Eds.), *Handbook of social and clinical psychology: The health perspective* (pp. 327-349). New York: Pergamon.

Coyne, J. C., & Whiffen, V. E. (1995). Issues in personality as diathesis for depression: The case of sociotropy-dependency and autonomy-self-criticism. *Psychological Bulletin, 118*, 358-378.

Denton, W. H., Golden, R. N., & Walsh, S. R. (2003). Depression, marital discord, and couple therapy. *Current Opinion in Psychiatry, 16*, 29-34.

Division 29 Task Force on Empirically Supported Therapy Relationships (2002). Conclusions and recommendations of the Division 29 Task Force. In J. C. Norcross (Ed.), *Psychotherapy relationships that work* (pp. 441-443). Oxford: Oxford University Press.

Elliott, R., Greenberg, L. S., & Lietaer, G. (2004). Research on experiential psychotherapies. In M. J. Lambert (Ed.), *Bergin and Garfield's handbook of psychotherapy change* (5th ed.) (pp. 493-539). New York: John Wiley & Sons.

Fonagy, P., Gergely, G., Jurist, E. L., & Target, M. (2004). *Affect regulation, mentalization, and the development of the self*. London/New York: Karnac.

Gabbard, G. O. (2000). A neurobiologically informed perspective on psychotherapy. *British Journal of Psychiatry, 177*, 117-122.

Geddes, J. R., Carney, S. M., Davies, C., Furukawa, T. A., Kupfer, D. J., Frank, E., & Goodwin, G. M. (2003). Relapse prevention with antidepressant drug treatment in depressive disorders: A systematic review. *The Lancet, 361*, 653-661.

Gilmer, W. S., & McKinney, W. T. (2003). Early experience and depressive disorders: Human and non-human primate studies. *Journal of Affective Disorders, 75*, 97-113.

Gold, P. W., & Chrousos, G. P. (2002). Organization of the stress system and its dysregulation in melancholic and atypical depression: High vs low CRH/NE states. *Molecular Psychiatry, 7*, 254-275.

Goldapple, K., Segal, Z., Garson, C., Lau, M., Bieling, P., Kennedy, S., & Mayberg, H. (2004). Modulation of cortical-limbic pathways in major depression. *Archives of General Psychiatry, 61*, 31-41.

Greenberg, L., & Watson, J. (1998). Experiential therapy of depression: Differential effects of client-centered relationship conditions and process experiential interventions. *Psychotherapy Research, 8*, 210-224.

Guthrie, E. (2000). Psychotherapy for patients with complex disorders and chronic symptoms. The need for a new research paradigm. *British Journal of Psychiatry, 177*, 131-137.

Gutman, D. A., & Nemeroff, C. B. (2003). Persistent central nervous system effects of an adverse early environment: Clinical and preclinical studies. *Physiology & Behavior, 79*, 471-478.

Hammen, C. (2003). Interpersonal stress and depression in women. *Journal of Affective Disorders, 74*, 49-57.

Harrington, R. C. (2001). Childhood depression and conduct disorder: Different routes to the same outcome? *Archives of General Psychiatry, 58*, 237-238.

Henderson, A. S. (1998). Social support: Its present significance for psychiatric epidemiology. In B. P. Dohrendwend (Ed.), *Adversity, stress, and psychopathology* (pp. 390-397). New York: Oxford University Press.

Ingram, R. E., & Price, J. M. (2001). Preface. In R. E Ingram & J. M. Price (Eds.), *Vulnerability to psychopathology. Risk across the lifespan* (p. ix-xii). New York/London: The Guilford Press.

Joiner, T. E., Jr. (2001). Nodes of consilience between interpersonal-psychological theories of depression. In S. R. H. Beach (Ed), *Marital and family processes in depression. A scientific foundation for clinical practice* (pp. 129-138). Washington, DC: American Psychological Association.

Joiner, T. E., Jr., Metalsky, G. I., Katz, J., & Beach, S. R. H. (1999). Depression and excessive reassurance-seeking. *Psychological Inquiry, 10,* 269-278.

Jones, E. E., & Pulos, S. M. (1993). Comparing the process of psychodynamic and cognitive-behavioral therapies. *Journal of Consulting and Clinical Psychology, 61,* 306-316.

Judd, L. L., Akiskal, H. S., & Paulus, M. P. (1997). The role and clinical significance of subsyndromal depressive symptoms (SSD) in unipolar major depressive disorder. *Journal of Affective Disorders, 45,* 5-17.

Kandel, E. R. (1999). Biology and the future of psychoanalysis: A new intellectual framework for psychiatry revisited. *American Journal of Psychiatry, 156,* 505-524.

Kasen, S., Cohen, P., Skodol, A. E., Johnson, J. G., Smailes, E., & Brook, J. S. (2001). Childhood depression and adult personality disorder. Alternative pathways of continuity. *Archives of General Psychiatry, 58,* 231-236.

Kendler, K. S. (1997). Social support: A genetic-epidemiologic analysis. *American Journal of Psychiatry, 154,* 1398-1404.

Kendler, K. S. (2001). Twin studies of psychiatric illness. An update. *Archives of General Psychiatry, 58,* 1005-1014.

Kendler, K. S., & Gardner, C. O. (1998). Boundaries of major depression: An evaluation of DSM-IV criteria. *American Journal of Psychiatry, 155,* 172-177.

Kendler, K. S., Gardner, C. O., & Prescott, C. A. (2003). Personality and the experience of environmental adversity. *Psychological Medicine, 33,* 1193-1202.

Kendler, K. S., & Karkowski-Shuman, L. (1997). Stressful life events and genetic liability to major depression: Genetic control of exposure to environment? *Psychological Medicine, 27,* 539-547.

Kendler, K. S., Kuhn, J., & Prescott, C. A. (2004). The interrelationship of neuroticism, sex, and stressful life events in the prediction of episodes of major depression. *American Journal of Psychiatry, 161,* 631-636.

Kendler, K. S., Neale, M., Kessler, R., Heath, A., & Eaves, L. (1993). A longitudinal twin study of personality and major depression in women. *Archives of General Psychiatry, 50,* 853-862.

Kessler, R. C., Merikangas, K. R., Berglund, P., Eaton, W. W., Koretz, D. S., & Walters, E. E. (2003). Mild disorders should not be eliminated from the DSM-V. *Archives of General Psychiatry, 60,* 1117-1122.

Klein, D. N., Lewinsohn, P. M., Seeley, J. R., & Rohde, P. (2001). A family study of major depressive disorder in a community sample of adolescents. *Archives of General Psychiatry, 58,* 13-20.

Kupfer, D. J., & Frank, E. (2001). The interaction of drug- and psychotherapy in the long-term treatment of depression. *Journal of Affective Disorders, 62,* 131-137.

Kwon, P. (1999). Attributional style and psychodynamic defense mechanisms: Toward an integrative model of depression. *Journal of Personality, 67,* 645-658.

Laakso, A., Wallius, E., Kajander, J., Bergman, J., Eskola, O., Solin, O., Ilonen, T., Salokangas, R. K. R., Syvälahti, E., & Hietala, J. (2003). Personality traits and striatal dopamine synthesis capacity in healthy subjects. *American Journal of Psychiatry, 160,* 904-910.

Lambert, M. J., & Ogles, B. M. (2004). The efficacy and effectiveness of psychotherapy. In M. J. Lambert (Ed.), *Bergin and Garfield's handbook of psychotherapy and behavior change* (5th ed.) (pp. 139-193). New York: John Wiley & Sons.

Leichsenring, D., & Leibling, E. (2003). The effectiveness of psychodynamic therapy and cognitive behavior therapy in the treatment of personality disorders: A meta-analysis. *American Journal of Psychiatry, 160,* 1223-1232.

Lewinsohn, P. M., Rohde, P., Seeley, J. R., Klein, D. N., & Gotlib, I. H. (2003). Psychosocial functioning of young adults who have experienced and recovered from major depressive disorder during adolescence. *Journal of Abnormal Psychology, 112,* 353-363.

Lewinsohn, P. M., Shankman, S. A., Gau, J. M., & Klein, D. N. (2004). The prevalence and co-morbidity of subthreshold psychiatric conditions. *Psychological Medicine, 34,* 613-622.

Linehan, M. M. (1993). *Cognitive-behavioral treatment of borderline personality disorder.* New York: The Guilford Press.

Main, M., Kaplan, N., & Cassidy, J. (1985). Security in infancy, childhood, and adulthood: A move to the level of representation. In I. Bretherton & E. Waters (Ed.), Growing points in attachment theory and research. *Monographs of the Society for Research in Child Development, 50,* 66-104.

281

McCullough, J. P. (2003). *Treatment for chronic depression: Cognitive Behavioral Analysis System of Psychotherapy (CBASP).* London: The Guilford Press.

Messer, S. (1986). Behavioral and psychoanalytic perspectives at therapeutic choice points. *American Psychologist, 41,* 1261-1272.

Monroe, S. C., & Simons, A. D. (1991). Diathesis-stress theories in the context of life stress research: Implications for the depressive disorders. *Psychological Bulletin, 110,* 406-425.

Moore, R. G., & Blackburn, I.-M. (1993). Sociotropy, autonomy and personal memories in depression. *British Journal of Clinical Psychology, 32,* 460-462.

Morrison, K. H., Bradley, R., & Westen, D. (2003). The external validity of controlled clinical trials of psychotherapy for depression and anxiety: A naturalistic study. *Psychology and Psychotherapy: Theory, Research and Practice, 76,* 109-132.

National Institute of Mental Health (2003). *Breaking ground, breaking through: The Strategic Plan for Mood Disorders Research.* Retrieved September 3, 2004, from http://www.nimh.nih.gov/strategic/mooddisorders.pdf

Nemeroff, C. B. (2002). Editorial. Comorbidity of mood and anxiety disorders: The rule, not the exception? *American Journal of Psychiatry, 159,* 3-4.

Nunn, J. D., Mathews, A., & Trower, P. (1997). Selective processing of concern-related information in depression. *British Journal of Clinical Psychology, 36,* 489-503.

Ormel, J., & de Jong, A. (1999). On vulnerability to common mental disorders: An evidence-based plea for a developmental perspective. In M. Tansella & G. Thornicroft (Eds.), *Common mental disorders in primary care* (pp. 34-52). London: Routledge.

Ormel, J., Oldehinkel, A. J., & Brilman, E. I. (2001). The interplay and etiological continuity of neuroticism, difficulties, and life events in the etiology of major and subsyndromal, first and recurrent depressive episodes in later life. *American Journal of Psychiatry, 158,* 885-891.

Ormel, J., Stewart, R., & Sanderman, R. (1989). Personality as modifier of the life change-distress relationship: A longitudinal modelling approach. *Social Psychiatry and Psychiatric Epidemiology, 24,* 187-195.

Ottens, A. J., & Hanna, F. J. (1998). Cognitive and existential therapies: Toward an integration. *Psychotherapy: Theory, Research, Practice, Training, 35,* 312-324.

Parker, G. (1999). Clinical trials of antidepressant medications are producing meaningless results. *British Journal of Psychiatry, 183,* 102-103.

Parker, G. (2000). Classifying depression: Should paradigms lost be regained? *American Journal of Psychiatry, 157,* 1195-1203.

Parker, G., Hadzi-Pavlovic, D., Roussos, J., Wilhelm, K., Mitchell, P., Austin, M.-P., Hickie, I., Gladstone, J., & Eyers, K. (1998). Non-melancholic depression: The contribution of personality, anxiety and life events to subclassification. *Psychological Medicine, 28,* 1209-1219.

Parker, G., Roy, K., & Eyers, K. (2003). Cognitive behavior therapy for depression? Choose horses for courses. *American Journal of Psychiatry, 160,* 825-834.

Parker, G., Roy, K., Wilhelm, K., Mitchell, P., Austin, M.-P., Hadzi-Pavlovic, D., & Little, C. (1999a). Subgrouping non-melancholic depression from manifest clinical features. *Journal of Affective Disorders, 53,* 1-13.

Parker, G., Roy, K., Wilhelm, K., Mitchell, P., Austin, M.-P., & Hadzi-Pavlovic, D. (1999b). Subgrouping non-melancholic major depression using both clinical and aetiological features. *Australian and New Zealand Journal of Psychiatry, 33,* 217-225.

Paykel, E. S. (2003). Editorial. Life events: Effects and genesis. *Psychological Medicine, 33,* 1145-1148.

Pier, M. P. B. I., Hulstijn, W., & Sabbe, B. (2004). Differential patterns of psychomotor functioning in unmedicated melancholic and nonmelancholic depressed patients. *Journal of Psychiatric Research, 38,* 425-435.

Raison, C. L., & Miller, A. H. (2003). When not enough is too much: The role of insufficient glucocorticoid signaling in the pathophysiology of stress-related disorders. *American Journal of Psychiatry, 160,* 1554-1565.

Rose, S. (2001). Moving on from old dichotomies: Beyond nature-nurture towards lifeline perspective. *British Journal of Psychiatry, 178* (Suppl 40), s3-s7.

Rutter, M. (2002). The interplay of nature, nurture, and developmental influences. The challenge ahead for mental health. *Archives of General Psychiatry, 59,* 996-1000.

Rutter, M., Dunn, J., Plomin, R., Simonoff, E., Pickles, A., Maughan, B., Ormel, J., Meyer, J., & Eaves, L. (1997). Integrating nature and nurture: Implications of person-environment correlations and interactions for developmental psychopathology. *Development and Psychopathology, 9*, 335-364.

Safran, J. D., & Segal, L. S. (1990). *Interpersonal process in cognitive therapy.* New York: Basic Books.

Saudino, K. J., Pedersen, N. L., Lichtenstein, P., McClearn, G. E., & Plomin, R. (1997). Can personality explain genetic influences on life events? *Journal of Personality and Social Psychology, 72*, 196-206.

Segal, Z. V., Williams, J. M. G., & Teasdale, J. D. (2002). *Mindfulness-based Cognitive Therapy for Depression: A new approach to preventing relapse.* New York: The Guilford Press.

Segerstrom, S. C., & Miller, G. E. (2004). Psychological stress and the human immune system: A meta-analytic study of 30 years of inquiry. *Psychological Bulletin, 130*, 601-630.

Segrin, C. (2000). Social skills deficits associated with depression. *Clinical Psychology Review, 20*, 379-403.

Shafran, R., & Mansell, W. (2001). Perfectionism and psychopathology: A review of research and treatment. *Clinical Psychology Review, 21*, 879-906.

Shahar, G., Blatt, S. J., Zuroff, D. C., Krupnick, J. L., & Sotsky, S. M. (2004). Perfectionism impedes social relations and response to brief treatment for depression. *Journal of Social and Clinical Psychology, 23*, 140-154.

Shaw, B. F., Elkin, I., Yamaguchi, J., Olmsted, M., Vallis, T. M., Dobson, K. S., Lowery, S., Sotsky, S. M., Watkins, J. T., & Imber, S. D. (1999). Therapist competence ratings in relation to clinical outcome in cognitive therapy of depression. *Journal of Consulting and Clinical Psychology, 60*, 441-449.

Shedler, J., & Westen, D. (2004). Refining personality disorder diagnosis: Integrating science and practice. *American Journal of Psychiatry, 161*, 1350-1365.

Silberg, J., Pickles, A., Rutter, M., Hewitt, J., Simonoff, E., Maes, H., Carbonneau, R., Murrelle, L., Foley, D., & Eaves, L. (1999). The influence of genetic factors and life stress on depression among adolescent girls. *Archives of General Psychiatry, 56*, 225-232.

Slade, M., & Priebe, S. (2001). Editorial. Are randomised controlled trials the only gold that glitters? *British Journal of Psychiatry, 179,* 286-287.

Solomon, A., Haaga, D. A. F., & Arnow, B. A. (2001). Is clinical depression distinct from subthreshold depressive symptoms? A review of the continuity issue in depression research. *Journal of Nervous and Mental Disease, 189*, 498-506.

Stern, D. N. (1985). *The interpersonal world of the infant: A view from psychoanalysis and developmental psychology.* New York: Basic Books.

Stiles, W. B., & Shapiro, D. A. (1989). Abuse of the drug metaphor in psychotherapy process-outcome research. *Clinical Psychology Review, 9*, 521-543.

Sullivan, P. F., Neale, M. C., & Kendler, K. S. (2000). The genetic epidemiology of major depression: Review and meta-analysis. *American Journal of Psychiatry, 157*, 1552-1562.

Teasdale, J. D., Segal, Z. V., Williams, J. M. G., Ridgeway, V. A.., Soulsby, J. M., & Lau, M. A. (2000). Prevention of relapse/recurrence in major depression by mindfulness based cognitive therapy. *Journal of Consulting and Clinical Psychology, 68*, 615-623.

Thapar, A., Harold, G., & McGuffin, P. (1998). Life events and depressive symptoms in childhood – shared genes or shared adversity?: A research note. *Journal of Child Psychology and Psychiatry, 39*, 1153-1158.

Thompson-Brenner, H., & Westen, D. (2004). *A naturalistic study of psychotherapy for bulimia nervosa: Comorbidity, outcome, and therapeutic interventions in the community.* Unpublished manuscript, Boston University, Boston.

Tse, W. S., & Bond, A. J. (2004). The impact of depression on social skills. A review. *Journal of Nervous and Mental Disease, 192*, 206-268.

Tsigos, C., & Chrousos, G. P. (2002). Hypothalamic-pituitary-adrenal axis, neuroendocrine factors and stress. *Journal of Psychosomatic Research, 53*, 865-871.

Uchino, B. N., Cacioppo, J. T., & Kiecolt-Glaser, J. K. (1996). The relationship between social support and physiological processes: A review with emphasis on underlying mechanisms and implications for health. *Psychological Bulletin, 119*, 488-531.

Van Houdenhove, B., & Egle, U. T. (2004). Fibromyalgia: A stress disorder? Piecing the biopsychosocial puzzle together. *Psychotherapy and Psychosomatics, 73*, 267-275.

Van Os, J., & Jones, B. P. (1999). Early risk-factors and adult person-environment relationships in affective disorders. *Psychological Medicine, 29*, 1055-1067.

Van Os, J., Park, S. B., & Jones, P. B. (2001). Neuroticism, life events and mental health: Evidence for person-environment correlation. *British Journal of Psychiatry, 178* (Suppl 40), s72-s77.

Van Praag, H. M., de Kloet, R., & van Os, J. (2004). *Stress, the brain and depression.* Cambridge:

Cambridge University Press.

Wachtel, P. L. (1997). *Psychoanalysis, behavior therapy, and the relational world.* Washington, DC: American Psychological Association.

Waddington, L. (2002). The therapy relationship in cognitive therapy: A review. *Behavioural and Cognitive Psychotherapy, 30,* 179-191.

Wampold, B. E. (1997). Methodological problems in identifying efficacious psychotherapies. *Psychotherapy Research, 7,* 21-43.

Weissman, M., Wolk, S., Goldstein, R. B., Moreau, D., Adams, P., Greenwald, S., Klier, C. M., Ryan, N. D., Dahl, R. E., & Wickramaratne, P. (1999a). Depressed adolescents grown up. *Journal of the American Medical Association, 281,* 1707-1713.

Weissman, M., Wolk, S., Wickramaratne, P., Goldstein, R. B., Adams, P., Greenwald, S., Ryan, N. D., Dahl, R. E., & Steinberg, D. (1999b). Children with prepubertal-onset major depressive disorder and anxiety grown up. *Archives of General Psychiatry, 56,* 794-801.

Westen, D. (2000). Integrative psychotherapy: Integrating psychodynamic and cognitive-behavioral theory and technique. In C. R. Snyder & R. E. Ingram (Eds.), *Handbook of psychological change* (pp. 217-242). New York: Wiley.

Westen, D. (2002). *Manual for the Social Cognition and Object Relations Scales (SCORS).* Emory University, Atlanta, GA.

Westen, D., & Morrison, K. (2001). A multidimensional meta-analysis of treatments for depression, panic, and generalized anxiety disorder: An empirical examination of the status of empirically supported therapies. *Journal of Consulting and Clinical Psychology, 69,* 875-899.

Westen, D., Novotny, C. M., & Thompson-Brenner, H. (2004a). The empirical status of empirically supported psychotherapies: Assumptions, findings, and reporting in controlled clinical trials. *Psychological Bulletin, 130,* 631-663.

Westen, D., Novotny, C. M., & Thompson-Brenner, H. (2004b). The next generation of psychotherapy research: Reply to Ablon and Marci (2004), Goldfried and Eubanks-Carter (2004), and Haaga (2004). *Psychological Bulletin, 130,* 677-683.

Westen, D., & Shedler, J. (2000). A prototype matching approach to diagnosing personality disorders: Toward DSM-V. *Journal of Personality Disorders, 14,* 109-126.

Widiger, T. A., & Anderson, K. G. (2003). Personality and depression in women. *Journal of Affective Disorders, 74,* 59-66.

Young, J. E. (1999). *Cognitive therapy for personality disorders: A schema-focused approach* (3th ed.). Sarasota, FL: Professional Resource Exchange.

Zuroff, D. C., & Blatt, S. J. (2002). Vicissitudes of life after the short-term treatment of depression: Roles of stress, social support, and personality. *Journal of Social and Clinical Psychology, 21,* 473-496.

Zuroff, D. C., Blatt, S. J., Krupnick, J. L., & Sotsky, S. M. (2003). Enhanced adaptive capacities after brief treatment for depression. *Psychotherapy Research, 13,* 99-115.

Zuroff, D. C., Mongrain, M., & Santor, D. (2004). Conceptualizing and measuring personality vulnerability to depression: Comment on Coyne and Whiffen (1995). *Psychological Bulletin, 130,* 489-511.

Author Index

Subject Index

Questionnaire)

Developmental psychopathology, 11, 74, 88, 163-165, 168, 184-185, 189-196, 200-205, 208-210, 216-220, 254, 260

Diagnostic and Statistical Manual of Mental Disorders (DSM), 1, 2, 10, 12, 18-19, 23, 25, 34-37, 70, 74, 89-90, 99, 166, 168, 227, 244-245, 253-260, 267-268, 270, 272, 276

Drug treatment, 7, 119

DSM (*See* Diagnostic and Statistical Manual of Mental Disorders)

Dynamic interactionism, 1, 4, 11-12, 104, 106, 108, 110, 153-154, 253-257, 260, 265, 270, 274, 277-278

Dysfunctional Attitudes Scale (DAS), 142, 162

Dysthymia (*See* Dysthymic Disorder)

Dysthymic disorder, 34, 99, 168, 170-172

Efficacy factor, 141, 145-146, 149

Endogenous depression, 89, 109, 119, 264

Gender differences, 71, 98, 183

Gene-environment correlations and interactions, 265

Genes, 11, 238-239, 243, 265-266, 272

Glucocorticoids, 33, 239, 241

Guilt, 3, 68, 70, 77-79, 82, 98, 138, 140-145, 153, 166-167, 173, 198-199, 202, 204, 207, 212

Helplessness, 3, 68, 76, 141, 143-144, 201-207, 211

Hopelessness, 3, 51, 58, 145

HPA axis, 33, 89, 229-245, 258-259, 266, 273, 277

Interpersonal relationships, 69, 73, 81, 84, 107, 117-118, 122, 139-151, 174, 206-207, 256, 262, 264

Interpersonal therapy (IPT), 6, 67, 115, 122, 148, 264, 269, 271, 273, 277

Interpretation, 44, 49, 82-83, 96, 108, 117-119, 192, 216, 235, 272, 275

Introjective (self critical) depression, 60, 68, 70, 90, 194, 206-212

IPT (*See* Interpersonal therapy)

Life events, 8, 27-28, 76, 78, 81, 95, 98, 103-109, 112, 146-147, 171-173, 184, 228, 245, 256, 258, 260, 265

Life stress
current, 4, 89, 108, 277
early, 89, 228-229, 238, 240, 242-245, 258, 268

Loss, 2-3, 8, 29-33, 36, 62, 72-73, 76-78, 81-82, 88, 112, 140-144, 147, 149, 154, 166, 168-169, 173

Major Depressive Disorder (MDD), 17-26, 29-37, 53-54, 74, 99, 165, 172, 227-229, 232-245, 256

MDD (*See* Major Depressive Disorder)

Mediating model, 107-108

Melancholia, 2, 104-141, 195

Memory (autobiographic), 10, 17, 20, 23, 29-33, 43-63, 169, 227, 262, 267

Mental representations (*See also* Object representations), 253, 260-263, 267, 275, 278

Mindfulness based cognitive therapy, 10, 62, 275

Mortality, 17, 20-23, 36-37, 165, 227, 234

Narcissistic depression, 196, 201-202, 206, 208

National Institute of Mental Health (NIMH), 5-8, 24-25, 27, 115, 119-122, 148, 165, 268-271

Neuroticism, 117, 228, 265-266

NIMH (*See* National Institute of Mental Health)

Object loss, 78, 140, 207

Object relationship, 201

Object representations, 78, 81, 152